Forelimb Lameness

Editors

KEVIN BENJAMINO
KENNETH A. BRUECKER

VETERINARY CLINICS OF NORTH AMERICA: SMALL ANIMAL PRACTICE

www.vetsmall.theclinics.com

March 2021 • Volume 51 • Number 2

ELSEVIER

1600 John F. Kennedy Boulevard • Suite 1800 • Philadelphia, Pennsylvania, 19103-2899
http://www.vetsmall.theclinics.com

**VETERINARY CLINICS OF NORTH AMERICA: SMALL ANIMAL PRACTICE Volume 51, Number 2
March 2021 ISSN 0195-5616, ISBN-13: 978-0-323-76246-5**

Editor: Stacy Eastman
Developmental Editor: Nicole Congleton

Photocopying

Single photocopies of single articles may be made for personal use as allowed by national copyright laws. Permission of the Publisher and payment of a fee is required for all other photocopying, including multiple or systematic copying, copying for advertising or promotional purposes, resale, and all forms of document delivery. Special rates are available for educational institutions that wish to make photocopies for non-profit educational classroom use. For information on how to seek permission visit www.elsevier.com/permissions or call: (+44) 1865 843830 (UK)/(+1) 215 239 3804 (USA).

Derivative Works

Subscribers may reproduce tables of contents or prepare lists of articles including abstracts for internal circulation within their institutions. Permission of the Publisher is required for resale or distribution outside the institution. Permission of the Publisher is required for all other derivative works, including compilations and translations (please consult www.elsevier.com/permissions).

Electronic Storage or Usage

Permission of the Publisher is required to store or use electronically any material contained in this periodical, including any article or part of an article (please consult www.elsevier.com/permissions). Except as outlined above, no part of this publication may be reproduced, stored in a retrieval system or transmitted in any form or by any means, electronic, mechanical, photocopying, recording or otherwise, without prior written permission of the Publisher.

Notice

No responsibility is assumed by the Publisher for any injury and/or damage to persons or property as a matter of products liability, negligence or otherwise, or from any use or operation of any methods, products, instructions or ideas contained in the material herein. Because of rapid advances in the medical sciences, in particular, independent verification of diagnoses and drug dosages should be made.

Although all advertising material is expected to conform to ethical (medical) standards, inclusion in this publication does not constitute a guarantee or endorsement of the quality or value of such product or of the claims made of it by its manufacturer.

Veterinary Clinics of North America: Small Animal Practice (ISSN 0195-5616) is published bimonthly by Elsevier Inc., 360 Park Avenue South, New York, NY 10010-1710. Months of issue are January, March, May, July, September, and November. Business and Editorial Offices: 1600 John F. Kennedy Blvd., Ste. 1800, Philadelphia, PA 19103-2899. Customer Service Office: 3251 Riverport Lane, Maryland Heights, MO 63043. Periodicals postage paid at New York, NY and additional mailing offices. Subscription prices are $358.00 per year (domestic individuals), $933.00 per year (domestic institutions), $100.00 per year (domestic students/residents), $451.00 per year (Canadian individuals), $998.00 per year (Canadian institutions), $488.00 per year (international individuals), $998.00 per year (international institutions), $100.00 per year (Canadian students/residents), and $220.00 per year (international students/residents). To receive student/resident rate, orders must be accompanied by name of affiliated institution, date of term, and the *signature* of program/residency coordinator on institution letterhead. Orders will be billed at individual rate until proof of status is received. Foreign air speed delivery is included in all *Clinics* subscription prices. All prices are subject to change without notice. **POSTMASTER:** Send address changes to *Veterinary Clinics of North America: Small Animal Practice*, Elsevier Health Sciences Division, Subscription Customer Service, 3251 Riverport Lane, Maryland Heights, MO 63043. Customer Service (orders, claims, online, change of address): Elsevier Periodicals Customer Service, Elsevier Health Sciences Division Subscription **Customer Service 3251 Riverport Lane Maryland Heights, MO 63043. Tel: 1-800-654-2452 (U.S. and Canada); 314-447-8871 (outside U.S. and Canada). Fax: 314-447-8029. E-mail: journalscustomerservice-usa@elsevier.com (for print support); journalsonlinesupport-usa@elsevier.com (for online support).**

Reprints. For copies of 100 or more of articles in this publication, please contact the Commercial Reprints Department, Elsevier Inc., 360 Park Avenue South, New York, NY 10010-1710. Tel.: 212-633-3874; Fax: 212-633-3820; E-mail: reprints@elsevier.com.

Veterinary Clinics of North America: Small Animal Practice is also published in Japanese by Inter Zoo Publishing Co., Ltd., Aoyama Crystal-Bldg 5F, 3-5-12 Kitaaoyama, Minato-ku, Tokyo 107-0061, Japan.

Veterinary Clinics of North America: Small Animal Practice is covered in *Current Contents/Agriculture, Biology and Environmental Sciences, Science Citation Index, ASCA, MEDLINE/PubMed (Index Medicus), Excerpta Medica,* and *BIOSIS.*

Contributors

EDITORS

KEVIN BENJAMINO, DVM
Diplomate, American College of Veterinary Surgeons; MedVet Medical and Cancer Centers for Pets, Columbus, Columbus, Ohio, USA

KENNETH A. BRUECKER, DVM, MS
Diplomate, American College of Veterinary Surgeons; Diplomate, American College of Veterinary Sports Medicine and Rehabilitation; Founder/Director, Continuing Orthopedic Veterinary Education, Moorpark, California, USA

AUTHORS

LUCAS HENRY BEIERER, BVSc, GradDipEd, MVetSurg
Diplomate, American College Veterinary Surgeons – Small Animal; Queensland Veterinary Specialists, Stafford Heights, Queensland, Australia

KEVIN BENJAMINO, DVM
Diplomate, American College of Veterinary Surgeons; MedVet Medical and Cancer Centers for Pets, Columbus, Columbus, Ohio, USA

JENNIFER A. BROWN, DVM
Diplomate, American College of Veterinary Sports Medicine and Rehabilitation, Board-Certified American College of Veterinary Surgeons – Large Animal

KENNETH A. BRUECKER, DVM, MS
Diplomate, American College of Veterinary Surgeons; Diplomate, American College of Veterinary Sports Medicine and Rehabilitation; Founder/Director, Continuing Orthopedic Veterinary Education, Moorpark, California, USA

LOÏC M. DÉJARDIN, DVM, MS
Diplomate, American College of Veterinary Surgeons; Professor, Head of Orthopaedic Surgery, Department of Small Animal Clinical Sciences, College of Veterinary Medicine, Michigan State University, East Lansing, Michigan, USA

DAVID DYCUS, DVM, MS, CCRP
Diplomate, American College of Veterinary Surgeons (Small Animal); Department of Orthopedic Surgery, Nexus Veterinary Bone & Joint Center, Baltimore, Maryland, USA

CHRISTELLE M. FOLLETTE, DVM
VCA Animal Specialty Group, Los Angeles, California, USA

DEREK B. FOX, DVM, PhD
Diplomate, American College of Veterinary Surgeons; Small Animal Orthopedic Surgery, Department of Veterinary Medicine and Surgery, University of Missouri, Veterinary Health Center Hospital, Columbia, Missouri, USA

REUNAN GUILLOU, Doc Vét
Diplomate, American College of Veterinary Surgeons; ACCESS Bone & Joint Center, Culver City, California, USA

KRYSTA JANAS, DVM
University of Tennessee College of Veterinary Medicine, Knoxville, Tennessee, USA

SHARON C. KERWIN, DVM, MS
Diplomate, American College of Veterinary Surgeons; Diplomate, American College of Veterinary Internal Medicine (Neurology); Professor, Department of Small Animal Clinical Sciences, College of Veterinary Medicine & Biomedical Sciences, Texas A&M University, College Station, Texas, USA

NINA R. KIEVES, DVM
Diplomate, American College Veterinary Surgeons – Small Animal; Diplomate, American College of Veterinary Sports Medicine and Rehabilitation; Assistant Professor, Small Animal Orthopedic Surgery, The Ohio State University, Columbus, Ohio, USA

RYAN KING, DVM
Diplomate, American College of Veterinary Radiology; Cummings School of Veterinary Medicine, Tufts University, North Grafton, Massachusetts, USA

JANIS LAPSLEY, DVM
Clinical Assistant Professor, Department of Veterinary Clinical Sciences, College of Veterinary Medicine, The Ohio State University, Columbus, Ohio, USA

DARRYL MILLIS, DVM
Diplomate, American College of Veterinary Surgeons; Diplomate, American College of Veterinary Sports Medicine and Rehabilitation; University of Tennessee College of Veterinary Medicine, Knoxville, Tennessee, USA

ANDY P. MOORES, BVSc, FRCVS
Diploma in Small Animal Surgery (Orthopaedics); Diplomate, European College of Veterinary Surgeons; Anderson Moores Veterinary Specialists, Hursley, Winchester, United Kingdom

ALESSANDRO PIRAS, DVM, ISVS
Senior Surgical Educational Advisor for IVC-Evidensia Finland, National Coordinator of Sporting Dog Clinics, Canine Sports Medicine and Orthopedics, Espoo, Finland

LAURA E. SELMIC, BVetMed (Hons), MPH
Diplomate, American College of Veterinary Surgery (Small Animal); Diplomate, European College of Veterinary Surgery; Founding Fellow, Surgical Oncology and Oral and Maxillofacial Surgery, Department of Veterinary Clinical Sciences, College of Veterinary Medicine, The Ohio State University, Columbus, Ohio, USA

REBECCA STOKES, DVM
Department of Small Animal Clinical Sciences, College of Veterinary Medicine, Iowa State University, Ames, Iowa, USA

AMANDA R. TAYLOR, DVM
Diplomate, American College of Veterinary Internal Medicine (Neurology); Neurologist, MedVet Dayton, Moraine, Ohio, USA; BluePearl North Hills, Pennsylvania, USA

JULIA TOMLINSON, BVSc, MS, PhD
Diplomate, American College of Veterinary Sports Medicine and Rehabilitation;
Diplomate, American College of Veterinary Surgeons; Twin Cities Animal Rehab and
Sports Medicine, Burnsville, Minnesota, USA

ALDO VEZZONI, DVM, SCMPA
Diplomate, European College of Veterinary Surgery; Clinica Veterinaria Vezzoni srl,
Cremona, Italy

CHARLES WALLS, DVM
Diplomate, American College Veterinary Surgeons; Sage Centers, Founder, Clayton,
California, USA

KIRK L. WENDELBURG, DVM
VCA Animal Specialty Group, Los Angeles, California, USA

Contents

> This article contains a guide for small animal practitioners to use when confronted with the challenge of diagnosing a forelimb lameness. The examination begins by monitoring the dog at a stance and a visual gait assessment. A hands-on evaluation includes the initial examination, checking for asymmetry and muscle atrophy while the dog is standing, and step-by-step instructions for a thorough forelimb examination.

> Diagnosis of forelimb lameness may be challenging, as it not only can be due to multiple common orthopedic diseases but also may occasionally be caused by neurologic disease. A thorough orthopedic and neurologic examination is key to determining which disease category is the likely culprit. Deficits identified on the neurologic examination, such as proprioceptive deficits, changes in reflexes, and presence of spinal hyperesthesia, are key in identifying neurologic causes of forelimb lameness.

> Fractures and ligamentous injuries of the front paw are common in small animals and usually result from direct trauma, such as vehicular accident, collision with a stationary object, falls from a height, or entrapment of the paw with leverage (eg, stepping in a hole while running). Metacarpal and phalangeal fractures may be associated with concurrent ligamentous injury. Tendon and paw injuries are generally associated with direct traumatic etiologies, such as laceration. Treatment of digit injuries follows the principles of surgery associated with similar injuries at other anatomic locations. External coaptation may be necessary to protect undersized implants.

> The canine and feline carpus is a complex arrangement of bones, ligaments, and joint spaces that functions as a ginglymus joint to provide carpal flexion and extension. Given the demanding biomechanical demands

on the carpus during weight bearing, a variety of region-specific pathology, often secondary to trauma, are reported. This review details carpal anatomy, biomechanical understandings, and current evidence surrounding carpal pathology and its management. Partial carpal arthrodesis and pancarpal arthrodesis outcomes are reviewed in detail.

Physeal injuries are common in the developing small animal and can result in growth disturbances of the forelimb. Resulting deformities can include limb shortening, joint incongruity, angulation, and alterations in joint loading with subsequent osteoarthritis, remodeling, and debilitation. Because of the unique paired bone configuration, the antebrachium is the main source for malalignment resulting from physeal disturbance in the forelimb. Successful correction of deformities requires in-depth understanding of normal physeal activity; careful consideration of patient signalment; and the ability to quantify the location, magnitude, and plane of the deformity or deformities.

The shoulder is a complex joint composed mostly of static and dynamic capsuloligamentous structures and plays an important role in forelimb lameness. Its complex anatomy and biomechanics necessitate thorough examination and diagnostic work-up for accurate diagnosis. This article provides an updated review of common canine shoulder pathologies, including osteochondrosis, bicipital and supraspinatus tendinopathies, infraspinatus contracture, medial shoulder syndrome, and luxation.

Lameness, new swelling, or mass occurrence are the most common reasons for presentation when neoplasia affects the limbs. Tumors of the skin or subcutaneous tissues, joints, muscles, bones, or digits of the forelimb are reported. Diagnosis with fine needle aspiration or biopsy is necessary before treatment to allow staging, planning of treatment, and prognostication. The planning of surgical treatment of limb tumors is essential to maximize the chance of a complete resection on the first surgery, given that less skin is available for primary closure in subsequent revision or recurrence surgeries.

Although lameness of the thoracic limb typically is due to orthopedic disease, there are several important neurologic conditions that result in lameness. Neurologic diseases cause lameness due to disease of the nerves, nerve roots, spinal cord, or muscles. Common differentials include lateralized intervertebral disc extrusions, caudal cervical spondylomyelopathy (wobbler disease), brachial plexus avulsion, neuritis, and peripheral nerve sheath tumors. Many of these diseases compress or destroy the nerve roots of the cervical intumescence, resulting in nonweight-bearing lameness, or root signature. Advanced diagnostics, such as magnetic resonance imaging, are necessary in these cases to determine the underlying cause.

Juvenile Disease Processes Affecting the Forelimb in Canines

Nina R. Kieves

Several juvenile diseases affect the canine forelimb. The most common are hypertrophic osteodystrophy, panosteitis, and retained cartilaginous core. Panosteitis and hypertrophic osteodystrophy tend to be self-limiting, with a good long-term prognosis, although severe cases can develop. These diseases may recur during growth. Severe cases of hypertrophic osteodystrophy can lead to angular limb deformities and may even be fatal. Retained cartilaginous cores can be benign with no evidence of clinical signs and be found incidentally on radiographs. However, if they disrupt the distal ulnar physis significantly, angular limb deformities may persist requiring surgical intervention with a corrective osteotomy.

Advanced Imaging of the Forelimb: Use of Musculoskeletal Ultrasound and MRI of the Shoulder and Brachial Plexus

Ryan King

Advanced imaging (ultrasound, computed tomography, MRI) is a key component in defining and localizing the underlying cause of forelimb lameness. Given the propensity of soft tissue injury/disease of the shoulder and brachial plexus, ultrasound and MRI are of particular utility in defining tendinous, muscular, and nerve lesions. An advanced knowledge of shoulder and brachial plexus anatomy is necessary for both image acquisition and interpretation. To determine clinical significance, interpretation of both normal anatomy and suspected pathology must be correlated with clinical signs and orthopedic examination findings.

Rehabilitation of the Canine Forelimb

Jennifer A. Brown and Julia Tomlinson

The goal of rehabilitation is to restore function and mobility and reduce pain associated with chronic disease. Physical therapy for humans is standard of care for acute and chronic injuries and an integral component of postoperative recovery. Although there is a dearth of evidence-based veterinary medical studies in rehabilitation therapy and modalities for forelimb injuries in dogs, some extrapolation from other species can be made and applied. When developing a rehabilitation and therapeutic plan, the biomechanics of the affected limb and timeline of tissue healing of the target tissue and/or joint are important to consider.

Humeral intracondylar fissure (HIF) was first described as incomplete ossification of the humeral condyle. It is now known that the fissure is a stress
fracture in some dogs. The descriptive term HIF is therefore preferred. In
young dogs an incomplete ossification cause may still be valid. Symptomatic HIF is treated surgically with a transcondylar implant. The aim is to
alleviate lameness and avoid condylar fracture. Choosing an appropriate
surgical approach and implant can reduce complications. HIF is not always symptomatic and, in these cases, surgical management is more
controversial, because a minority of such cases become lame or fracture.

Elbow dysplasia is a major cause of front limb lameness in medium to large
dog breeds. Underlying causes include ununited anconeal process, medial
coronoid process disease, and osteochondritis dissecans. When a definitive diagnosis of elbow dysplasia is made, the surgeon can improve elbow
function but cannot entirely prevent progression of osteoarthrosis. Conventional surgical treatment with joint debridement and removal of loose
osteocartilaginous bodies is not rewarding if joint incongruity persists;
the result is overloading and subchondral bone exposure with erosion of
the cartilage of the medial humeral condyle and medial coronoid area of
the ulna leading to medial compartment disease.

Erosion of the articular cartilage of the medial compartment of the elbow
(the humeroulnar articulation) secondary to incongruency associated
with elbow dysplasia or traumatic injury has been termed, medial compartment disease. When nonsurgical strategies to manage osteoarthritis (OA)
fail, surgical solutions may be warranted. Surgical strategies to reduce
pain include osteotomies of the humerus or ulna to shift the weight bearing
axis laterally off the medial compartment of the elbow. Other strategies
involve replacement of portions or all of the articular surface of the medial
compartment. With global elbow joint OA (medial and lateral compartment), a total elbow replacement may be required.

VETERINARY CLINICS OF NORTH AMERICA: SMALL ANIMAL PRACTICE

FORTHCOMING ISSUES

May 2021
Small Animal Nutrition
Dottie Laflamme, *Editor*

July 2021
Working Dogs: An Update for Veterinarians
Maureen McMichael and Melissa
Singletary, *Editors*

September 2021
**Effective Communication in Veterinary
Medicine**
Christopher A. Adin and Kelly D.
Farnsworth, *Editors*

RECENT ISSUES

January 2021
Advances in Gastroenterology
Frédéric P. Gaschen, *Editor*

November 2020
**Emergency and Critical Care of Small
Animals**
Elisa M. Mazzaferro, *Editor*

September 2020
**Feline Practice: Integrating Medicine and
Well-Being (Part II)**
Margie Scherk, *Editor*

SERIES OF RELATED INTEREST

Veterinary Clinics of North America: Exotic Animal Practice
https://www.vetexotic.theclinics.com/

Preface

Decoding Forelimb Lameness: Acquiring the Techniques to Diagnose and Treat

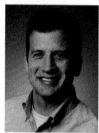
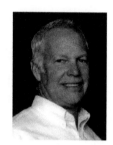

Kevin Benjamino, DVM Kenneth A. Bruecker, DVM, MS
Editors

The ability to appropriately diagnose and treat many forelimb issues in the canine (and feline) has been a source of contention for many in veterinary medicine, from those early on in their career to those advanced. The main objective of this issue is to unlock the mystery. Albeit this an arduous task, a collection of veterinary specialists contributed in agreement with this vision. The collection of contributors is an international mix of the highest caliber.

This edition of *Veterinary Clinics of North America: Small Animal Practice* has been developed to take the reader through a journey of the most and least common causes of forelimb lameness and pathology. The articles follow a systematic approach starting from a general examination to differentiation of orthopedic, neurologic, and oncologic causes. Next, each segment of the limb is explored from the digits to the scapula. Imaging of the forelimb is also reviewed within the individual articles, and advanced imaging of the forelimb (MRI) is covered.

One of the most challenging orthopedic conditions that clinicians face is congenital disease processes, in particular, elbow dysplasia. Elbow dysplasia is many times a damning condition to both the patient and the owner, and there is still so much that we do not know about the disease. Two articles have been devoted to this disease process (likely a whole book dedicated to elbow dysplasia could be written) as we try to undo some of the fallacies and mystery surrounding its diagnosis and treatment. In these articles, a full review of the disease process is evaluated, as well as an algorithm for treatment, and overall prognosis. In the more progressed patient, advanced procedures, such as the canine unicompartment arthroplasty, sliding humeral osteotomy, proximal abduction ulnar osteotomy, and unicompartment or total elbow replacement, may be indicated. Overview of these procedures (and more) is reviewed.

Vet Clin Small Anim 51 (2021) xiii–xiv
https://doi.org/10.1016/j.cvsm.2020.12.009
0195-5616/21/© 2020 Published by Elsevier Inc.

We want to thank each and every contributor in this issue for lending their expertise on this very important contribution to the veterinary profession and literature. We are also very appreciative of everyone's sacrifice in collaborating for this issue, especially in the midst of the current COVID-19 global pandemic. We are very cognizant of the challenges this may have caused and the added stress. It is our desire that this edition is of great benefit to all who read this issue and gives the clinician added confidence and tools to be used on a daily basis. Enjoy and gain from the knowledge and insight of some of the most experienced clinicians!

Kevin Benjamino, DVM
MedVet Medical and Cancer Centers
for Pets, Columbus
300 East Wilson Bridge Road
Worthington, OH 43085, USA

Kenneth A. Bruecker, DVM, MS
Continuing Orthopedic Veterinary Education
6370 Grimes Canyon Road
Moorpark, CA 93021, USA

E-mail addresses:
kevin.benjamino@medvet.com (K. Benjamino)
kbruecker@me.com (K.A. Bruecker)

Forelimb Examination, Lameness Assessment, and Kinetic and Kinematic Gait Analysis

Darryl Millis, DVM*, Krysta Janas, DVM

KEYWORDS

- Thoracic limb • Forelimb • Lameness • Gait • Examination • Kinetics • Kinematics

KEY POINTS

- Subtle forelimb lameness can be difficult to evaluate.
- A complete orthopedic examination is essential when diagnosing a forelimb lameness.
- Regardless of lameness lateralization, an examination should be performed bilaterally.
- The range of motion of joints should be assessed and recorded during each examination.

INTRODUCTION

Forelimb lameness in dogs can be difficult to subjectively assess. Often, forelimb issues are bilateral, which can effectively reduce the asymmetry of gait abnormalities. Some practices have force plates or pressure walkways to objectively measure the amount of weight a dog places on each limb, whereas others must rely on a subjective visual lameness evaluation. In either case, a thorough orthopedic examination of the forelimb is necessary to determine the next appropriate diagnostic tools and the cause of the lameness.

Lameness Evaluation

A good orthopedic examination begins by determining which limb or limbs are lame. Symmetry of the stance should be critically evaluated before ambulation for redistribution of weight. Dogs with forelimb discomfort and muscle atrophy often stand asymmetrically, with the less affected limb held closer to the midline, or they may shift their weight off the painful limb. The placement of the elbows can also be an important indicator of pain. Elbows held in adduction against the thoracic wall, with the distal

University of Tennessee College of Veterinary Medicine, 2407 River Drive, Knoxville, TN 37996, USA
* Corresponding author.
E-mail address: dmillis@utk.edu

Vet Clin Small Anim 51 (2021) 235–251
https://doi.org/10.1016/j.cvsm.2020.10.001
0195-5616/21/© 2020 Elsevier Inc. All rights reserved.

antebrachium and paw externally rotated, could indicate muscle contracture of the proximal forelimb. Elbows in abduction with the antebrachium internally rotated may be trying to alter weight-bearing in the elbows. Bilaterally affected dogs may shift their weight toward the pelvic limbs.

A flat, even surface with good traction is essential for gait evaluation. Both the walk and the trot should be observed from different angles (from both sides, the front, and behind the dog). Each limb strikes the ground separately at a walk, making it somewhat easier to distinguish which limb or limbs are lame. Although it is easier to observe and detect abnormalities at a walk, a subtle lameness may not be detectable at a slower speed because of reduced forces placed on the limb at a walk compared with a trot. Diagonal fore and pelvic limbs strike the ground simultaneously at a trot, making it somewhat more difficult to determine which limb is more lame. In the digital age, it is helpful to record the dog and watch the gait in slow motion. The adage, "down on the sound," can be used while evaluating a forelimb lameness. Dogs lift their head and transfer forces to the pelvic limb when the injured limb strikes the ground and lower their head when the unaffected limb is on the ground.[1] Dogs with forelimb lameness frequently have a shortened stride length and may have a shuffling-type gait because they maintain the joints in a more extended position with limited flexion of the elbows and carpi during gait.

A visual analog scale (VAS) or numeric rating score (NRS) may be used to describe limb function. The VAS consists of a measured line (usually 10 cm), with 1 end representing non-weight-bearing lameness and the opposite end representing an orthopedically sound dog. The observer makes a mark on the line based on their interpretation of the gait. The NRS assigns a numeric score to the lameness, with 0 being orthopedically sound, and the highest number on the scale representing a non-weight-bearing lameness.

It is important to remember that these measurements are subjective evaluations. Previous studies evaluating subjective gait analysis of induced hindlimb lameness have found that there is significant interobserver variability and low agreement when compared with objective gait analysis.[2] A recent article comparing interobserver and intraobserver agreement on VAS and NRS in dogs with elbow osteoarthritis (OA) found that both were similar before and after orthopedic examination.[3]

If the lameness is not obvious while walking or trotting, the dog can be walked down stairs or a hill. The braking required by the forelimbs during the descent may accentuate the issue. Dogs can also be walked over Cavaletti rails to evaluate elbow and carpal flexion.[4] OA of these joints can limit flexion, and dogs may compensate by swinging the limb out to clear the obstacle. If the dog is a competition or working dog, it is beneficial to watch them perform their specific tasks.

Kinetics and Kinematics

Kinetic gait analysis is performed with a force plate or walkway system. These tools can detect the peak vertical force (maximum force the dog places on each limb) and vertical impulse (area under the force-time curve). Force plates can also determine braking and propulsion forces. A study evaluating the agreement between NRS, VAS, and force plate analysis in dogs undergoing a right tibial osteotomy repair model found that agreement between the 3 analysis systems was most accurate when lameness was severe, but overall agreement was low.[5] This finding suggests that the ability to subjectively evaluate lameness is low unless the lameness is obvious. Force plate gait analysis is very sensitive and considered to be the gold standard, but subjective visual analysis should not be ignored.

Kinematic gait evaluation objectively assesses joint motion and stride characteristics, including joint range of motion (ROM), velocity, acceleration, swing time, stance time, and stride length in a 3-dimensional field. Evaluation of walking, trotting, and various exercises has been performed by applying reflective markers around individual joints and using a series of cameras to record and analyze the amount of flexion and extension. The approximate ROM of the shoulder, elbow, and carpus at a walk is 30°, 45°, and 90°, respectively. Trotting increases joint excursions by 5° in most joints, whereas the stifle increases approximately 20°.[6]

The kinematics of the major joints during various exercises were described by Carr and colleagues.[7] They found that the maximum flexion, extension, and ROM of the elbow and carpus, and shoulder flexion and ROM, significantly increased when walking up a 35° ramp or standard stairs compared with trotting on level ground. Others have found no changes in joint motion while ascending a 6.3° slope compared with walking.[8] Walking over low Cavalettis significantly increases elbow flexion.[7,8] Dogs with a fragmented medial coronoid process have decreased ROM of the elbow, carpus, and metacarpophalangeal joints of the affected limb.[9]

Initial Evaluation

During initial evaluation of the forelimbs, dogs should be in a standing position with the limbs located squarely beneath them to accurately assess for muscle atrophy. An asymmetrical stance (eg, with 1 limb ahead of another) causes asymmetrical stretching of muscle bellies, which may give the false impression of muscle atrophy. The limbs are assessed for pain, inflammation, swelling, and anatomic asymmetry. Both hands should be used to palpate and compare the limbs simultaneously working in a proximal to distal direction.

The scapulae should be palpated simultaneously to assess for symmetry of muscle mass and prominence of the scapular spine. Next, assess the relative positions of the greater tubercles in comparison with the acromial processes of the scapulae. If muscle atrophy is present, there will be less muscle between the 2 bony prominences. This area is also evaluated for shoulder luxation by determining if one of the greater tubercles is asymmetrical compared with the contralateral limb.

The elbow is one of the most complex joints in the body. Both elbows should be carefully assessed for the presence of effusion in the craniomedial and caudolateral quadrants. Because there is also a significant amount of soft tissue (the flexors and extensors of the carpi and digits originate from the epicondyles) in a small area, it is difficult to appropriately evaluate for subtle joint effusion with the dog laying on its side. Having the dog in a standing position increases the amount of loading pressure on the joint, and palpating both joints simultaneously makes it easier to appreciate effusion. The craniomedial quadrant of the elbow can be identified by first finding the medial epicondyle and moving craniodistally and palpating the joint region just behind the pronator teres muscle. The caudolateral compartment can be located by identifying the space between the lateral epicondyle and olecranon of the ulna.

The shafts of the radius and ulna should be palpated for pain and swelling, working distally toward the manus. The long bones should always be assessed for pain to rule out panosteitis, hypertrophic osteodystrophy, and fractures in young dogs, and neoplasia or fractures in older dogs. The carpi should be evaluated for any effusion or anatomic asymmetry suggestive of fracture or subluxation of the carpal bones.

The carpus should be observed at a standing angle and evaluated for the presence of hyperextension. The carpus is the only joint in the body that has a greater angle than 180° while standing.[10] Dogs with greater than 200° of extension should be evaluated for carpal hyperextension injury. Varus or valgus positioning of the lower limb may indicate an angular limb deformity. Carpal laxity syndrome and carpal flexural deformity may occur in puppies.

ORTHOPEDIC EXAMINATION

After the standing evaluation is complete, and you have a general idea where the disorder is, the dog can be placed in lateral recumbency with the less affected (less lame) side up. Evaluating this side first will help prevent the dog from becoming tense and resistant as a result of pain and discomfort. Often, forelimb disease is bilateral, so this will also help prevent missing conditions in the contralateral limb. The examination may begin distally and work proximally, or vice versa. The important thing is to always perform the orthopedic examination the same way every time to avoid missing conditions.

Joint Measurements

The ROM of the joints should be measured while performing an orthopedic examination. Joint measurement is performed with a goniometer. Full flexion and extension of joints are determined using specific landmarks, as previously described.[10] The joints of both limbs can then be compared with each other and a database to determine if disease is present, and if it is unilateral or bilateral. Remember that OA is one of the most common conditions diagnosed in older dogs, with approximately half of adult dogs having OA, usually in more than 1 joint,[11] and dogs with OA often have decreased ROM.

Digits and Metacarpals

The nails, interdigital space, and paw pads should be assessed for abnormalities and asymmetry. Abnormal wearing of the nails suggests neurologic conditions or trauma. The base of the nail should be evaluated for infections (paronychia) and tumors. Squamous cell carcinoma and melanoma, especially in darker dogs, are the most common tumors associated with the digits.[12,13] The toes should be spread apart to look for interdigital pyoderma, characterized by swelling, focal alopecia, pruritis, or nodules.[14] The digital and metacarpal pads are susceptible to abrasions, lacerations, cracking, thermal injury, corns, and foreign bodies. The paw pads of indoor dogs can also become soft if they are not frequently exercised, making them more likely to become sore if their exercise suddenly increases.

The digits can be flexed and extended as 1 unit, paying close attention to the dog for any signs of discomfort or a decreased ROM; if abnormalities are noted, the area should be assessed more closely (**Figs. 1** and **2**). The dewclaw (phalanx I) should not be overlooked if present. Owners may forget to trim this nail, and it can grow until it irritates the soft tissues. Sporting and working dogs are more prone to digit injuries, so each digit and joint should be palpated separately. The digits should be evaluated for soft tissue and joint swelling, decreased ROM, pain on palpation of the diaphysis of the phalanges or sesamoid bones, and instability/crepitus owing to fractures. The collateral stability of the interphalangeal and metacarpophalangeal joints should also be assessed by applying varus and valgus stresses to each joint. If abnormalities are noted, radiographs should be performed. OA is especially common in the digits of sporting and working dogs, and the interphalangeal and metacarpophalangeal joints can be swollen and painful and have a decreased ROM.

The common digital extensor, superficial digital flexor, and deep digital flexor tendons attach to extensor processes of the distal phalanges, the palmar surface of the base of the second phalanges of digits II–V, and the flexor tubercle on the palmar

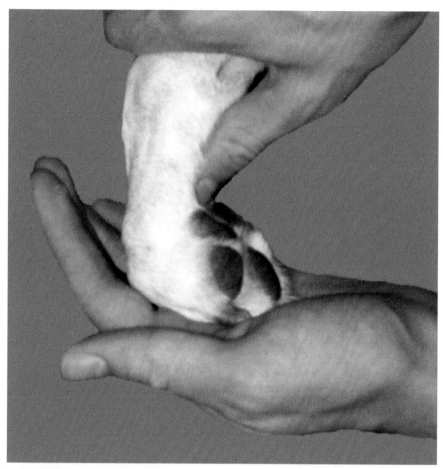

Fig. 1. Flexion of the canine digits.

surface of the distal phalanges of the digits, respectively.[15] Flexor tendon injury most commonly affects the deep digital flexor tendon because it is more superficial at the level of the metacarpophalangeal joint and results in a dropped toe (hyperextension of the distal interphalangeal joint).[16] The nails of affected digits can be excessively long because they are not worn while the dog is walking. Valgus deformities of the digit are rare but can occur secondary to immune-mediated conditions (eg, rheumatoid arthritis) and give the appearance that the foot is externally rotated.

The metacarpal bones should be individually palpated to assess for swelling and pain, which can indicate fractures and occasionally neoplastic processes. Fractures occur most commonly in the body of the metacarpals.[17]

Carpus

The carpus should be flexed and extended while monitoring the dog for pain and abnormal ROM (**Figs. 3** and **4**). The ROM for a normal dog is approximately 200° of extension and 31° to 34° of flexion; however, this can be affected by breed.[10,18] In general, dogs with normal carpi should be able to touch their manus to the antebrachium

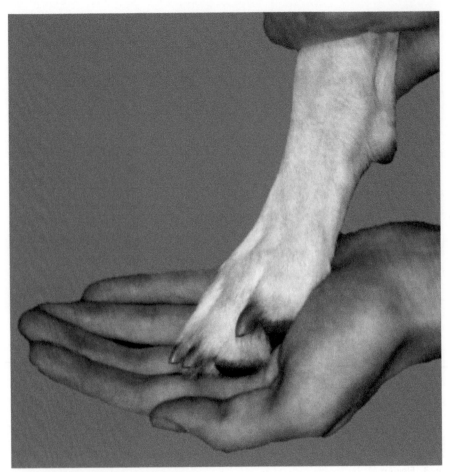

Fig. 2. Extension of the canine digits.

when the carpus is fully flexed. Often, older dogs will have a minor loss of flexion; however, this is usually not clinically relevant because dogs do not fully flex their carpus for normal daily function. Carpal hyperextension injury, with damage to the palmar fibrocartilage and carpal ligaments, occurs secondary to a jump, fall, or degenerative process.[19] Affected dogs have increased joint extension (>200° at a stance), and often soft tissue swelling, joint effusion, and pain on manipulation of the carpus. If suspected, stress radiographs should be obtained. Special attention should be paid to the carpus of 4- to 7-month-old dogs to evaluate for carpal laxity syndrome and carpal flexural deformity.[20]

The carpus should next be extended and varus and valgus stresses applied to assess for collateral ligament injuries. There is more varus-valgus motion in the carpus than other joints. Approximately 6° to 8° of varus and up to 10° to 14° of valgus can be obtained in the extended carpus of normal Labrador retrievers.[10]

The radiocarpal, ulnar, numbered carpal, and accessory carpal bones should be individually palpated to assess for pain. Fractures of the carpal bones can occur as a result of trauma. Joint luxation can occur at the level of the proximal

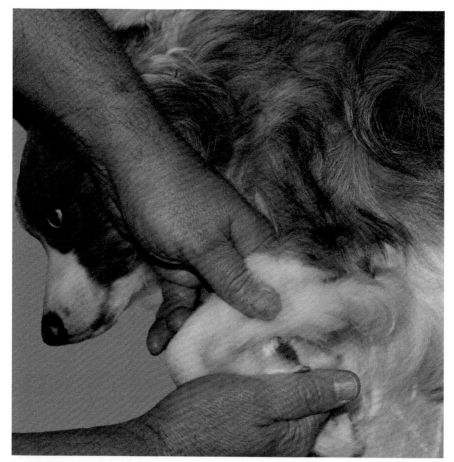

Fig. 3. Flexion of the canine carpus.

(antebrachiocarpal), middle, or distal (carpometacarpal) carpal joint, so any asymmetry between the carpi should be noted. If suspected, stress radiographs should be obtained.

All of the carpal joints can develop arthritis, but OA of the antebrachiocarpal joint may be most noted because it normally has greater ROM than the other joints. Clinical signs may include pain and inflammation, joint effusion, decreased ROM, and/or bony deformation at one or more levels of the carpus.

Radius and Ulna

The radius and ulna should be palpated individually. Starting at the styloid process of the ulna on the caudolateral antebrachium, palpate proximally to the dorsal aspect of the olecranon while assessing for pain. The radius can be similarly palpated on the cranial aspect of the antebrachium from the antebrachiocarpal joint to the head of the radius. The abductor pollicis longus runs cranially through the radial and ulnar groove, obliquely crosses the radius and ulna, and inserts on the proximal aspect of the first metacarpal bone. This tendon should be palpated separately to assess for

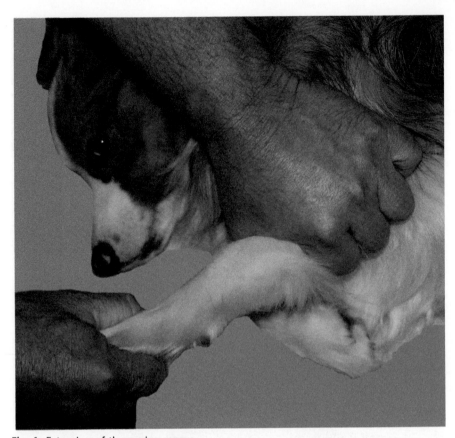

Fig. 4. Extension of the canine carpus.

pain and a firm swelling at the distal medial aspect of the antebrachium, suggestive of stenosing tenosynovitis.[21]

Differentials for pain on palpation of the antebrachium vary based on location, age, and breed of the dog. Each bone should be palpated directly, as opposed to attempting to feel the bone through the muscles. Pain associated with the diaphysis of the radius and ulna of large and giant breed dogs, particularly German shepherds, is frequently associated with panosteitis. Discomfort at the metaphysis of large dogs may occur with hypertrophic osteodystrophy, or retained cartilage cores of the distal ulna, whereas older dogs are more likely have a neoplastic process in this location.[22–24]

Traumatic fractures can occur at any location along the radius and ulna, but most commonly occur at the middiaphysis to distal one-third of the radius and ulna in toy or miniature breed dogs.[25] The radius has minimal soft tissue coverage, and if a fracture is suspected, this area should be closely inspected to rule out an open fracture.

Angular limb deformity of the antebrachium is common when skeletally immature dogs have trauma to the distal ulnar or, occasionally, radial physis. As the normal distal radial growth plate continues to lengthen, the damaged ulna restricts normal growth, resulting in radial procurvatum and external rotation of the paw. This type of injury can also lead to incongruity of the elbow.[26]

Elbow

The elbow should be flexed and extended to evaluate the ROM. The remaining joints in the forelimb should not be manipulated during the elbow examination, because this can cause confounding pain. Dogs without elbow disease should have 35° of flexion and 165° of extension.[10] Clinically, they should be able to touch their carpus to the greater tubercle of their shoulder during elbow flexion. When putting the elbow through these movements, monitor for resistance, discomfort, and crepitus, particularly at end flexion and extension. Any loss of ROM is associated with significant degenerative radiographic changes and decreased weight-bearing as measured on a force plate.[27] While extended, the elbow should have varus and valgus stress applied to evaluate the collateral ligaments.

Joint effusion is most easily palpated while standing; however, effusion can still be appreciated in dogs with moderate to severe disease when laterally recumbent. Both the craniomedial and the caudolateral joint compartments should be palpated. It is extremely important to include this aspect of the examination in young dogs to identify elbow dysplasia early, before the onset of clinical OA. Dogs with fragmented medial coronoid processes often have effusion in the craniomedial compartment, whereas dogs with ununited anconeal processes frequently have caudolateral effusion.

The bony prominences of the elbow should be individually identified and palpated for symmetry, pain, and stability. At the most proximal aspect of the elbow joint, the olecranon should be palpated. Moving distally, on the medial aspect of the elbow, the medial epicondyle is the first projection craniodistal to the tip of the olecranon; the flexor tendons arise from this area (**Figs. 5** and **6**). Just craniodistal to the medial epicondyle, the region of the medial coronoid process may be assessed. The medial coronoid can be difficult to accurately palpate because of the overlying soft tissue. To find the medial coronoid, the elbow should be flexed to relax the muscles and allow palpation of the medial coronoid process area. Discomfort during palpation of this area while supinating and pronating the antebrachium is suggestive of a fragmented medial coronoid process.[28]

On the lateral aspect of the elbow, the lateral epicondyle is craniodistal to the tip of the olecranon and should be in the same plane as the medial epicondyle (**Fig. 7**). The extensor tendons and the ulnaris lateralis originate from the lateral epicondyle. Asymmetry of the bony prominences can indicate traumatic luxation if the dog has an acute or traumatic history of forelimb lameness. Dogs most commonly develop a lateral elbow luxation, whereby the anconeal process slides over the lateral epicondyle, because it is significantly smaller than the medial epicondyle.[29] If the owners describe a more gradual onset or if the lameness waxes and wanes, anatomic abnormalities may be secondary to progressive degenerative joint disease.

The soft tissues surrounding the elbow are also susceptible to injury and should be evaluated, especially in dogs with a chronic forelimb lameness. All 4 heads of the triceps insert on the olecranon, and pain associated with direct palpation of the tendon may indicate a triceps insertion tendinopathy or olecranon fracture. Hygromas are commonly associated with the olecranon in large and giant breed dogs.[30] The biceps tendon inserts on the cranial aspect of the proximal radius and ulna, at the radial and ulnar tuberosities. To assess for a biceps insertion tendinopathy, the elbow should be extended to increase tension while the tendon insertion is directly palpated for pain.

Humerus

As with the antebrachium, the humerus should be palpated from distal to proximal. The humerus is enveloped by muscles, so it may be difficult to palpate the shaft of

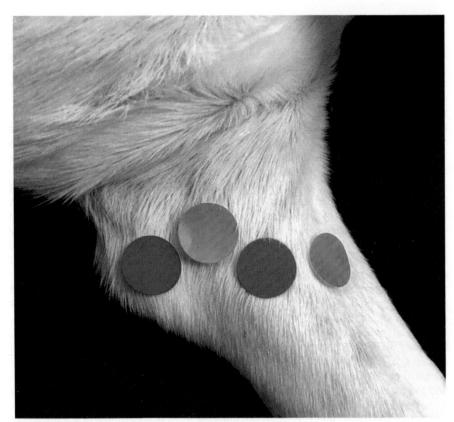

Fig. 5. Medial aspect of the left canine elbow. Dots are labeled from left to right. Red: olecranon; blue: medial epicondyle of the humerus; red: medial coronoid process of the ulna; blue: biceps tendon of insertion.

the bone without compressing muscle bellies. The radial nerve also crosses over the craniolateral aspect of the distal one-third of the humerus, and direct palpation of the nerve can cause discomfort.

Similar to the radius and ulna, the diaphysis of the humerus in young, large, and giant breed dogs is susceptible to panosteitis.[22] Pain associated with the proximal metaphysis in older dogs is frequently caused by osteosarcoma.[31]

Fractures can occur at any location but are more common in the middle and distal one-third of the humerus.[32] Significant pain on palpation of the humerus as well as fragment instability can be appreciated on examination. If a fracture is suspected, the neurologic function of the limb must be assessed to rule out radial nerve damage; this can be accomplished with toe-pinches and skin pricks to assess sensation. The lateral condyle of the humerus often fractures in young dogs after a fall or jump from a height.[33] Fractures of the medial condyle and bicondylar fractures are less frequent. These dogs are usually non-weight-bearing lame, with significantly decreased ROM and crepitus present on palpation and manipulation of the elbow. Spaniels, Labrador retrievers, Rottweilers, and other breeds are susceptible to incomplete ossification of the humeral condyle. If presented early, these dogs may have forelimb lameness with elbow effusion. However, if this pathologic condition is not corrected, they can develop unicondylar or bicondylar fractures of the humeral condyle.[34]

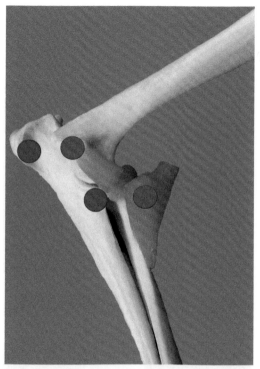

Fig. 6. Bony prominences of the left canine elbow. Dots are labeled from left to right. Red: olecranon; blue: medial epicondyle of the humerus; red: medial coronoid process of the ulna; blue: biceps tendon of insertion.

Shoulder

Passive ROM should be evaluated by flexing and extending the shoulder while assessing for limitations, pain, and crepitus. Normal dogs should have 55° of flexion and 165° of extension; however, a normal ROM does not mean that the shoulder is without issue.[10] Trigger points (muscle pain and fasciculations elicited by palpation) are commonly found during palpation of the muscles surrounding the shoulder, particularly the deltoideus, when shoulder abnormalities are present.

The shoulder is surrounded by muscles, tendons, and ligaments that act to stabilize the joint, and all are susceptible to injury. The associated soft tissues make it difficult to detect effusion, so assessment of the shoulder relies on manipulation of the joint and soft tissue palpation. Pathologic conditions affecting the shoulder structures include biceps tenosynovitis, supraspinatus tendinopathy, medial glenohumeral instability, and infraspinatus contracture. Working and performance animals seem to be particularly prone to injuring these tissues. Young, large breed dogs should be evaluated for osteochondritis dissecans.

The biceps tendon originates from the supraglenoid tubercle and can be identified as it crosses the joint just medial to the greater tubercle. The biceps tendon maneuver is used to detect biceps pain, suggestive of biceps tenosynovitis (**Fig. 8**). The biceps maneuver can be performed by flexing the shoulder while simultaneously extending the elbow; pain is associated with inflammation of the biceps and tendon sheath. The biceps tendon should also be palpated while performing this procedure to detect early pathologic condition or pathologic condition in stoic dogs.

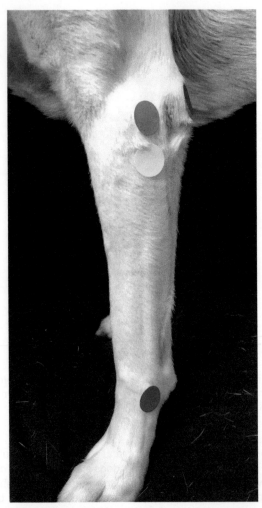

Fig. 7. Lateral aspect of the left canine elbow and antebrachium. Proximal red: olecranon of the ulna; blue: lateral epicondyle of the humerus; yellow: head of the radius; red: styloid process of the ulna.

The supraspinatus muscle lies cranial to the spine of the scapula and inserts on the greater tubercle of the humerus. Sporting dogs that overwork their shoulder by applying torsional stresses around the shoulder joint with rapid turning and pivoting seem to be at risk for injuring the supraspinatus tendon.[35,36] The tendon may feel firm and fibrotic with pain on shoulder flexion and palpation when compared with the contralateral limb. If untreated, the tendon is susceptible to develop chronic changes and calcification. Inflammation of the supraspinatus tendon can cause painful impingement of the biceps tendon. Flexion and internal rotation of the shoulder increase the amount of impingement and discomfort associated with this disease.

Medial shoulder instability (MSI) may result from injury to the medial glenohumeral ligament and/or subscapularis muscle and tendon. Similar to the supraspinatus tendon, it is most susceptible to damage when sporting dogs make rapid turns or jump down, and often these dogs have multiple muscles and tendons affected.

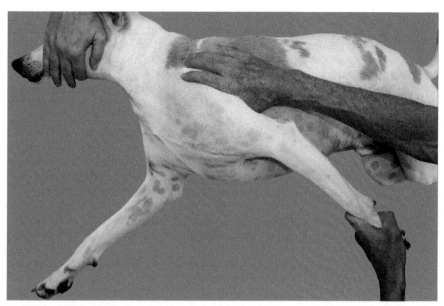

Fig. 8. Biceps maneuver.

Both structures are intraarticular and cannot be directly palpated. Historically, measurement of the shoulder abduction angle, the angle between the spine of the scapula and the lateral brachium during extension of the shoulder and elbow, has been recommended to diagnose MSI (**Fig. 9**).[37] If the shoulder is not extended, the angle of

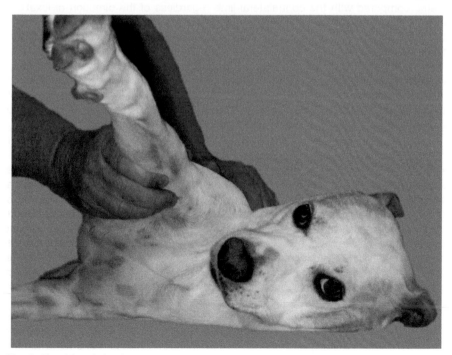

Fig. 9. Shoulder abduction.

abduction will be falsely high. The angle of the affected limb is then compared with the contralateral limb, and if MSI is present, the angle of abduction will be significantly higher with pain at the end of abduction. Normal abduction angles should be approximately 30°; however, the angle should be compared with the contralateral limb. More recently, studies have found poor interobserver repeatability of goniometric measurements.[38] Many dog breeds that participate in sporting events (eg, border collies) are stoic and may only show discrete signs of discomfort, such as lip licking or a temporary pause in panting.

The infraspinatus muscle lies caudal to the spine of the scapula and inserts distal to the greater tubercle. Contracture of the infraspinatus muscle can develop and is most frequently diagnosed in hunting dogs. Presentation of these dogs is often biphasic. Acutely, there is pain and soft tissue swelling associated with the infraspinatus muscle, suspected to be caused by traumatic compartment syndrome; however, this stage is rarely identified, as signs resolve with conservative management. In the following weeks to months after the initial injury, the damaged infraspinatus undergoes fibrosis and contracture, and the muscle atrophies. The fibrosis of the muscle and tendon prevents full extension of the shoulder. Dogs have a distinctive gait and posture that make them easy to identify. At a stance, the shoulder is held in abduction, while the elbow is adducted against the body wall. The fibrosis and contraction results in abduction and external rotation of the paw, even when placed in lateral recumbency. During ambulation, there is a weight-bearing lameness, and the limb is circumducted with a flip of the paw just before placement.[39]

Luxations of the shoulder are uncommon but can occur in any direction. Traumatic luxations can occur in any breed, whereas toy and mini-breed dogs are susceptible to congenital shoulder laxity or malformation leading to luxation. On examination of these dogs, the spatial relationship between the acromion and greater tubercle is asymmetric compared with the contralateral limb regardless of the direction of luxation. Dogs with medial shoulder luxation may hold the elbow flexed and adducted, with the antebrachium held in abduction. Dogs with a lateral shoulder luxation may adduct the antebrachium.[40]

Osteochondrosis dissecans can develop on the caudal aspect of the humeral head in skeletally immature large and giant breed dogs.[22] Dogs with this condition are often in pain with either shoulder extension, or shoulder flexion and internal rotation. OA of the shoulder is common in adult and geriatric dogs; however, these dogs seem to do well clinically.

Scapula

Although the scapula is covered by soft tissue, several bony prominences can be appreciated. The acromial process, spine of the scapula, and dorsal border of the scapula should be palpated, while monitoring for stability and the presence of crepitus. Fractures can occur anywhere along the acromion, glenoid, supraglenoid tubercle, scapular neck, scapular spine, and body of the scapula. A scapular luxation occurs when the serratus ventralis is torn from the thoracic wall or the scapula. These dogs are relatively easy to identify, with the scapula proximally displaced dorsal to the spine of the dog. The muscles cranial and caudal to the spine of the scapula, including the supraspinatus, infraspinatus, and long head of the triceps, should be assessed for firm, fibrous tissue.

During the examination, one should always keep in mind that there could be a primary or underlying neurologic component. The axillary region should be palpated as far medially and proximally as possible while the shoulder is abducted. Brachial plexus tumors are uncommon but can be a primary cause of forelimb lameness.

SUMMARY

Thorough lameness and orthopedic examinations are essential to properly evaluate and diagnose a patient with a forelimb lameness. A systematic method of evaluation will result in a precise and efficient examination.

CLINIC CARE POINTS

- Forelimb lameness is difficult to detect, so if there is any suspicion, a full examination and relevant workup are indicated.
- A complete orthopedic examination should always be performed bilaterally, regardless of where pain is identified.
- Always be systematic in your examination.
- A full orthopedic examination should be performed in young, growing dogs at their last vaccination visit to evaluate for elbow dysplasia and osteochondritis dissecans.
- A complete neurologic examination should be performed to rule out underlying neurologic disease.

DISCLOSURE

No proprietary interest or funding was provided for this article.

REFERENCES

1. Carr BJ, Dycus DL. Canine gait analysis. Today Vet Pract 2016;93–100.
2. Waxman AS, Robinson DA, Evans RB, et al. Relationship between objective and subjective assessment of limb function in normal dogs with an experimentally induced lameness. Vet Surg 2008;37(3):241–6.
3. Aulakh KS, Dongaonkar KR, Barnes K, et al. Influence of orthopedic examination on lameness scores and interobserver and intraobserver agreement in dogs with naturally occurring elbow osteoarthritis. Vet Surg 2020;49(3):455–62.
4. Weigel JP, Millis DL. Biomechanics of physical rehabilitation and kinematics of exercise. In: Millis DL, Levine D, editors. Canine rehabilitation and physical therapy. St Louis (MO): Elsevier; 2014. p. 401–30.
5. Quinn MM, Keuler NS, Lu Y, et al. Evaluation of agreement between numerical rating scales, visual analog scoring scales, and force plate gait analysis in dogs. Vet Surg 2007;36(4):360–7.
6. Allen K, DeCamp CE, Braden TD, et al. Kinematic gait analysis of the trot in healthy mixed breed dogs. Vet Comp Orthop Traumatol 1994;7(4):148–53.
7. Carr JG, Millis DL, Weng HY. Exercises in canine physical rehabilitation: range of motion of the forelimb during stair and ramp ascent. J Small Anim Pract 2013; 54(8):409–13.
8. Holler PJ, Verena B, Dal-Bianco B, et al. Kinematic motion analysis of the joints of the forelimbs and hind limbs of dogs during walking exercise regimens. Am J Vet Res 2010;71(7):734–40.
9. Burton NJ, Dobney JA, Owen MR, et al. Joint angle, moment and power compensations in dogs with fragmented medial coronoid process. Vet Comp Orthop Traumatol 2008;21(2):110–8.
10. Jaegger G, Marcellin-Little DJ, Levine D. Reliability of goniometry in Labrador retrievers. Am J Vet Res 2002;63(7):979–86.

11. Millis DL, Tichenor MG, Hecht S, et al. Prevalence of osteoarthritis in dogs undergoing routine dental prophylaxis. Oral Presentation at: World Small Animal Veterinary Association World Congress proceedings; September 16-19, 2014; Cape Town, South Africa.

12. Henry CJ Jr, Brewer WG, Whitley EM, et al. Canine digital tumors: a Veterinary Cooperative Oncology Group retrospective study of 64 dogs. J Vet Intern Med 2005;19(5):720–4.

13. Wobeser BK, Kidney BA, Powers BE, et al. Diagnoses and clinical outcomes associated with surgically amputated canine digits submitted to multiple veterinary diagnostic laboratories. Vet Pathol 2007;44(3):355–61.

14. Mason IS. Canine pyoderma. J Small Anim Pract 1991;32(8):381–6.

15. Evans HE, de Lahunta E. Guide to the dissection of the dog. In: Withrow SJ, MacEwen EG, editors. The skeletal and muscular systems. 7th edition. St Louis (MO): Saunders Elsevier; 2010. p. 32–9.

16. Williams N, Payne JT, Tomlinson JL, et al. Deep digital flexor tendon injuries in dogs. Compend Contin Educ Vet 1998;19:853–60.

17. Failing K, Matis U, Kornmayer M. Long-term prognosis of metacarpal and metatarsal fractures in dogs. Vet Comp Orthop Traumatol 2014;27(01):45–53.

18. Laura LH, Geoffrey TF, Weh M. Comparison of range of motion in Labrador retrievers and border collies. J Vet Med Anim Health 2015;7(4):122–7.

19. Whitelock R. Conditions of the carpus in the dog. In Pract 2001;23(1):2–13.

20. Yardimci C, Sağlam M, Çetinkaya MA. Carpal laxity syndrome in forty-three puppies. Vet Comp Orthop Traumatol 2007;02(02):126–30.

21. Grundmann S, Montavon PM. Stenosing tenosynovitis of the abductor pollicis longus muscle in dogs. Vet Comp Orthop Traumatol 2001;14(02):95–100.

22. Scott H. Non-traumatic causes of lameness in the forelimb of the growing dog. In Pract 1998;20(10):539–54.

23. Kushwaha RB, Aithal HP, Kinjavedakar P, et al. Incidence of skeletal diseases affecting long bones in growing dogs–a radiographic survey. Intas Polivet 2012;13(2):337–44.

24. Dernell WS, Straw RC, Withrow SJ, Piermattei DL, Flo GL, DeCamp CE. Tumors of the skeletal system. In: Small animal clinical oncology. Philadelphia: WB Saunders; 2001. p. 262–96.

25. Cooley S, Warnock JJ, Nemanic S, et al. Augmentation of diaphyseal fractures of the radius and ulna in toy breed dogs using a free autogenous omental graft and bone plating. Vet Comp Orthop Traumatol 2015;28(02):131–9.

26. Krotscheck U, Bottcher P. Surgical diseases of the elbow. In: Johnston SA, Tobias KM, editors. Veterinary surgery small animal. 2nd edition. St Louis (MO): Elsevier; 2018. p. 836–55.

27. Whitlock D, Millis DL, Odoi A. Can goniometry be used to detect the presence of lameness in dogs with chronic elbow osteoarthrosis? Vet Comp Orthop Traumatol 2010;23(4):A14.

28. Fitzpatrick N, Yeadon R. Working algorithm for treatment decision making for developmental disease of the medial compartment of the elbow in dogs. Vet Surg 2009;38(2):285–300.

29. Mitchell K. Traumatic elbow luxation in 14 dogs and 11 cats. Aust Vet J 2011; 89(6):213–6.

30. Angelou V, Papazoglou LG, Tsioli V, et al. Complete surgical excision versus Penrose drainage for the treatment of elbow hygroma in 19 dogs (1997 to 2014). J Small Anim Pract 2020;61(4):230–5.

31. Culp WTN, Olea-Popelka F, Sefton J, et al. Evaluation of outcome and prognostic factors for dogs living greater than one year after diagnosis of osteosarcoma: 90 cases (1997–2008). J Am Vet Med Assoc 2014;245(10):1141–6.
32. Harari J, Roe SC, Johnson AL, et al. Medial plating for the repair of middle and distal diaphyseal fractures of the humerus in dogs. Vet Surg 1986;15(1):45–8.
33. Denny HR. Condylar fractures of the humerus in the dog; a review of 133 cases. J Small Anim Pract 1983;24(4):185–97.
34. Langley-Hobbs SJ. Fractures of the humerus. In: Johnston SA, Tobias KM, editors. Veterinary surgery small animal. 2nd edition. St Louis (MO): Elsevier; 2018. p. 820–36.
35. Soslowsky L, Thomopoulos S, Tun S, et al. Overuse activity injures the supraspinatus tendon in an animal model: a histologic and biomechanical study. J Shoulder Elbow Surg 2000;9(2):79–84.
36. Lafuente MP, Fransson BA, Lincoln JD, et al. Surgical treatment of mineralized and nonmineralized supraspinatus tendinopathy in twenty-four dogs. Vet Surg 2009;38(3):380–7.
37. Cook JL, Renfro DC, Tomlinson JL, et al. Measurement of angles of abduction for diagnosis of shoulder instability in dogs using goniometry and digital image analysis. Vet Surg 2005;34(5):463–8.
38. Jones SC, Howard J, Bertran J, et al. Measurement of shoulder abduction angles in dogs: an ex vivo study of accuracy and repeatability. Vet Comp Orthop Traumatol 2019;32(06):427–32.
39. Tangner CH, Taylor J. Acquired muscle contractures in the dog and cat. A review of the literature and case report. Vet Comp Orthop Traumatol 2007;02(02):79–85.
40. DeCamp CE, Johnston SA, Dejardin LM, et al. The shoulder joint. In: Brinker, Piermattei, and Flo's handbook of small animal orthopedics and fracture repair. 5th edition. St Louis (MO): Elsevier; 2006. p. 260–97.

Assessment of Orthopedic Versus Neurologic Causes of Gait Change in Dogs and Cats

Sharon C. Kerwin, DVM, MS[a], Amanda R. Taylor, DVM[b],*

KEYWORDS

- Forelimb • Lameness • Root signature

KEY POINTS

- The most common causes of thoracic limb lameness are orthopedic diseases.
- The elbow joint is the source of most orthopedic disease resulting in lameness.
- Neurologic disease resulting in a gait change often causes other changes in the neurologic examination.
- Dogs may be affected by both orthopedic and neurologic disease, making determination of the underlying cause of gait change challenging.

INTRODUCTION

A change in gait is a common cause for clients to present their pet to a veterinarian for assessment. Determination of the underlying cause can be challenging even with full investigation of gait change with examination and diagnostics. In this article, the authors review examinations, both orthopedic and neurologic, specific to assessing the thoracic limb (forelimb) for underlying causes of gait change. The causes are reviewed in other articles included in this issue.

CLIENT HISTORY

Before examination, a discussion with the client regarding their pet is a helpful piece of evidence in determining the underlying reason for a gait change. Orthopedic disease is more likely to be present at all times and will look worse at faster speeds. Neurologic disease may be more intermittent in presentation and tends to appear worse at slower speeds. Clients should be asked whether they have noticed knuckling of the affected limb or limbs, abnormal toenail wear, and sores on the toes or pads (**Fig. 1**). Home video recordings provided by the client are a helpful tool, particularly for cats, and for dogs that are uncooperative for examination in the clinic.

[a] Department of Small Animal Clinical Sciences, College of Veterinary Medicine & Biomedical Sciences, Texas A&M University, TAMU 4474, College Station, TX 77843-4474, USA; [b] Pittsburgh Veterinary Specialty & Emergency Center, 807 Camp Horne Road, Pittsburgh, PA 15237, USA
* Corresponding author.
E-mail address: Amanda.taylor@bluepearlvet.com

Vet Clin Small Anim 51 (2021) 253–261
https://doi.org/10.1016/j.cvsm.2020.11.001
vetsmall.theclinics.com

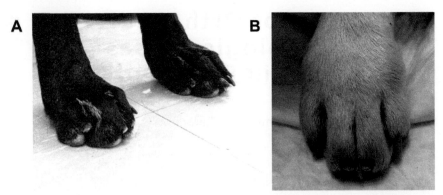

Fig. 1. Lateral (*A*) and dorsal (*B*) views of thoracic paws with worn nails consistent with proprioceptive deficits resulting in dragging of the limb.

GAIT EXAMINATION

A gait assessment is an essential first step for any cause of gait change and should be performed before other examination of the patient. Dogs should be walked with a slip lead on a surface with traction. Their gait should be observed from the front, back, and side. Cat examinations may need to be more creative for gait assessment, but often a cat will walk around a small, closed room as they explore their environment, finding interest in following their carrier or a laser pointer. Gait should be assessed at a walk and a trot, if possible, as different speeds can make a lameness more obvious.

When walking a dog for examination, it is important that the dog not be pulling at the leash or diving off to the left and right. It takes some practice to gain experience at walking a dog correctly so that the observer can see the gait from all angles and at several different speeds. Adjusting the slip lead higher up the cervical region may give the examiner more control; however, take care with dogs with neck pain. If there is any discomfort, consider walking with a harness or leash looped around 1 forelimb (**Fig. 2**). At the walk, one may observe a "head bob" with the head moved up as the painful affected forelimb strikes the ground. Typically, the more proximal (and more severe) the disease process, the more pronounced the head bob. Some lameness may not show up at the walk but is more apparent at the trot; conversely, some lameness may be most obvious at a slow walk.

The key differentiating factor between orthopedic and neurologic disease is assessing whether the patient is aware of limb position in space. A digital video (smartphone) camera is helpful, as the examination played back in slow motion can allow identification of relatively subtle lameness, particularly for small dogs with long-haired coats that obscure limb motion. While watching the animal move, the examiner should note which joint or joints have an increased or decreased flexion/extension, evaluate stride length for each limb, and compare right versus left. Circumduction in an affected limb may be apparent when viewing from the front or rear. Orthopedic disease will result in shortened stride, may limit motion of a joint, and may cause the weight of the patient to shift to the sound limb. The examiner should also listen to detect dragging toenails that may indicate a neurologic problem. Patients with decreased proprioception owing to neurologic disease may exhibit knuckling, scuffing, and crossing over midline with the affected limb. Although a short-strided, shuffling gait can indicate lower motor neuron disease (ie, polyneuropathy), it can also be indicative of orthopedic disease in multiple limbs (ie, hip plus elbow dysplasia or polyarthropathy) or

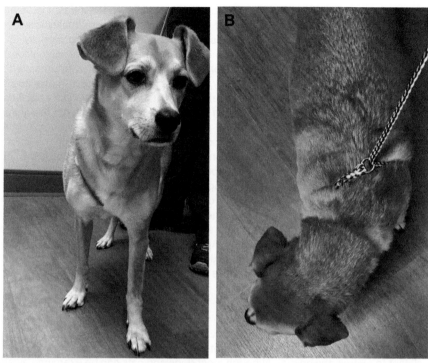

Fig. 2. Cranial (*A*) and dorsal view (*B*) of leash placement over 1 limb to avoid placing pressure on cervical region in dogs with neck pain.

diffuse, severe spinal pain without neurologic deficits (discospondylitis). In addition, limbs crossing over midline may also be observed in patients with orthopedic disease, but will not be accompanied by ataxia.

When possible, the animal should be observed going up and down steps, circling, going over curbs or small obstacles to detect subtle lameness, ataxia, or propriocep-tive deficits. For the cat, observing the gait as it jumps down from a low chair or stool may be valuable in differentiating orthopedic versus neurologic gait abnormality. An-imals with proprioceptive deficits may miss a step or hit the dorsal surface of a paw against the step as they go up.

Head and neck posture and mobility should also be assessed. Animals with neck pain may hold the neck low and straight and will move their eyes only, while keeping the head still, to observe things going on around them. Most animals without spinal pain will hold their heads up and move the neck about freely while observed on or off leash. If knuckling, scuffing, or ataxia is noted on gait evalua-tion, the authors recommend that neurologic evaluation be prioritized over ortho-pedic examination in cats and very nervous dogs, although typically they are done concurrently.

ORTHOPEDIC EXAMINATION
Standing

With the animal standing squarely, the head restrained by an assistant, and the exam-iner standing behind the patient, the examiner should carefully palpate and examine all of the major muscle masses of both forelimbs (as well as the rear limbs and spine). One of the easiest ways to detect muscle atrophy is by comparing the infraspinatus and supraspinatus muscles along the spine of the scapula. The triceps muscles should also be compared as well as the muscles of the antebrachium. Occasionally, one can detect more subtle differences, such as a difference in width or distension of the elbow or carpal joints, and joint effusion in general is much better appreciated in standing as opposed to lateral recumbency, while the joints are loaded. In challenging animals that resent lateral recumbency, evaluating joint range of motion and palpation of the long bones and muscles for signs of tenderness may be done with the animal standing. Although uncommon, peripheral nerve sheath tumors may be palpable on a standing examination as a mass in the axillary region or peripherally on the limb.

With the animal standing, proprioception should be assessed by flipping the foot and observing the amount of time it takes for the patient to replace the foot in a normal position (paw replacement reaction), making sure to support the patient under the pelvic limbs or chest to help them avoid falling or forcing all of their body weight on a painful or weak limb. In a normal dog or cat, the paw is replaced immediately.[1] Although orthopedic pain may slow this response, even in animals with orthopedic disease, normal paw replacement should occur. Appropriate support of the patient should allow even very painful animals to knuckle appropriately. Delayed or absent paw replacement may indicate a proprioceptive deficit, and a complete neurologic examination should be performed.

Lateral Recumbency

A complete orthopedic examination cannot be done without the help of a competent assistant to restrain the animal. Although most dogs and cats can be examined awake in lateral recumbency, occasionally sedation may be needed to complete the examination, and for the cat, much of what can typically be done in lateral recumbency for the dog can be done standing.

First, the nails and digits should be evaluated for abnormal wear or damage, saliva staining, or swelling around the nail beds. The area between the toes and pads should be closely examined for foreign bodies, draining tracts, skin lesions, and thickening. Each interphalangeal joint should be individually flexed and extended. Many normal dogs resent having their feet examined; however, this is usually an initial reaction, and the dog will relax as the examination continues. Each metacarpal should be palpated up to the carpus.

The carpus should be completely flexed and extended. In many (but not all) dogs and cats, the carpal pad can be touched to the caudal aspect of the antebrachium (**Fig. 3**) and the carpus can be extended past 180°. However, some dogs have more limited flexion of the carpus (eg, greyhounds); careful comparison of both sides is important. Average flexion/extension angles for the Labrador retriever have been reported as 32°/196° in dogs and 22°/198° in cats.[2,3] The tendons crossing the carpus should be palpated as well as the antebrachiocarpal, intercarpal, and carpometacarpal joints for instability and effusion. The integrity of the collateral ligaments is assessed by stressing the carpus medially and laterally.

The radius and ulna should be palpated separately, traveling from distal to proximal up the antebrachium, looking for bony changes or pain. The muscles of the antebrachium are also palpated separately from the bones, assessing for pain, hypertrophy, atrophy, or tendon thickening. Occasionally, small nerve sheath tumors or other soft tissue masses causing lameness can be found with careful muscle palpation.

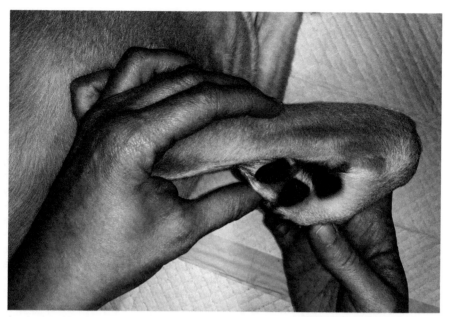

Fig. 3. Complete flexion of carpus with digital and metacarpal pads making contact with antebrachium.

The elbow is flexed and extended, and internally and externally rotated, which puts pressure on the coronoid processes of the ulna. Average flexion and extension angles for the elbow of Labrador retrievers are 36°/165° and 22°/162° in the cat.[2,3] The joint capsule should be palpated medially and laterally for evidence of thickness or effusion. It may be difficult to differentiate elbow from shoulder pain, as manipulation of 1 joint may affect the other, particularly in extension. As for the proximal limb, the humeral shaft should be individually palpated and the muscles of the upper forelimb palpated separately, evaluating for muscle and bone pain or deformity.

The shoulder has a very wide range of motion, with flexion and extension reported as 57°/165° in the Labrador retriever and 32°/162° in the cat.[2,3] It is important to fully manipulate the shoulder not just in flexion and extension but also in abduction/adduction and internal/external rotation. If shoulder instability is suspected, it may be useful to hold the distal scapula fixed and attempt to manipulate the proximal humerus in a "drawer"-type motion cranially and caudally. Although joint effusion is difficult to detect in the shoulder, joint pain can be detected by palpating the caudal joint capsule, particularly in dogs with osteochondritis dissecans of the shoulder. The best way to find this area is to "walk" down the spine of the scapula until the acromial process is reached; just below and caudal to this is the caudal aspect of the humeral head. Carefully palpate the biceps tendon with the shoulder in extension but also in full flexion, with the limb pulled almost parallel to the trunk to put maximum stress on the biceps brachii tendon, which runs just medial to the greater tubercle of the humerus. There are several publications evaluating whether medial shoulder instability is present based on measuring shoulder abduction angles in the dog; however, it is not clear how repeatable this test is in general practice.[4] Despite this, shoulder abduction can be helpful in detecting intermittent luxation, sometimes seen in toy breed dogs. As a routine part of the examination, the axilla should be palpated deeply, checking for muscle atrophy and masses and attempting to palpate the brachial plexus. A normal animal should not resent even deep palpation of the axillary area. Although rare, scapular avulsion (separation of the scapula from the thoracic body wall) has been reported in both dogs and cats. Excessive mobility of the scapula may also be noted on gait examination.

Once the examination in lateral recumbency is completed, there are 2 more important steps: spinal palpation and rectal examination. For spinal palpation, the animal is restrained as above for standing examination. In a normal dog or cat, the animal should be able to comfortably extend the cervical spine so that the nose points up at the ceiling, can flex down to almost touch the chest, and extend laterally from side to side to touch the thorax. Use caution with cervical flexion in patients with neck pain, especially toy breed dogs, as instability associated with atlantoaxial subluxation could damage the spinal cord. It is also important to deeply palpate the bones of the cervical vertebral column, from the wings of the atlas back to the ventral and lateral processes of C6-7. Animals with neck pain may have noticeable muscle fasciculation or spasm. For the thoracolumbar spine, many examiners will locate the spinous process, and then put firm, even pressure with the finger and thumb from T1 back to the lumbosacral space. The tail should be elevated dorsally, and the lumbosacral space should be palpated on rectal examination (dogs) as well (reserve as needed for cats under sedation), while the pelvic canal is evaluated for any masses, pain, or deformity of bony structures (pelvis, hips) and anal tone is assessed.

NEUROLOGIC EXAMINATION
Postural Reaction Testing

Paw replacement (knuckling) reaction has been discussed above. Wheelbarrowing (supporting the pelvic limbs just above the ground and moving the animal forward to evaluate forelimb gait) can be helpful in detecting more subtle proprioceptive deficits, and many examiners will repeat that maneuver with the head up or with the eyes covered. In smaller dogs and sometimes in cats, it is possible to test proprioception by bringing the dorsal surface of the paw gently up beneath the edge of examination table until it touches the table: a normal animal will place the paw on the table automatically (placing test). The animal should also be hopped back and forth on each forelimb individually, always with support to the rest of the body (keep in mind that normal cats may just flop down and will not always play this game). Carefully evaluate the pelvic limbs as well. Some dogs with cervical spinal cord involvement presenting for thoracic limb lameness will have proprioceptive or reflex abnormalities in the pelvic limbs associated with spinal cord compression that were not detected in the gait evaluation.

Forelimb Reflexes

Although the withdrawal reflex is the only consistently reliable forelimb reflex in small animals, it can be worthwhile to do the others if only to better evaluate muscle tone and orthopedic status and to compare between sides. These reflexes are typically done with the animal in lateral recumbency along with that portion of the orthopedic examination; however, the withdrawal reflex may be assessed with the animal standing and the thorax supported.

Extensor carpi reflex

With the limb supported and the carpus relaxed (it must be somewhat flexed or the reflex is impossible to see), the proximal, central portion of the extensor carpi radialis muscle is struck with the point of the reflex hammer, stimulating the radial nerve and causing a brief extension of the carpus. Hand positioning can be seen as in **Fig. 4**.

Biceps brachii reflex

The shoulder is flexed, making the insertion of the biceps brachii tendon taut and easily palpable at the level of the medial elbow. One or 2 fingers, depending on the size of the animal, are placed directly over the tendon and the fingers struck with the point of the hammer. The biceps muscle, innervated by the musculocutaneous nerve, is usually observed contracting along its length from shoulder to elbow. Hand positioning can be seen in **Fig. 5**.

Triceps reflex

Triceps reflex is the most difficult to observe. The elbow is flexed and slightly rotated to make the tendon taut. The examiner places a finger over the tendon and strikes it with the hammer or strikes the tendon with the flat side of the hammer, looking for contraction of the muscle belly and a brief elbow extension.

Withdrawal reflex

Withdrawal reflex is a general test of the entire brachial plexus and relies on both the sensory and the motor components of the nerves stimulated to be effective. Finger pressure can be effective, but some larger dogs may require pressure with a pair or hemostats to stimulate an effective response. The degree of flexion of the shoulder, elbow, and carpus should be assessed, and subjectively the strength of the limb should be assessed as well. A normal limb should fully flex each joint with this stimulus. Care should be taken not to apply too much counteractive force in small dogs and cats, as this may prevent withdrawal.

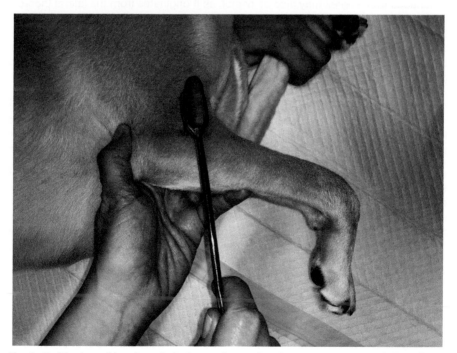

Fig. 4. Positioning of hands and pleximeter for performing extensor carpi radialis reflex.

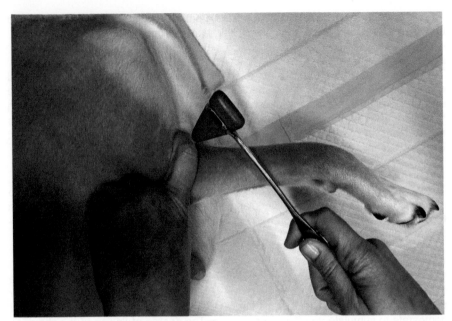

Fig. 5. Positioning of hands and pleximeter for performing biceps reflex.

Cutaneous trunci reflex

Cutaneous trunci reflex may also be useful, as it originates from the lateral thoracic nerve, which exits at the level of C7-T2 intervertebral foramen. The sensory arm of the reflex is the individual dorsal spinal nerves, which travel from lateral to midline and caudal to cranial, typically traversing 1 to 2 vertebral body lengths. The reflex typically starts in the midlumbar region, and hemostats are often required to generate sufficient sensory stimulus, particularly in larger dogs. The skin is pinched, and if the reflex arc is intact, the cutaneous trunci muscle will quickly contract bilaterally. Any lesion affecting the lateral thoracic nerve will eliminate this reflex on 1 side as the efferent arm of the reflex arc is affected. It should be kept in mind that occasionally there are normal dogs that do not have a cutaneous trunci reflex.

Cranial nerve examination and Horner syndrome

Brachial plexus injuries involving the outflow tracts of T1-T3 may cause Horner syndrome (loss of sympathetic innervation to the ipsilateral eye), resulting in ptosis, miosis, enophthalmos, and third eyelid elevation. A careful cranial nerve examination, focusing on assessment of pupil size and position, should be included in the case of forelimb dysfunction and is a part of a complete neurologic examination.

DISCUSSION

As a general rule, orthopedic disease is a far more common cause of forelimb gait abnormality in dogs and cats than neurologic disease. However, they often coexist, particularly in older animals, and orthopedic disease may get most of the attention, resulting in a lost opportunity for early diagnosis and treatment of important neurologic disease.

Some disorders, particularly foraminal extrusion of disc with cervical intervertebral disc disease, and disorders of the brachial plexus can look like orthopedic disease early on and may present without any neurologic abnormalities. These cases eventually present for referral with multiple sets of normal radiographs of the bones and joints of the affected limb, and advanced imaging and electrodiagnostics may be needed to make the diagnosis. Many of these disease processes will eventually result in obvious neurologic deficits.

Performing the orthopedic and neurologic examination simultaneously is an efficient way of getting the most diagnostic information possible in 1 visit. With practice, a combination examination can be done quickly and effectively, even in cats or challenging dogs. When orthopedic and neurologic abnormalities are both present, the neurologic problem should be prioritized when planning diagnostics to include imaging, although a thorough knowledge of any orthopedic abnormalities will be helpful in setting owner expectations for outcome and in designing and evaluating an appropriate treatment plan.

SUMMARY

Diagnosis of forelimb lameness may be challenging, as it not only can be due to multiple common orthopedic diseases but also may occasionally be caused by neurologic disease. A thorough orthopedic and neurologic examination is key to determining which disease category is the likely culprit. Deficits identified on the neurologic examination, such as proprioceptive deficits, changes in reflexes, and presence of spinal hyperesthesia, are key in identifying neurologic causes of forelimb lameness.

CLINICS CARE POINTS

- Combining all, or elements of, the orthopedic and neurologic examination for every patient with thoracic limb lameness will improve diagnostic capability.

- Attention to whether the animal knows where the limb is in space (proprioception) is key in differentiating neurologic versus orthopedic gait abnormalities.

- Orthopedic disease and neurologic disease often present together, with the neurologic disease taking diagnostic precedence.

DISCLOSURE

The authors of this article have no commercial or financial conflicts of interest.

REFERENCES

1. de LaHunta A, Glass E, Kent M. Veterinary neuroanatomy and clinical neurology. Elsevier; 2015.
2. Jaeger GH, Marcellin-Little DJ, Depuy V, et al. Validity of goniometric joint measurements in cats. Am J Vet Res 2007;68(8):822–6.
3. Jaegger G, Marcellin-Little DJ, Levine D. Reliability of goniometry in Labrador retrievers. Am J Vet Res 2002;63(7):979–86.
4. Franklin SP. Editorial: diagnosis of medial shoulder instability. Vet Comp Orthop Traumatol 2019;32:v–vi.

Common Pathology Associated with the Digits and Metacarpal Region

Alessandro Piras, DVM, MS[a],*, Kenneth A. Bruecker, DVM, MS[b]

KEYWORDS

- Metacarpal • Phalangeal • Digit • Fracture • Ligament • Sprain • Tendon • Corn

KEY POINTS

- Fractures and ligamentous injury of the paw are common injuries in small animal.
- The principles of fracture repair are similar as for long bones in other areas of the body.
- The principles of ligament repair are similar for other joints.
- Corns are thickened areas of tissue in the digital pad caused by repeated mechanical injury.

INTRODUCTION

Fractures and ligamentous injuries of the front paw are common in small animals and usually result from direct trauma, such as a vehicular accident, collision with a stationary object, falls from a height, or entrapment of the paw with leverage (eg, stepping in a hole while running).[1–4] Metacarpal and phalangeal fractures may be associated with concurrent ligamentous injury. Tendon and paw injuries are generally associated with direct traumatic etiologies, such as laceration.

FRACTURES

Fractures of the metacarpal and phalangeal bones are classified according to their anatomic location as fractures of the base, fractures of the shaft, and fractures of the head[5] (**Fig. 1**).

Diagnostic Imaging Evaluation

Orthogonal radiographs, dorsopalmar (DP) and lateral views, from carpus to toes are the standard. In addition, DP 15° oblique views and lateral 45° oblique views or stress views are often necessary to isolate individual bones or to evaluate complex multiple fractures and ligamentous injuries. When assessing the digits, separation of the toes

a Sporting Dog Clinic, Kurjenkellontie 14, Espoo 02270, Finland; b Continuing Orthopedic Veterinary Education, Ventura County, Moorpark, CA 93021, USA
* Corresponding author.
E-mail address: alexpvet@mac.com

Vet Clin Small Anim 51 (2021) 263–284
https://doi.org/10.1016/j.cvsm.2020.12.001
0195-5616/21/© 2020 Elsevier Inc. All rights reserved.

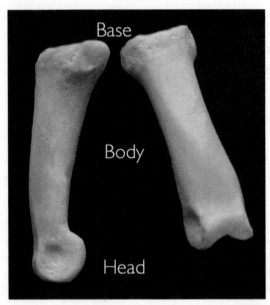

Fig. 1. Phalangeal fracture anatomic location. (*Courtesy* A. Piras, DVM, IVIS, Sporting Dog Clinic- Espoo, Finland.)

on the lateral and DP views with the aid of stirrups of tape on the second and fifth digits is beneficial (fan lateral and DP views) (**Fig. 2**). A computed tomography scan is quicker, provides a more detailed evaluation of the fracture configuration and is especially useful for assessment of articular fractures.

Metacarpal Fractures

Fractures of the base
Basilar fractures are generally avulsions of the ligamentous or tendinous insertions and usually involve the second and the fifth metacarpal. [6–13] Conservative treatment is an acceptable treatment option for nondisplaced and inherently stable fractures.

Owing to the tendency of the fragment to displace, there is risk of malunion and angular deviation in unstable fractures. In these selected cases, open reduction and internal fixation represents the treatment of choice. Fixation can be achieved with a small diameter Kirschner wire (K wire) and a figure-of-8 tension band wire. As an alternative, multiple lag screws are inserted after anatomic fracture reduction (**Fig. 3**). If a plate is used to buttress the fractures, some screws can be inserted through the plate (**Fig. 4**).

Fractures of the shaft
Metacarpal shaft fractures can be treated either conservatively or surgically. The decision between these methods is based on the configuration and location of fractures, the number of bones involved, and the inherent stability of the fractures. The most commonly used implants are locking compression plates, usually 1.5 or 2.0 mm, and can be used in standard, locking, or hybrid mode. A range of miniaturized plates and 1.1-mm screws are available, tackling the challenge related to the small bone size in toy breed dogs and feline patients. Another practical option is to use cuttable plates. They are available in different design, thickness, and screw

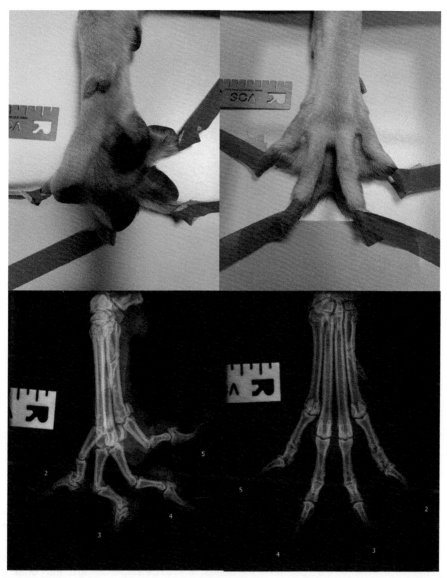

Fig. 2. Radiographic positioning and corresponding x-ray imagines of ML and DP "fan" views. These views are very helpful to clearly identify the anatomic structures of the digits. (*Courtesy of* E. Syrjanen, DVM, Espoo, Finland.)

sizes. The screw holes are round and can accommodate 2 screws sizes (1.5/2.0, 2.0/ 2.4, 2.4/2.7); although they do not allow interfragmentary compression, this is not considered necessary in the majority of the cases. The fracture configuration usually dictates the modality of application of the implant (interfragmentary compression vs neutralization or bridging), but it is possible to apply exceptions to the rule, particularly when dealing with multiple metacarpal fractures. In this case, prioritization and fracture alignment are more important than perfect anatomic reconstruction and

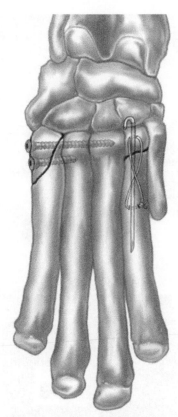

Fig. 3. Fracture of the base of the second metacarpal bone stabilized with K wire and tension band, and of the base of the fifth metacarpal bone with lag screws. (*From* Piras A and Dee JF. Repair of fractures involving metabones and phalanges, In: Bojrab MJ, Waldron DR, Toombs JP, eds. Current Techniques in Small Animal Surgery. Jackson, WY: Teton NewMedia; 2014:965-972; with permission.)

fixation modality. If adjacent metacarpal bones are intact or stable after repair, these bones can have a splinting effect, such that bridging of nonreducible fractures can be successful (**Fig. 5**).

Transverse, nondisplaced fractures of either 1 or 2 metacarpal bones, located at the proximal and middle third portion of the bones, tend to be stable owing to the containing effect of the adjacent intact metacarpals, and can be treated with closed reduction and external coaptation.

Fractures located in the distal portion of the shaft tend to displace and are more difficult to maintain in a reduced position with external coaptation. Internal fixation of shaft fractures is usually indicated when there are multiple bones fractured, when the 2 central weight-bearing bones (third and fourth) are fractured, or fracture fragments are severely displaced. Open reduction and internal fixation should be considered to achieve the best functional results especially in canine athletes and working dogs. Plate application in transverse fractures ensures a very stable fixation. The plate is applied to the dorsal aspect of metacarpals III and IV, to the medial aspect of metacarpal II and to lateral aspect of metacarpal V.

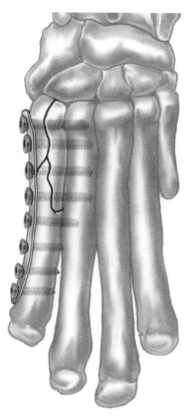

Fig. 4. A comminuted fracture of the base and shaft of the metacarpal bone V have been treated with a veterinary cuttable plate (1.5/2.0 mm), applied on the lateral aspect of the bone. The first 4 screws are applied in lag fashion. (*From* Piras A and Dee JF. Repair of fractures involving metabones and phalanges, In: Bojrab MJ, Waldron DR, Toombs JP, eds. Current Techniques in Small Animal Surgery. Jackson, WY: Teton NewMedia; 2014:965-972; with permission.)

Intramedullary pinning has been described as a successful method of treatment and its indications are fractures involving only 1 or 2 meta-bones that are stable after reduction and fractures in young non-athletic breeds. Although intramedullary pinning improves angular alignment, torsional stability is not achieved. External coaptation is thus required.

A small diameter K wire is inserted, starting distally, close to the dorsal attachment of the joint capsule and driven into the proximal fragment, up to the base of the bone. A slot can be created in the dorsal cortex at the insertion point for the wire with a high-speed burr to facilitate the insertion of the wire. The protruding portion of the wire is bent over into a hook and lodged in the slot (**Fig. 6**). Micromotion, pin migration, and nonunion are common complications. Rigid external coaptation (splint or cast) is required to limit micromotion.

Long oblique and spiral fractures are generally repaired with multiple lag screws. If screws are used as the only form of fixation, the length of the fracture has to be at least twice the diameter of the metacarpal and a minimum of 2 screws need to be placed (**Fig. 7**). If required, the repair can be supported with a neutralization plate. This point

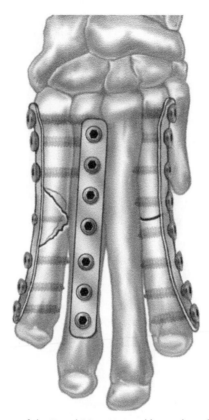

Fig. 5. Transverse fractures of the II and IV metacarpal bones have been treated with medial (MC II) and dorsal (MC IV) plating. A comminuted fracture of the V metacarpal bone has been treated with a bridging plate applied laterally. In this case, it is possible to stabilize the large butterfly fragment with a 1.5-mm screw applied through the plate. (*From* Piras A and Dee JF. Repair of fractures involving metabones and phalanges, In: Bojrab MJ, Waldron DR, Toombs JP, eds. Current Techniques in Small Animal Surgery. Jackson, WY: Teton NewMedia; 2014:965-972; with permission.)

is especially true in the case of fractures involving metacarpal III or IV. Comminuted fractures are best repaired with a combination of lag screws and plates. With large fragments, screws can be applied in lag fashion through the plate.

A biological approach is recommended for nonreconstructable, highly comminuted fractures. A bone plate can be applied in a bridging fashion, maintaining axial alignment, torsional alignment and length. An acrylic external fixation approach, nicknamed the "spider fixator" has been described.[14]

Fractures of the head
Fractures of the head (distal) are usually intra-articular, involving the condyles. Closed reduction is only advisable for incomplete fractures. Surgical treatment is indicated for monocondylar and for T or Y fractures. Simple fractures can be repaired with application of one or a combination of lag screws, usually 1.5 mm or 1.1 mm (see **Fig. 5**). Although repair by the use of a small cerclage wire has been described, the authors do not recommend this technique owing to its many limitations that range from soft

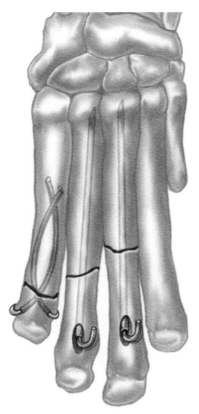

Fig. 6. Transverse fractures of the III and IV metacarpal bones repaired with intramedullary pins using the "slot" technique. A transverse fracture of the metaphysis of the V metacarpal bone repaired with 2 Rush pins. (*From* Piras A and Dee JF. Repair of fractures involving metabones and phalanges, In: Bojrab MJ, Waldron DR, Toombs JP, eds. Current Techniques in Small Animal Surgery. Jackson, WY: Teton NewMedia; 2014:965-972; with permission.)

tissues irritation and entrapment, wire breakage, and bulkiness of the wire twist that often risk to protrude through the scarce soft tissues coverage. In more complex fractures, it is possible to use appropriately sized T or lateral plates (**Fig. 8**).

Postoperative care. After surgery, a padded bandage is applied for approximately 3 to 4 weeks until radiographic signs of bone healing are seen. Kennel or cage confinement is necessary until the bandage removal. This period is followed by 4 to 8 weeks of restricted exercise. A molded splint is applied where the need for implant protection is deemed appropriate.

Conservative treatment. A padded bandage is reinforced with a molded splint or with a fiberglass cast. Kennel confinement and rest are required until there are radiographic signs of bone healing, which occurs usually within 4 to 8 weeks.

Phalangeal Fractures

Phalangeal fractures are common injuries, but often underestimated. As a consequence, their treatment is often suboptimal. Breed, age, type of activity, owner expectations, and compliance, as well as, injury characteristics, pattern of the fracture, and

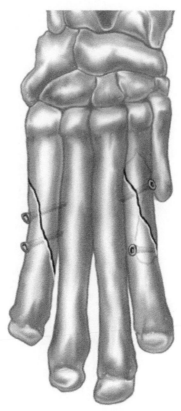

Fig. 7. Two oblique shaft fractures have been repaired with lag screws. It may be possible to reinforce the repair by adding a neutralizing plate. (*From* Piras A and Dee JF. Repair of fractures involving metabones and phalanges, In: Bojrab MJ, Waldron DR, Toombs JP, eds. Current Techniques in Small Animal Surgery. Jackson, WY: Teton NewMedia; 2014:965-972; with permission.)

soft tissue damage are all important factors that must be taken into account when establishing a treatment plan.

Phalangeal fractures of P1 and P2 can be classified similarly to metacarpal fractures according to location and configuration. Transverse, long oblique and spiral extra-articular fractures are common patterns, particularly for P1. Multifragmented fractures of the shaft can be extra-articular or extend to the joint level. Condylar fracture can be monocondylar, bicondylar, or comminuted (**Fig. 9**). Pediatric fractures usually affect the proximal growth plate and, less commonly, the shaft (**Fig. 10**).

Simple, stable, nondisplaced fractures, especially in young dogs, respond very well to conservative treatment by strapping the toes together with kinesiology tape, "buddy taping" (**Fig. 11**). The technique consists of taping the affected digit against the next intact digit (digits) taking advantage of the natural splinting action offered from intact adjacent digits. After the tape is applied, the extremity is protected with a padded bandage. The bandage is changed every 3 to 5 days until bone healing occurs, usually around 3 to 4 weeks.

Fractures with an unstable configuration are traditionally treated with open reduction and internal fixation with lag screws (1.5 mm or 1.1 mm) or miniplates (**Fig. 12**).

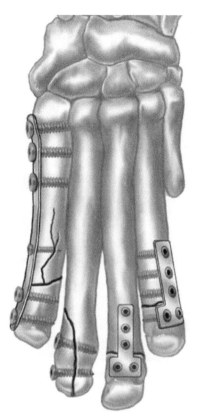

Fig. 8. Fractures of the metaphysis of the II and III metacarpal bones. These fractures are treated with a small lateral plate and a small T plate. Care should be taken to avoid the joint space and to avoid allowing the screws to protrude into the sesamoids. A fracture of the head of the IV metacarpal bone is repaired with 2 lag screws. Excessive countersinking of the head of the most distal screw can damage the insertion of the collateral ligament and can irritate the joint capsule. A fracture of the metaphyseal area of the V metacarpal bone presents several fissures extending proximally. This fracture is repaired with a Veterinary Cuttable Plate in a bridging fashion. Two proximal and 2 distal screws are usually sufficient. (*From* Piras A and Dee JF. Repair of fractures involving metabones and phalanges, In: Bojrab MJ, Waldron DR, Toombs JP, eds. Current Techniques in Small Animal Surgery. Jackson, WY: Teton NewMedia; 2014:965-972; with permission.)

Careful handling of the fracture fragments with appropriate instruments and gentle traction is required not to compromise the delicate vascular structures in this area. Failure to respect the blood supply can lead to severe complications from nonunion or necrosis of the toe.

Selected fractures in pediatric patients can be treated with a less invasive approach using a small diameter K wire (usually 0.8 mm) inserted in a Rush fashion from the base into the medullary canal of the bone with the purpose of maintaining alignment during the rapid bone healing (**Fig. 13**). The interphalangeal joint level is localized with an insulin needle. Through a small stab incision in the skin, with the edge of the base localized, the K wire is advanced while maintaining the digit in gentle traction and the fracture reduced by digital pressure. When the K wire is safely inserted, the protruding portion is bent slightly and cut adjacent to the bone. Buddy taping is applied and

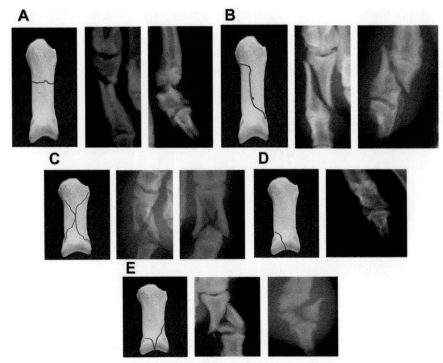

Fig. 9. Fractures of the phalanges. (*A*) Transverse, (*B*) long spiral oblique, (*C*) comminuted, (*D*) condylar, and (*E*) bicondylar. (*Courtesy* A. Piras, DVM, IVIS, Sporting Dog Clinic- Espoo, Finland.)

supported with a padded bandage. Frequent rechecks and bandage changes are necessary (typically every 3–5 days). As soon as there is radiographic evidence of callus formation, the K wire can be removed and the buddy taping reapplied for another 10 days.

Fractures of the base or of the head are articular and almost invariably involve the insertion of the collateral ligaments. Fractures of the condyles can be managed with

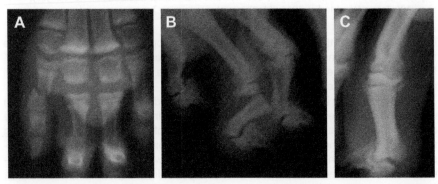

Fig. 10. Pediatric phalangeal fractures. (*A*) Transverse, (*B*) proximal physis, and (*C*) proximal condylar. (*Courtesy* A. Piras, DVM, IVIS, Sporting Dog Clinic- Espoo, Finland.)

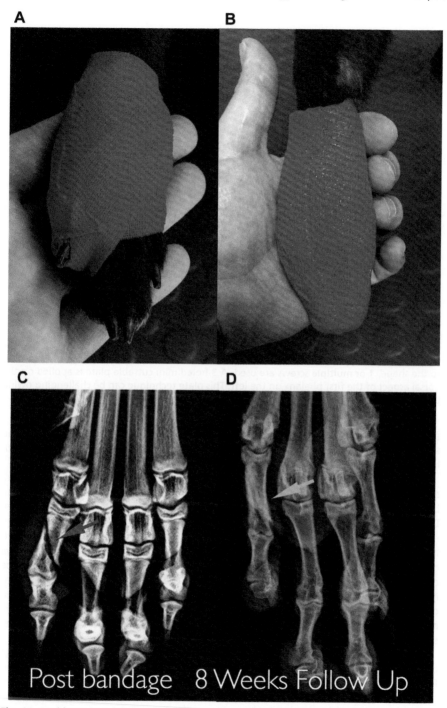

Fig. 11. Buddy taping. (*A*) Conservative treatment by buddy taping of a nondisplaced long oblique fracture of P1 of the II digit. (*B*) After application of the strips of tape, a padded bandage is applied. (*C*) Immediate postbandage radiograph. Note the minimal displacement owing to the containment of the periosteal sleeve in this 5-months-old Greyhound (*red arrow*). (*D*) The *yellow arrow* shows the healing and remodeling on a radiograph at 8 weeks of follow-up.

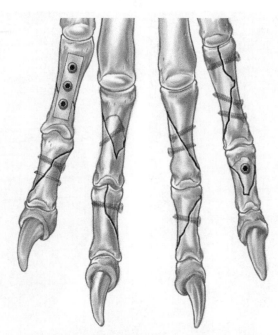

Fig. 12. Different phalangeal fracture patterns repaired with 1.5-mm lag screws. According to the shape, 1 or multiple screws are used. A 3-holed mini cuttable plate is applied on the dorsal aspect of the first phalanx on the left. This plate technique can be challenging owing to the presence of the extensor tendon and usually applies only on P1 in large patients.

application of lag screws or with a loop of cerclage wire unless the fragments are too small to be safely secured in place. Very small fragments can be excised. In cases with large unfixable fragments involving the joint, digit amputation may be advisable.

Traditionally, the lag screw technique has been the standard for fixation of oblique, spiral, and condylar fractures. This technique is relatively straightforward for most long bones fractures, but can be technically challenging for fracture fixation of small bones. Despite the availability of very small implants, the size of these screws remains large relative to the phalanges and the fragments to be fixed, leaving little room for error and increasing the chance of iatrogenic comminution. The advent of 1.1-mm microscrews dramatically improved the outcome in internal fixation of phalangeal fractures. The use of microimplants requires a certain degree of skill. The use of magnifying loops is highly recommended. The most common challenges are related to the drilling technique owing to the size of the drill bit (0.8 mm), the screw insertion and tightening because it is very easy to apply excessive force that can shear the head off the neck of the screw.

The application of bicortical (positional) self-tapping screws provides the advantage of elimination of a surgical step. There is less chance for the reduction to be lost and for splitting of the fragments. With bicortical screws, the proximal cortex is not overdrilled, and the screw threads achieve purchase in both cortices while reduction and compression are maintained with bone clamps.[15]

Open fractures are often comminuted and highly contaminated with severe soft tissue damage and avascular bone fragments protruding through the skin. In these cases, digit amputation is the best choice, offering a good prognosis even in sporting dogs with a rapid return to performance.

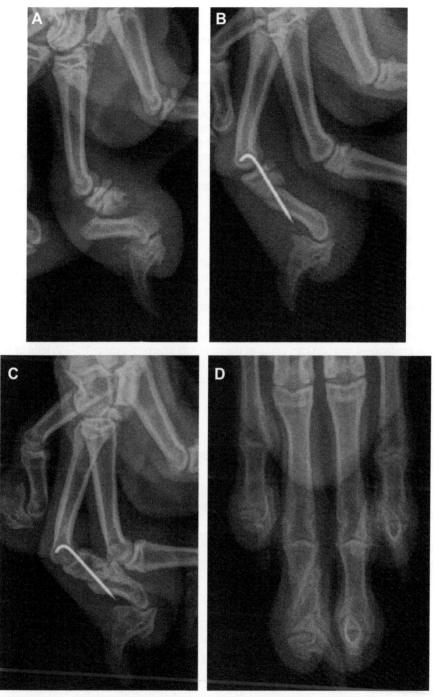

Fig. 13. Preoperative (*A*) and postoperative (*B*) Radiograph images of a fracture of P2 in a 3-months-old Sloughi. The fracture have been realigned and repaired with of a 1.0 mm K wire inserted through a stab incision and guided fluoroscopically. Follow-up radiographs at 4 weeks postoperative (*C*) and at 2 weeks after pin removal (*D*).

Fractures of P3 can involve the joint, split the phalanx obliquely, or involve the tuberosity of insertion of the deep flexor tendon or the ungual crest (**Fig. 14**). Owing to the small size of P3, attempts at internal fixation are unlikely to be successful and digit amputation is necessary.

Postoperative care after surgical repair consists of the application of a padded bandage for 3 to 4 weeks and confinement for a total of 6 to 8 weeks. The bandage can be reinforced with a palmar splint for the first 2 weeks. After bandage removal and when radiographs confirm that the bone is healed, 3 weeks of limited exercise on a lead and a gradual increase in activity should precede a return to full activity.

After amputation, a light bandage is applied for 2 weeks. As soon as the swelling decreases and the reflected digital pad is properly sealed, it is possible to gradually reintroduce the dog to exercise. For sporting dogs, the return to full training after amputation is expected by 5 to 6 weeks postoperatively. The prognosis for noncomplicated cases is usually good to excellent.

LIGAMENT INJURIES

Phalangeal subluxations and luxations are uncommon injuries in the canine pet population, but are very common injuries in sporting dogs, especially in racing, coursing, and agility athletes.[16] Uneven terrain (hard and soft surfaces, synthetic surfaces, holes), sudden changes in direction, and agility course A frames and tunnels, as well as digit conformation such as flat toes or spread toes and/or excessively long toe nails, are predisposing factors for ligamentous injuries.[17]

A phalangeal luxation can occur at the proximal interphalangeal (P1–P2) joint or the distal interphalangeal (P2–P3) joint. Farrow[18] has classified sprain injuries according to severity. A first-degree sprain consists of minimal tearing or stretching of the ligament fibers. A second-degree sprain is a partial rupture with evident structural damage. Third-degree sprains consist of a complete rupture of the ligament fibers and may

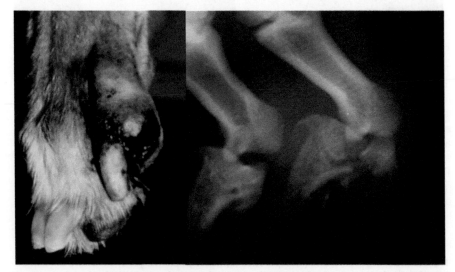

Fig. 14. Comminuted fracture of P3 confirmed by radiographic evaluation. Note the vast bruising and the skin laceration between the digital pad and the nail. These fractures are almost invariably open and contaminated.

include avulsion injuries of the origin or insertion of the ligament with one or more bone chips.

First- and Second-Degree Sprains

P1 to P2 and P2 to P3 collateral ligaments

Lameness is usually minimal or absent with bruising, joint effusion, and palpable swelling. To verify the stability of the joint, it is necessary to extend the phalanges and apply mediolateral movement. In first-degree injuries, there is a light pain response and good joint stability, whereas in a second-degree sprain, there is minimal lateral instability and it is often possible to palpate, with the tip of a finger, an increased joint space.

If joint laxity is detected, it is possible to apply a light bandage or phalangeal buddy taping. Shortening the nail is useful to decrease the leverage on the affected joint. Two to 3 weeks of confined activity followed by 3 weeks of controlled exercise are generally sufficient to allow healing of the lesion. Fibrosis of the joint can be expected, and recurrence is not unusual. In some second-degree sprains with excessive instability, surgical reinforcement of the stretched capsule and ligament is advised. One to 3 synthetic absorbable sutures can be placed over the ligament for stress protection during healing.

Third-Degree Sprain

In the case of complete ligament rupture with the joint in a reduced position, lameness can be from minimal to slight during weight-bearing. In dogs with a subluxated or luxated joint, lameness can be significant.[19] Swelling and bruising are consistent findings.

Palpation of the joint elicits pain, and it is possible to dislocate the joint with minimal mediolateral or varus–valgus pressure. In the case of a bilateral ligament rupture, the joint tends to stay in a subluxated position with the toe slightly rotated (**Fig. 15**). Radiographic or, preferably, computed tomography evaluation is necessary to evaluate the integrity of the condyles and/or the base of the phalanges because small avulsed chips are often detected with radiographs. These types of injuries necessitate surgical repair.

Surgical Technique

The dog is placed in lateral recumbency with the side of the toe to be operated facing up. With the patient in dorsal recumbency, the medial and lateral aspects of the metacarpal and phalangeal joints are accessible. A small direct surgical approach is sufficient to expose the ligament. The joint is explored to remove any small avulsion fragments. One to 3 modified Kessler loop sutures of 5-0 to 4-0 synthetic absorbable suture material are placed in the ligament and joint capsule (**Fig. 16**). A single large Connell suture to encompass the repair can be used for extra stability. The author's preferences regarding the suture material are polydioxanone or polyglactin 910. In bilateral repair, additional strength is achieved by adding some suture of nonabsorbable monofilament suture material. The nail is cut short to minimize leverage forces.

The repair is protected with a padded bandage for 2 to 3 weeks. Once the bandage is removed, controlled exercise such as swimming and leash-controlled walks are allowed until 6 to 8 weeks postoperatively. During reintroduction to training, the affected digit can be supported with toe strapping using kinesiology tape. Severe bilateral ligament ruptures with large articular chips, chronic ligament lesions, and gross instability are usually treated with toe amputation or arthrodesis.

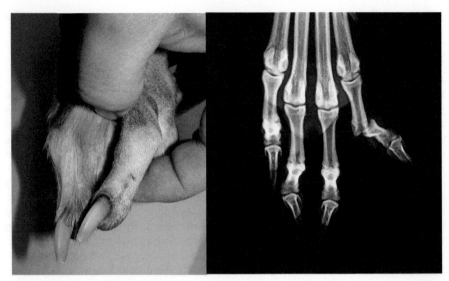

Fig. 15. Bilateral collateral instability affecting the P1 to P2 joint of the second digit confirmed by radiographic evaluation.

Metacarpophalangeal Instability Owing to Ligament Damage

In racing greyhounds, these injuries usually affect either the V or the II digit, more often the left V and right II. In acute injuries, the dog is generally lame, but weight bearing. The affected area is swollen with flexion and extension of the joint eliciting a pain response. Inward or outward rotation of the digit can dislocate the joint. Conservative treatment is not successful and surgical repair is preferred.

Some dogs with chronic injuries are occasionally able to perform with the application of a strapping of kinesiology tape around the distal metacarpophalangeal joints to provide additional support. Surgical treatment consists of the repair and support of the

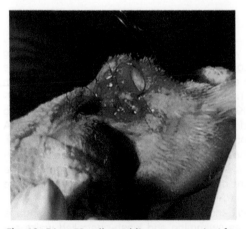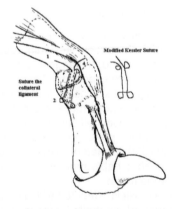

Fig. 16. P1 to P2 collateral ligament repair. After direct surgical exposure, the ruptured ligament is visualized and repaired with a series of modified Kessler loop sutures. (*Adapted from* DeCamp CE, Johnston SA, Dejardin LM, et al. Fractures and other orthopedic conditions of the carpus, metacarpus, and phalanges. In: DeCamp CE, Johnston SA, Dejardin LM, Schaefer SL, eds. Brinker, Piermattei, and Flo's Handbook of Small Animal Orthopedics and Fracture Repair. 5th ed. St. Louis, MO: Elsevier; 2016:389-433; with permission.)

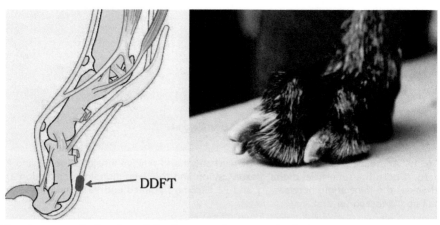

Fig. 17. Anatomic drawing of the flexor mechanism and relative insertions on P2 and P3 (*left*). If only the deep digital flexor tendon is affected, the joint angle between P1 and P2 remains normal around 135°. The third phalanx will flip up with the nail obviously elevated from the ground owing to the action of the extensor tendon and dorsal elastic ligaments ("knocked up toe").

damaged ligaments via a palmar or lateral approach. The same type of repair described for the interphalangeal ligaments is used.

After surgery, a padded bandage is applied for 3 weeks, followed by buddy taping for another 2 to 3 weeks. Mild activity is encouraged starting 5 to 6 weeks postoperatively. Return to training is expected between 8 and 10 weeks after surgery. These repairs have a high rate of failure and often amputation of the entire digit is the only choice. After digit amputation, the dog can restart training in 3 to 4 weeks.

TENDON INJURIES AND SESAMOID FRACTURES

Laceration of the deep or superficial digital flexor tendons represents the most common injury of tendons of the digits in these authors' experiences. Rupture or avulsion

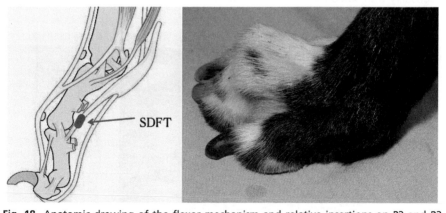

Fig. 18. Anatomic drawing of the flexor mechanism and relative insertions on P2 and P3 (*left*). If only the superficial digital flexor tendon is affected, the joint angle between P2 and P3 remains normal with the nail in contact with the ground. The joint angle between P1 and P2 becomes flattened owing to the increased extension.

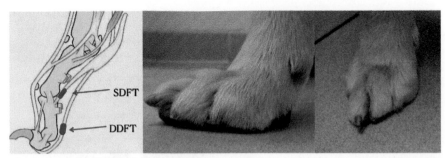

Fig. 19. Anatomic drawing of the flexor mechanism and relative insertions on P2 and P3 (*left*). If both the superficial digital flexor tendon and the deep digital flexor tendon are affected, the joint angle between P1 and P2 become flattened and P3 extends with the nail up ("knocked up toe").

of the insertion of the tendon is seen less frequently. The diagnosis is made largely on physical examination. The deep digital flexor tendon inserts on the palmar surface of P3. Thus, injury results in an elevated toe nail or a knocked up toe (**Fig. 17**). The superficial digital flexor tendon inserts on the palmar surface of the base of P2. Isolated injury of this tendon results in a flat foot appearance with the nail in contact with the ground (**Fig. 18**). The digit will be flattened and the nail elevated when both the superficial digital flexor tendon and deep digital flexor tendon are injured (**Fig. 19**). As with ligament injuries, the authors prefer a modified Kessler pattern using absorbable monofilament for repair of digital flexor tendon injuries in athletes and working dogs (**Fig. 20**).

Palmar sesamoid fractures are thought to result from repetitive excessive tension of the overlying digital flexor tendons during hyperextension of the metacarpophalangeal joints (**Fig. 21**). An over-representation in the Rottweiler may mean this breed is genetically predisposed to palmar sesamoid fractures. Pain can usually be elicited with focal palpation and is confirmed radiographically (see **Fig. 15**). In acute cases, splinting may result in osseous or fibrous union. Chronic cases often exhibit lameness only after heavy exercise. In some chronic cases, excision of the sesamoid fragments may be necessary with outcomes similar to digital flexor tendon injuries.[20]

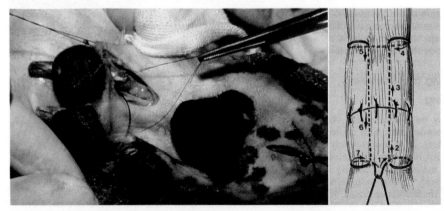

Fig. 20. The deep flexor tendon is repaired by end to end apposition and application of 2 Modified Kessler Loops sutures with 4-0 polydioxanone.

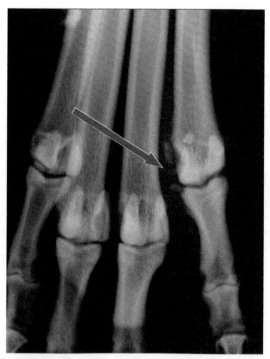

Fig. 21. Palmar sesamoid fracture (*red arrow*). (*Courtesy* A. Piras, DVM, IVIS, Sporting Dog Clinic- Espoo, Finland.)

INFECTIONS AND NEOPLASIA

Infection and osteomyelitis associated with injury of the toenail and nail bed is not uncommon. If the infection is accompanied by significant osteomyelitis of P3, amputation of the affected digit by disarticulation at P2 or P3 may be required for

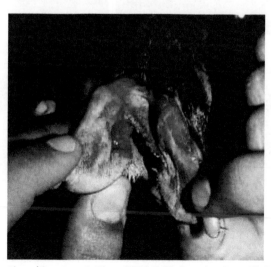

Fig. 22. Web laceration. (*Courtesy* A. Piras, DVM, IVIS, Sporting Dog Clinic- Espoo, Finland.)

resolution. As with infection, the nail bed of P3 is the most common location for neoplastic conditions. Neoplasia is discussed in more detail in chapter Common neoplastic diseases affecting the forelimb by Lapsley and Selmic.

PAW INJURIES AND CORNS

Pad lacerations and web lacerations result from direct injury to paws[21] (**Fig. 22**). In acute cases, a primary repair may be warranted. In more chronic cases, healing by secondary intention may be indicated. In either case, protecting the wound by rigid coaptation with a caudal spoon splint is indicated to prevent separation of the wound with every weight bearing step.

Corns are thickened areas of tissue in the digital pad caused by repeated mechanical injury (**Fig. 23**). Corns occur most commonly in Greyhounds retired from racing. Lameness is most pronounced on hard surfaces. Corns are quite painful to focal palpation pressure. Classically, hulling out the corn with a curette, dental instrument, or scalpel has been the treatment of choice. A recurrence rate of 80%, however, means lifelong management and a protective booty is generally necessary. Repeated recurrence may necessitate digit amputation. More recently, Guillard[22] described

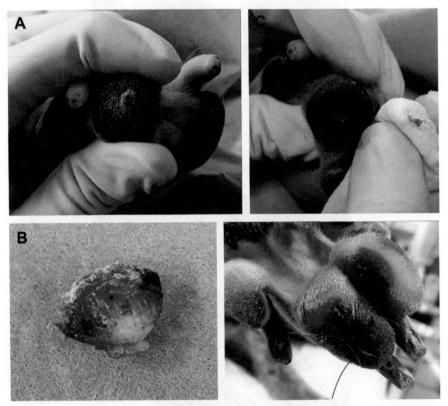

Fig. 23. A corn affecting the digital pad (*A*) has been removed full thickness with a number 11 blade (*B*). Once removed the wound is curetted deep enough to remove any remaining portion of corn from the pad (*C*), the wound is then sutured with interrupted nonresorbable monofilament nylon (*D*). (*Courtesy of* E. Syrjanen, DVM, Espoo, Finland.)

treatment of corns by superficial digital flexor tenotomy. Superficial digital flexor tenotomy causes the toe to tip up, off-loading the area of the corn, and the corn eventually exfoliates and disappears.

CLINICS CARE POINTS

- Injuries of the digits of the forelimb including fractures of the metacarpal bones and phalangeal bones, as well as ligament and tendon injuries are not uncommon.

- The principles of fracture management are similar to other long bones of the body. The bones of the digits are, however, very small and thus small implants are required. The need to use undersized implants often necessitates protecting the stabilization with external coaptation in the early postoperative period.

- Similarly, the principles of collateral ligament repair of the digits is the same as collateral ligament repair in other regions of the body. As with fractures, the need to use small or undersized suture material makes augmentation with external coaptation generally necessary.

- Tendon lacerations can be repaired surgically using techniques appropriate for tendon repair elsewhere in the body.

- Corns are not uncommon in retired greyhounds. The treatment for corns, including resection, can be unrewarding because recurrence is common. Transection of the deep digital flexor tendon causes the digit to raise and off-load the affected pad.

REFERENCES

1. Piras A, Dee JF. Repair of fractures involving metabones and phalanges. In: Bojrab MJ, Waldron DR, Toombs JP, editors. Current techniques in small animal surgery. 5th edition. Teton New Media; 2014. p. 965–72.
2. Eaton-Wells RD. The distal limb. In: Houlton JEF, Cook JL, Innes JF, et al, editors. BSAVA manual of canine and feline musculoskeletal disorders. Gloucester (England): Small Animal Veterinary Association; 2006. p. 292–308.
3. Phillips IR. A survey of bone fractures in the dog and cat. J Small Anim Pract 1979;20:661–74.
4. Boemo CM. Injuries of the metacarpus and metatarsus in: canine sports medicine and surgery. In: Bloomberg MS, Dee JF, Taylor RA, editors. W.B. Saunders; 1998. p. 150–73.
5. Dee JF. Fractures of metacarpal and metatarsal bones in: AO principles of fracture management in the dog and cat. In: Johnson AL, Houlton JEF, Vannini R, editors. AO Publishing; 2005. p. 361–9.
6. Muir P, Norris JL. Metacarpal and metatarsal fractures in dogs. J Small Anim Pract 1997;38(8):344–8.
7. Manley PA. Distal extremity fractures in small animals. J Vet Orthop 1981;2:38–48.
8. Benedetti LT, Berry K, Bloomberg M. A technique for intramedullary pinning of metatarsals and metacarpals in cats and dogs. J Am Anim Hosp Assoc 1986; 22:149–52.
9. Gentry SJ, Taylor RA, Dee JF. The use of veterinary cuttable plates: 21 cases. J Am Anim Hosp Assoc 1993;29:455–9.
10. Kapatkin A, Howe-Smith R, Shofer F. Conservative versus surgical treatment of metacarpal and metatarsal fractures in dogs. Vet Comp Orthop Traumatol 2000; 13:123–7.

11. Newton CD. Fracture and dislocation of metacarpal bones, metacarpophalangeal joints, phalanges, and interphalangeal joints. In: Textbook of small animal orthopaedics. Newton CD.

12. Okumura M, Watanabe K, Kadosawa T, et al. Surgical salvage from comminuted metatarsal fracture using a weight-bearing pin-putty apparatus in a dog. Aust Vet J 2000;78:95–8.

13. Brinker, Piermattei and Flo: Fractures of carpus, metacarpus and phalanges in: handbook of small animal orthopedics and fracture repair. 5th edition. Elsevier; 2016. p. 418–33.

14. Fitzpatrick N, Jerry OR, Thomas JS, et al. Combined intramedullary and external skeletal fixation of metatarsal and metacarpal fractures in 12 dogs and 19 cats. Vet Surg 2011;8:1015–22.

15. Roth JF, Auerback DM. Fixation of hand fractures with bicortical screws in. J Hand Surg Am 2005;30(1):151–3.

16. Sellon DC, Martucci K, Wenz JR, et al. A survey of risk factors for digit injuries among dogs training and competing in agility events. J Am Vet Med Assoc 2018;252:75–83.

17. Gillette RL. Nails: long or short. The Athletic and Working Dog Newsletter 2002;1(2).

18. Farrow CS. Sprain, strain, and contusion. Vet Clin North Am 1978;8(2):169–82.

19. Guillard MJ. Proximal interphalangeal joint instability in the dog. J Small Anim Pract 2003;44(9):399–403.

20. Robins GM, Read RA. Diseases of the sesamoid bones in: canine sports medicine and surgery. In: Bloomberg MS, Dee JF, Taylor RA, editors. W.B. Saunders; 1998. p. 255–61.

21. Eaton-Wells RD. Injuries of the digits and pads. In: Bloomberg MS, Dee JF, Taylor RAWB, editors. Canine sports medicine and surgery. Philadelphia: Saunders Company; 1998. p. 165–73.

22. Guilliard M. Flexor tenotomy for the treatment of corns. Greyhound health initiative. 2020.

Canine Carpal Injuries
From Fractures to Hyperextension Injuries

Lucas Henry Beierer, BVSc, GradDipEd, MVetSurg

KEYWORDS

- Carpus • Carpal • Hyperextension • Fracture • Arthrodesis • Instability

KEY POINTS

- Carpal joint injuries appear to be a somewhat frequent cause of lameness in dogs and may consist of ligamentous pathology, fractures, or a combination thereof.
- Independent carpal bone fractures have been reported, involving the radial carpal bone, ulna carpal bone, and accessory carpal bone.
- Carpal arthrodesis is a technically demanding procedure and is indicated for the management of major carpal pathology, with complication rates up to 50%.
- Carpal hyperextension injuries often result in multiligamentous pathology, necessitating carpal arthrodesis, which can be partial or complete, depending on the structures injured.
- Tenosynovitis of the abductor pollicis longus muscle is a reported cause of thoracic limb lameness in the dog, with treatment including peritendinous steroid and tendon resection.

INTRODUCTION

Carpal joint injuries anecdotally appear to be a somewhat frequent cause of lameness in dogs, although the epidemiology is poorly understood. Carpal injuries may consist of ligamentous pathology, fractures, or a combination thereof. The presenting history often is influenced by the dog's purpose, with racing greyhounds over-represented for certain fracture configurations.[1,2] Common historical events include trauma due to falling from an elevated position or other forms of direct carpal trauma. Strategies for management can vary from conservative therapy, to primary repair, and to salvage procedures, such as partial carpal arthrodesis (PtCA) or pancarpal arthrodesis (PCA). Although understanding of carpal kinematics and biomechanics is increasing, treatment algorithms and outcome assessments remain largely limited to observational studies.[3–5] Injuries to the carpus in cats appear to be a rare event, with a prevalence of 0.26%, with 72.6% of those cases attributed to falls from height.[6]

Queensland Veterinary Specialists, 263 Appleby Road, Stafford Heights, Queensland 4053, Australia
E-mail address: Lucas.beierer@qldvetspecialists.com.au

Vet Clin Small Anim 51 (2021) 285–303
https://doi.org/10.1016/j.cvsm.2020.12.002
0195-5616/21/© 2020 Elsevier Inc. All rights reserved.
vetsmall.theclinics.com

ANATOMY
Overview

The canine carpus is a ginglymus (hinged) joint, allowing flexion and extension, with a limited degree of lateral excursion.[7] It is composed of the antebrachiocarpal (AC), middle carpal, and carpometacarpal joints. Seven carpal bones contribute to multiple articulations. The AC joint is the articulation between the radius, ulna, and the proximal row of carpal bones. The middle carpal joint is between the proximal and distal rows of carpal bones. The metacarpophalangeal joint lies between the distal row of carpal bones and the joint surface at the base of the metacarpal bones.

Carpal Bones

The 7 carpal bones are arranged in 2 rows (**Figs. 1–5**). The proximal row is composed of the radial or intermedioradial carpal bone, ulnar carpal bone, and accessory carpal bone (ACB). The distal row is made of the 4 numbered carpal bones, beginning with 1 (most medial) and increasing to 4 at the lateral extent of the carpus.

Ligaments

Stability is provided by short extra-articular and intra-articular ligaments, an articular disc (also known as the dorsal radioulnar ligament), palmar fibrocartilage, and the joint capsule (see **Figs. 1–4**). Short medial and lateral collateral ligaments as well as the palmar carpal ligaments are the main stabilizers of the AC joint.[7] The collateral ligaments function to prevent medial and lateral opening of the AC joint, whereas the palmar carpal ligaments and the palmar interosseous ligament prevent hyperextension of the AC joint.[7] There are no continuous collateral ligaments that cross the 3

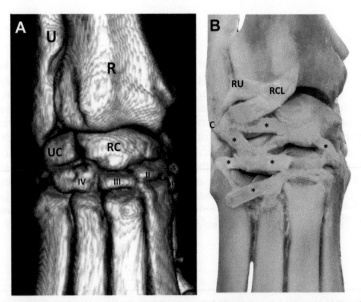

Fig. 1. Dorsal view of carpal bones and ligaments. (*A*) Metacarpal 1 2 3 4. Computed tomography (CT) 3-dimensional view from a 1-year-old border collie. R, radius; RC, radial carpal bone; S, sesamoid; U, ulna; UC, ulnar carpal bone. (*B*) Anatomic dissection of carpal ligaments. *, intercarpal ligaments; RU, dorsal radioulnar ligament; RCL, dorsal radiocarpal ligament. (*Courtesy of* Murdoch College of Veterinary Medicine, Anatomy Department, Murdoch, Western Australia.)

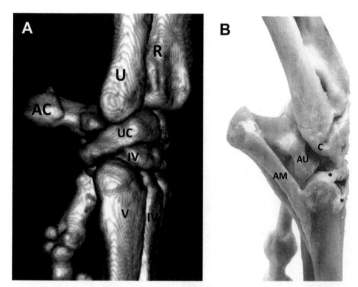

Fig. 2. Lateral view of carpal bones and ligaments. (*A*) CT 3-dimensional view from a 1-year-old border collie. AC, ACB; R, radius; RC, radial carpal bone; U, ulna; UC, ulnar carpal bone. (*B*) Anatomic dissection of carpal ligaments. *, intercarpal ligaments; AM, accessorometacarpal ligament V; AU, accessorio-ulnocarpal ligament; C, short ulnar collateral ligament. (*Courtesy of* Murdoch College of Veterinary Medicine, Anatomy Department, Murdoch, Western Australia.)

rows of the joint, but instead there are strategic thickenings of the periarticular fascia that provides ligamentous support. Multiple small dorsal ligaments unite the carpal bones transversely and are intimately associated with the joint capsule dorsally.

The palmar radiocarpal ligament starts on the palmar surface of the radial articular surface near the ulna, runs diagonally, and attaches to the lateral aspect of the radial carpal bone (see **Fig. 3**). The palmar ulnocarpal ligament runs diagonally from the radial side of the distal ulna, behind the articular disc, and attaches to the palmar surface of the radialcarpal bones as well as the radial side of the ACB. These 2 ligaments form the major deep ligaments of the carpus. It has been assumed that hyperextension is largely prevented by the palmar radiocarpal and ulnocarpal ligaments, the flexor retinaculum, and the very substantial palmar carpal fibrocartilage. The collateral ligaments, however, have been shown to have a role in protecting against hyperextension.[5]

MECHANICAL BEHAVIOR OF THE CARPUS

The normal angle of extension of the carpus in a standing dog assessed radiographically is reported as 13.66°.[8] Carpal joint angles at walk, at trot, and traversing jumps have been reported at up to 18°, 29.2°, and 44.1°, respectively.[9–11] The AC joint accounts for 58% to 70% of total carpal joint movement whereas the remaining intercarpal and carpometacarpal joints provide the residual.[3,12] Carpal stability is provided exclusively by soft tissue constraints, permitting extension beyond 180°, but the tolerance of carpal support structures before injury is unclear. Evaluation of the mechanical properties of the 6 major canine carpal ligaments (medial collateral, lateral collateral, palmar ulnocarpal, palmar radiocarpal, accessorometacarpal-V, and accessorometacarpal-IV) found that the accessorometacarpal ligaments had a high

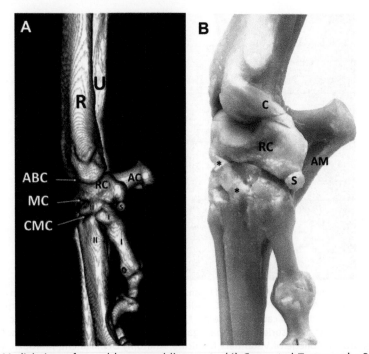

Fig. 3. Medial view of carpal bones and ligaments. (*A*) Computed Tomography 3-dimensional view from a 1-year-old border collie. ABC, AC joint; AC, ACB; MC, middle carpal joint, carpo-metacarpal joint; R, radius; RC, radial carpal bone; S, sesamoid; U, ulna. (*B*) Anatomic dissection of carpal ligaments. *, intercarpal ligaments; AM, accessorometacarpal ligament IV; C, short radial collateral ligament. (*Courtesy of* Murdoch College of Veterinary Medicine, Anatomy Department, Murdoch, Western Australia.)

elastic modulus whereas the medial and lateral collateral ligaments had the lowest elastic modulus of any of the ligaments tested.[13] The mode of failure of all 6 carpal ligaments tested showed that 58.3% failed midligament, 22.9% had an avulsion fracture, and 18.8% failed at the bone-ligament interface.

CARPAL BONE DISORDERS
Radial Carpal Bone Fractures

Radial carpal bone fractures are rare but have been reported in both racing greyhounds and other breeds, without a recognized traumatic etiology.[14–17] Similarities in presenting findings include a bilateral presentation and breed predilection (boxers, English springer spaniel, setters, and pointers).[14,15,18] Several studies indicate a predisposition for radial carpal bone fractures to occur along the lines of ossification.[14,15] Because the radial carpal bone represents a fusion of the primitive radial carpal bone with the central and intermediate carpal bones, radial carpal bone fractures have been proposed to be due to an incomplete fusion of the centers of ossification.[7,16] Histopathologic samples taken from 2 dogs with this pathology demonstrated the presence of persistent cartilaginous areas within immature cancellous bone and fibroconnective tissue on the fracture surfaces similar to changes identified with incomplete ossification of the humeral condyle.[16,19] A traumatic radial carpal bone fracture on the right side of racing greyhounds has been recognized. They often are oblique,

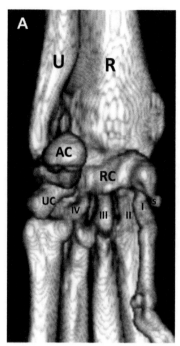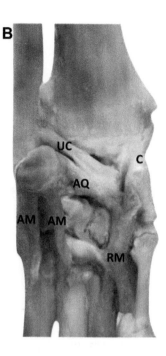

Fig. 4. Palmar view of carpal bones and ligaments. (*A*) CT 3-dimensional view from a 1-year-old border collie. AC, ACB; R, radius; RC, radial carpal bone; S, sesamoid; U, ulna; UC, ulnar carpal bone. (*B*) Anatomic dissection of carpal ligaments. *, intercarpal ligaments; AM, accessorometacarpal ligament IV and V; AQ, accessorio-quartile ligament; C, short radial collateral ligament; RM, palmar radiocarpal-metacarpal ligament; UC, accessorio-ulnocarpal ligament. (*Courtesy of* Murdoch College of Veterinary Medicine, Anatomy Department, Murdoch, Western Australia.)

midbody fractures that can be incomplete, making radiographic diagnosis difficult. Chip or avulsion fractures associated with ligamentous attachment (palmar carpometacarpal or short radial collateral ligament) also are reported.

Clinical signs associated with carpal bone fractures include mild to moderate lameness, joint swelling, and reduced carpal range of motion.[16] Three radiographic patterns visible on a dorsopalmar radiographic view are described15:

1. Sagittal fracture with a small medial fragment (approximately 25% of radial carpal bone width)
2. Oblique fracture, extending from midway beneath the radius in a medial direction to end above the second carpal bone, with a larger medial fragment (approximately 50% of radial carpal bone width)
3. Comminuted fracture of the radial carpal bone with an oblique, dorsopalmar fracture line combined with a mediolateral fracture line in the dorsal region of the bone

Computed tomography and arthroscopy have a role in the diagnosis and management of some cases when radiographic evidence is inconclusive.[16,18]

Management

Management has included medical therapy with exercise restriction and nonsteroidal anti-inflammatory drugs, fragment removal, lag screw application, and PCA.[15,16,18]

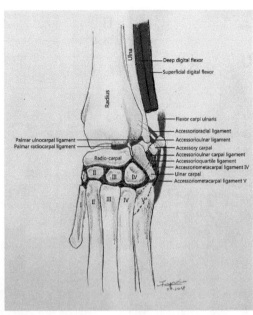

Fig. 5. Anatomy of the carpus illustrating the palmar carpal ligaments and the ligaments associated with the ACB. (*Courtesy of* D. K. Fung, Perth, Australia.)

Intuitively, a superior clinical outcome is expected with restoration of radial carpal joint surfaces and reduction in severity of osteoarthritis, although limited objective outcome data are published. Internal fixation in 5 dogs using a variably pitched headless cannulated compression screw (Acutrak, Acumed, Oregon, USA) placed via an open arthrotomy has been reported.[18] This was associated with resolution of lameness and evidence of progressive radiographic healing; however, there was inconsistent evidence of radiographic union. Concurrent carpal joint osteoarthritis is an inconsistent finding at diagnosis; however, osteoarthritis was observed in all dogs managed conservatively.[16]

Approaches for surgical fixation range from an open arthrotomy to minimally invasive techniques.[18,20,21] A dorsal surgical approach is indicated for repairing small dorsal slab fractures. If large dorsal slab fractures are present, the approach should be combined with opening the tendon sheath of the extensor carpi radialis muscle proximally. The palmaromedial approach allows exposure to repairing midbody radial carpal bone fractures. A combination of the palmaromedial approach and the dorsal approach reportedly increases exposure, facilitates fracture reduction, and allows better orientation for placing the lag screw to repair midbody fractures.

When internal fixation is performed, it typically is accepted to use external coaptation in the immediate convalescence period. A splint or cast has been advocated for 6 weeks to 8 weeks postoperatively to reduce patient demands on the repair, although objective evidence supporting this recommendation is lacking.

Radial Carpal Bone Luxation

Luxation of the radial carpal bone has been reported in limited numbers. Successful management with either open or closed reduction, followed by a period of external coaptation, is described.[22,23] Luxation is associated with failure of the radial collateral ligament and dorsal capsule, with preservation of, and rotation around, the palmar ligament connecting the radial carpal and the second and third metacarpals. Closed reduction is accomplished under anesthesia via digital pressure on the radial carpal bone associated with a combination of joint movements, including hyperflexion first, then supination, and lastly hyperextension of the carpus. Internal fixation has been reported using bone anchors to reconstruct the medial radial collateral ligament. Management with external coaptation is recommended for 5 weeks to 8 weeks postreduction. Chronic luxations and those associated with additional injury may not be amenable to reduction; instead, arthrodesis may be the most appropriate treatment. Although carpal osteoarthritis is an inevitable consequence of this injury, satisfactory limb function is expected.

Ulna Carpal Bone Fracture

There are 2 reports of an ulna carpal bone fracture in veterinary literature.[24–26] Both documented known trauma at the onset of lameness. Standard orthogonal projections may facilitate diagnosis, although a palmaromedial-dorsolateral hyperflexed oblique view is recommended for assessment of the palmar aspect of the bone. The optimal approach to this injury is unclear, given the paucity of published literature, but nonsurgical, internal fixation, fragment removal, and PCA all are potential treatments.

Accessory Carpal Bone Fracture

Research into ACB fractures has focused on the racing greyhound. Fractures are reported most frequently in the right carpus in dogs that race on elliptical tracks in a counterclockwise direction.[1,2] The proposed mechanism of injury at the track is excessive load on the ACB at the race track turn when the ACB is acting as a fulcrum for the palmar carpal ligaments and flexor tendons to prevent hyperextension. These injuries can occur in other breeds as a consequence of a traumatic overloading. Cases should be evaluated thoroughly for concurrent palmar ligamentous injury. ACB fractures have been classified into 5 types (**Table 1**).[1]

Clinical signs include reduced performance measures reported by the trainer, progressive weight bearing to non–weight-bearing lameness, carpal swelling, and carpal pain. Some degree of carpal collapse is evident during weight bearing depending on the fracture configuration. Some owners fail to present dogs acutely due to misdiagnosis or inappropriate advice from within the racing industry, resulting in chronic remodeling of fracture fragments.

Diagnosis is achieved with a lateral radiograph with the carpus in extension. An orthogonal projection always is obtained to survey for concomitant injury. Oblique or stress radiographs can be employed in some cases to better define the fracture configuration and make decisions regarding management. Computed tomography may be useful to survey for comminution that may alter treatment progression in select cases.

Management can be accomplished via either internal fixation and/or fragment removal and external coaptation. Treatment selection is influenced by fracture configuration, chronicity of injury, and performance expectations postoperatively. Internal fixation is accomplished via a palmarolateral approach to the carpus.[21] Type I and type II ACB fractures are intra-articular by classification, and close inspection of the articular surface for congruency postreduction and the presence of free fragments is advised. Given the small size of the involved fragments, a 1.5-mm or 2.0-mm screw placed in lag fashion or positional screw often is all that is possible. Use of an aiming device intraoperatively can facilitate accurate screw trajectory. Given the difficulty of access, screws typically are placed from distal to proximal for type I and type II ACB fractures. Type V ACB fractures (comminuted) are considered nonsurgical.

Table 1
Accessory carpal bone fracture classification

Type	Description	Incidence in a Study of 50 Greyhound Cases (%)
Type I, distal basilar	Avulsion fracture of the distal margin of the articular surface at the origin of the accessoroulnar carpal ligaments	67
Type II, proximal basilar	Avulsion fracture of the proximal margin at the insertion of the ligaments to the radius, ulna, and radial carpal bone	13
Type III, distal apical	Avulsion fracture of the distal margin of the palmar end of the bone at the origin of the 2 palmar accessorometacarpal ligaments	3
Type IV, proximal apical	Avulsion fracture of the tendon of insertion of the flexor carpi ulnaris muscle at the proximal surface of the palmar end of the bone	5
Type V, comminuted fracture of the body	May extend into the articular surface	12

Adapted from Johnson KA. Accessory carpal bone fractures in the racing greyhound. Classification and pathology. *Vet Surg.* 1987;16(1):60-64; with permission.

Conventional wisdom indicates management with external coaptation should focus on unloading of the ACB from the flexor carpi ulnaris via varying degrees of carpal flexion. This can be accomplished by creating an initial cast with the carpus in moderate flexion, then progressively straightening the carpus every 10 days to 14 days until extension is reached at 6 weeks. It may be possible to promote increasing loading of the fracture line as bone healing matures. Bone healing may be slow to document radiographically despite satisfactory clinical progression. Given the variety of presenting configurations and clinical factors influencing outcome, long-term data predicting outcome are insufficient. Dogs should be able to resume good pet function with appropriate management, and some may return to competitive racing.

Avascular Necrosis of the Carpal Bones

Avascular necrosis has been reported in canine carpal bones, including the accessory carpal and radial carpal bone without a clear etiology.[27–29] Radiographic changes include mottled osteolysis, increased opacity, and trabecular consolidation. Magnetic resonance imaging (MRI) can be used in the diagnosis and is considered a sensitive and specific test for avascular necrosis. The histologic findings in this disease are consistent with ischemic necrosis, which may predispose to fracture. Clinical signs are consistent with a thoracic limb lameness localized to the carpus, with or without associated swelling, and with variable response to analgesics. PCA is associated with resolution of lameness.

LIGAMENTOUS INJURIES

A sprain is the overstretching or tearing of ligaments, commonly classified into 3 grades. Grade I sprain injuries are mild and associated with an overstretching of the ligament without disruption or loss of function. Grade II sprains are moderate in severity, associated with a partial tear of the ligament. Grade III sprain injuries are complete failure or avulsion of the ligament. Ligamentous injury to the carpus can occur at the level of the collateral support or ACB and more globally associated with the palmar ligaments. Although the accessibility of radiography makes it a standard tool in the assessment of carpal stability, MRI has shown superiority in detecting carpal sprains in dogs compared with computed tomography.[30]

Carpal Stress Radiography

Stress radiography is the mainstay of diagnosis and guiding treatment of carpal ligamentous injury. Given the variety between patients, it is essential that left and right comparative films are obtained. Standard orthogonal projections of the carpus are obtained of both limbs, followed by applying a unidirectional quasiphysiologic load to assess 3 distinct regions, including the medial and lateral collateral ligaments and palmar ligaments. The limb should be rigidly immobilized proximal to the carpus while the stressed load is applied to the distal aspect of the metacarpals. Instability is confirmed when joint space widening is detected compared with the contralateral limb.

Collateral Ligament Injuries

Isolated collateral ligament injuries rarely are documented in the pet population. There have been limited reports in the racing greyhound.[31] Guidelines for management are based largely on textbook or review article descriptions. Clinical signs are as expected for a collateral ligament injury, including varying degree of lameness, soft tissue swelling, pain on manipulation, and varying degrees of visual or palpable instability. Grade I sprains are unlikely to result in detectable instability and may be diagnosed on clinical suspicion or confirmed via MRI or ultrasound.[32] Chronic lateral collateral ligament sprain resulting in carpal varus has been reported in a case series of 10 dogs and case report of 2 dogs.[33] Although conservative treatment of collateral ligament injuries has been reported with success, the absence of detailed outcome measures and limited published evidence means definitive guidelines are lacking.

A case series of 14 dogs treated for unidirectional carpal instability with a carpal brace found improved stability and lameness, with a majority of dogs returning to normal function.[34] Surgical therapy ranges from primary repair to synthetic ligament techniques. Most recommendations advocate for synthetic suture stabilization techniques, given the limited purchase available in the torn ligament remnants. Synthetic ligament techniques include bone tunnels, bone anchors, and screws, with the prosthetic ligament comprising wire, nylon, or braided materials. Rigid external coaptation with either splints or casts are recommended for 4 weeks to 8 weeks postoperatively. PCA is reserved for chronic instability with significant degenerative changes.

A retrospective case series of shearing injuries found that 9 of 18 carpi had joint instability.[35] Shearing injuries most commonly involve the medial aspect of the limb with variable loss of soft tissue support, often involving the radial styloid process and short radial collateral ligament. The severity of soft tissue and bone loss determines whether the joint can be stabilized by reconstruction using bone anchors and prosthetic ligament support or, when more severe damage is present, by arthrodesis. It is unclear if managing instability with ligament reconstruction techniques, transarticular external skeletal fixators, or PCA immediately, compared with delaying stabilization until the wound is healthy, affects clinical results.[36]

Flexor Tendon Disease

ACB enthesopathy has been documented in agility and working dogs. The mechanism proposed is a chronic grade I sprain, resulting in bone remodeling at the origin and insertion sites of the accessorometacarpal ligaments causing subclinical carpal laxity resulting in carpal osteoarthritis.[37] Optimal treatment is unclear.

Hyperextension Injuries

It is accepted that disruption to the flexor retinaculum and palmar fibrocartilage results in pathologic hyperextension. Cadaveric in vitro modeling indicates that both the medial and lateral collateral ligaments play a role in preventing hyperextension injury as well as the palmar carpal ligaments, although the implications for management are unclear.[5] Causes of hyperextension injuries include fall from heights, injury during athletic activity, trauma, and inflammatory diseases. Carpal disruption and luxation may occur at the AC, intercarpal, or carpometacarpal level. Clinical signs include a weight bearing to non–weight-bearing lameness, varying degrees of visible carpal hyperextension, and carpal swelling. Sometimes profound acute joint swelling can hamper efforts to detect instability, and misdiagnosis of the severity of injury and joint level involved can result. Investigation should include stressed radiography typically under sedation/general anesthesia. The role for MRI in clinical decision making remains unclear. Treatment via conservative management usually is unsuccessful, resulting in continued and progressive hyperextension of the carpus with progressive joint instability, degenerative changes, and lameness. Individual ligament reconstruction for hyperextension injuries is not performed routinely; instead, treatment usually constitutes arthrodesis given the multiligamentous involvement and challenging biomechanical loading conditions of the carpus.

ARTHRODESIS OF THE CARPUS

Carpal arthrodesis is a salvage procedure to address significant carpal pathology. Indications are varied and include ligamentous injury, hyperextension trauma, luxation, shearing injury, articular fractures, severe degenerative joint disease, immune-mediated arthritis leading to joint collapse, congenital abnormalities, and neurogenic injury involving the distal limb.[38–40] PCA spans the antebrachium to metacarpal bones whereas PtCA extends from the proximal row of carpal bones to the metacarpal bones. Selecting the level of arthrodesis is based on the nature and location of the underlying pathology.

Pancarpal Arthrodesis

Technique
The principles of arthrodesis include complete articular cartilage removal, autogenous cancellous bone grafting, and rigid long-lasting fixation.[41] Approaches to the carpus vary and include palmar, medial, and dorsal techniques, with the dorsal approach most common due to the ease of soft tissue access. The historically recommended angle of fusion is 10° to 12° of extension but studies comparing clinical outcome with varying angles of extension are lacking. Implant options are extensive with a variety of different manufactures offering dedicated dorsal plate options. Common to dedicated implants are a varied screw size between the radius and metacarpal to avoid excessively large implants in the smaller metacarpal bone, and screw holes

positioned to engage the radius, radial carpal bone, and 3rd metacarpal. Orthogonal plate fixation has been described for complex PCA when a single plate may be inadequate.[42]

Outcomes

Long-term assessment of PCA has been reported in 12 working dogs.[43] Six dogs reportedly were able to complete normal work duties whereas 4 were able to perform most duties, with a majority of owners satisfied with the outcome postsurgery. A second report describing retrospective owner questionnaires in 22 dogs found 70% of dogs returned to full function, whereas 17% remained severely lame and 13% had minor ongoing lameness.[44] Long-term outcomes assessed by owner questionnaire after PCA in cats has been reported as excellent in 7 of 11 cats, with the remainder achieving a satisfactory result.[45] The apparent importance of supination and protonation in the cats has been proposed as a reason to avoid PCA in cats.[46] PCA seems supported, however, as a procedure with minimal disability and satisfactory success rates.[45] The major reported limitation postoperatively is a reduced willingness to jump and climb.[45]

Complications

Complications post–carpal arthrodesis are numerous. including implant breakage or loosening, infection, persistent discomfort, fracture, and wound dehiscence. Complication rates reported throughout the literature range from 14% to 50% and are recorded in **Table 2**. Cast-related complications post-PCA has been reported in up to 44.4% of cases.[38,47] The decision to pursue external coaptation post–carpal arthrodesis is not borne out by evidence but instead appears practiced as a historical, anecdotally accepted best practice.[48] Adjunctive external coaptation does not appear to have a measurable clinical benefit but is associated with morbidity. The high postoperative infection rate reported (7%–66%) is of particular note to clinicians because PCA carries a high risk of surgical site infection compared with other orthopedic procedures. Possible reasons for this likely relate to limited soft tissue coverage, wound dehiscence, length of surgery, or thermal damage from burring. All these factors could be exacerbated further by dressing application and subsequent compromise to local blood flow.

Metacarpal fractures appear to be a common complication post-PCA, reported in 11% of dogs in one retrospective series.[49] Screw diameter was not a significant factor in cases with metacarpal fractures, but the length of the metacarpal bone covered by the bone plate did affect the frequency of metacarpal fracture, with fewer fractures occurring when greater than 53% of the bone length was covered by the plate.[49] It has been suggested that to reduce the likelihood of fracture, the plate should cover more than 50% of the length of the plated metacarpal bone. Implant removal seems to be a common requirement post-PCA, reported in 21% of cases in 1 retrospective study.[50] Comminuted articular fractures of the distal radius and ulna managed by PCA is associated with a high risk of complication and a guarded prognosis for a full functional outcome.[42]

Biomechanics

The AO/ASIF 3.5-mm dynamic compression plate (DCP) historically was the plate of choice for large dog PCA until the 2.7/3.5-mm hybrid DCPs (HDCPs) were manufactured. Comparison of the 2.7/3.5-mm HDCP and the 3.5-mm DCP of approximately equal lengths in 4-point bending showed a small but significant difference between bending moments at failure, favoring the HDCP.[57] Additionally, mechanical properties of a 3.5-mm limited contact DCP or a 3.5/2.7-mm HDCP were compared in

Table 2
Pancarpal arthrodesis case series reported in the literature

Case Number	Indication	Implant Locations and Types	Rigid Postoperative Coaptations Use (Yes/No)	Intraoperative Complications (%)	Postoperative Infections Rate (%)	Postoperative Complications (Total, Including Infection [%])	Study Type
9 dogs (10 limbs)[51]	Carpal injury	CESF	No		Not recorded	40	Retrospective case series
15 dogs[52]	Carpal injury	Dorsal 2.7/3.5 mm locking and DCP, HDCP	No		20	40	Retrospective case series
9 dogs[39]	Carpal injury	Dorsal DCP (2.7 mm, 3.5 mm, or 4.5 mm)	Yes (3–9 wk)		22	33	Retrospective case series
11 dogs (13 limbs)[53]	Traumatic or degenerative injury	Dorsal CLP (2.7/3.5 mm)[a]	Variable	28	7	14	Retrospective case series
231 dog limbs[38]	Variable	Dorsal HDCP (2.7/3.5 mm)[b] or CLP (2.7/ 3.5 mm)[a]	Variable	12 HDCP 22 CLP	18	34 HDCP 18 CLP	Multicenter, retrospective, cohort study
9 dogs (10 limbs)[54]	Traumatic injury	Medial 2.7 mm DCP	Yes (6–8 wk)		11	33	Retrospective case series
3 cats[55]	Traumatic injury	Medial Compact 2.0 LOCK system[c,d]	Yes (1–6 wk)			33	Retrospective case series
40 dogs (43 limbs)[56]	Hyperextension injury	Dorsal DCP (2.7 mm, 3.5 mm, or 4.5 mm)	Yes (6 wk)		18	44	Retrospective case series

44 dogs (52 limbs)[50]	Carpal trauma	Dorsal SHCP (2.7/2.0 mm, 3.5/2.7 mm, 3.5/3.5 mm)		15	8	48	Multicenter, retrospective, cohort study
8 dogs (9 limbs)[42]	Distal antebrachial fracture	Variable Orthogonal plate fixation Single dorsal plate fixation ESF	Variable	0	66	87	Retrospective case series
14 dogs[47]	Carpal trauma	Dorsal HDCP (2.7/3.5 mm or 3.5/3.5 mm)[b]	Yes (6 wk)		28	35	Prospective case series
12 dogs[43]	Carpal trauma	Dorsal DCP (3.5 mm) or HPCP (2.7/3.5 mm)[b]	Yes		33	50	Retrospective case series
18 cats (20 limbs)[45]	Varied	Variable VCP[c] ±cross-pins HDCP[b] (1.5/2.0 mm or 2.0/2.7 mm) Cross-pins ESF	Variable		5	20	Retrospective case series

When complication rates could not be determined, the entry was left empty.
Abbreviations: CESF, circular external skeletal fixator; ESF, external skeletal fixator; SHCP, stepped hybrid carpal arthrodesis plate; VCP, veterinary cuttable plate.
[a] CLP, Orthomed Ltd (Halifax, UK).
[b] Hybrid dynamic compression plate (HDCP), Veterinary Instrumentation (Sheffield, UK).
[c] Synthes GmbH (Oberdorf, Switzerland).
[d] Insorvet (Spain, Barcelona).
Data from Refs. 38,39,42,43,45,47,50–56

nondestructive bending, and the HDCP was found to have superior mechanical properties.[58] These studies suggest the HDCP offers superior mechanical properties to conventional multipurpose AO bone plates for canine PCA.

Due to the complications associated with bandage application post–carpal arthrodesis, some implant manufacturers have marketed implants as castless, the assumption being that plates not marketed as castless may have inferior biomechanical properties, necessitating additional support in the form of external coaptation. The Veterinary Instrumentation HDCP, and the Orthomed arthrodesis castless plate (CLP) were compared in a single-cycle load to failure and cyclical loading until failure (or 10^6 cycles).[48] The investigators found bending stiffness was higher for the HDCP but no difference in bending strength and no plate failures, suggesting no mechanical advantage within the limitations of the study design for the CLP design. The same HDCP was compared as a stand-alone implant or reinforced with cross-pins (1.6-mm Kirschner wires) in an ex vivo model axially loaded to failure.[59] Stiffness and failure load were not different between the 2 constructs whereas the cross-pin reinforcement afforded higher yield loads.

Partial Carpal Arthrodesis

Technique

The principles of PtCA are identical to those of PCA but the AC joint is preserved. The unique challenge of PtCA is linked with the limited proximal bone stock available for fixation, avoiding implant impingement during preserved AC joint extension and accurately selecting appropriate cases where the AC joint is normal. Like PCA, approaches include medial, dorsal, and palmar techniques. Fixation has been accomplished with a variety of implants, including plates, cross-pins, and retrograde metacarpal intramedullary pinning.[60] Clinical superiority of technique is unclear. Long-term risks with PtCA include progressive degeneration of the AC joint, which has been reported in 36% of cases.[61]

Outcome and complications

The sparsity of literature around PtCA makes determining outcome difficult (**Table 3**). Client questionnaires in a retrospective case series of 39 dogs reported improvement or great improvement, with all owners pleased or very pleased with the final result.[60] This was in contrast to the 1 case series that compared both PtCA and PCA and reported 50% satisfactory results for PtCA and 70% for PCA.[56] Degenerative joint disease in the adjacent AC joint is reported in 15.5% to 36% of cases whereas 9% to 11% had persistent hyperextension.[60,61] The average range of motion post-PtCA was approximately half that of the normal unaffected limb; however, it still was adequate to allow functional use of the limb. This variation in outcome suggests that unidentified injury at the antebrachial carpal joint, poor patient selection, errors in technique, or the effect of stress concentration at the nonfused antebrachial carpal joint influences success post-PtCA. Use of a straight DCP for PtCA is associated with an unacceptable complication rate associated with interference with the radial-carpal joint space and cannot be recommended.[56]

Biomechanics

The Orthomed PtCA CLP (2.7 mm) was compared ex vivo to a cross-pin technique (two 1.6-mm Kirschner wires) and Synthes T-plate (7-hole, 2.7 mm) by measuring micromotion and load to failure.[62] No differences in load to failure were detected between the 3 constructs whereas less micromotion was detected in the plated limbs.

Table 3
Partial carpal arthrodesis case series reported in the literature

Case Number	Indication	Implant Location and Type	Rigid Postoperative Coaptation Use (Yes/No)	Intraoperative Complications (%)	Postoperative Infection Rate (%)	Postoperative Complication (Total, Including Infection [%])	Study Type
39 dogs (45 limbs)[60]	Traumatic grade 3 sprains	Varied T-Plate[a] Retrograde intramedullary pins Cross-pins Wire Lag screw	Yes (4–18 wk)	20	2		Retrospective case series
21 animals (19 dogs, 2 cats)[61]	Hyperextension injury	Cross-pin fixation	Yes	61		47	Retrospective case series
10 dogs (13 limbs)[56]	Hyperextension injury	Dorsal DCP (2.7 or 3.5 mm)	Yes (6 wk)			76	Retrospective case series
2 cats[45]	Hyperextension injury	Cross-pin fixation	Varied			100	Retrospective case series

When complication rates could not be determined, the table was left empty.
[a] Synthes LTD USA (Paoli, PA).
Data from Refs.[45,56,60,61]

ABDUCTOR POLLICUS LONGUS TENOSYNOVITIS

Tenosynovitis of the abductor pollicis longus muscle is a reported cause of thoracic limb lameness in the dog.[63–65] It often occurs in medium to large breed dogs that present with a firm swelling at the medial aspect of the AC joint and varying degrees of weight bearing lameness. The abductor pollicis longus muscle originates on the lateral surface of the radius and ulna. Its fibers blend into a strong tendon toward the carpus, crossing the tendon of the extensor carpi radialis muscle, and passing into the medial sulcus of the radius under the short medial collateral ligament. A tendon sheath of varying length is located in this segment. Clinical examination reveals pain on carpal hyperflexion and palpable thickening of the tendon sheath. There is limited information in the literature to definitely guide treatment recommendations. Therapy with peritendinous injection of corticosteroid (Methylprednisone, 20 mg) and post-treatment external coaptation has been described.[63] If a positive response to medical therapy was witnessed, repeat treatment was performed. If results were unsatisfactory, surgical débridement of the tendon was completed. Post-intervention diffuse carpal osteoarthritis has been reported and may be secondary to progressive carpal instability due to postsurgical management or the chronic effects of regional corticosteroids.

CLINICS CARE POINTS

- Both medial and lateral collateral ligaments play a role in preventing hyperextension injuries as well as the flexor retinaculum and palmar fibrocartilage.
- Infection rates post-PCA are reported in 7% to 66% of cases.
- Evidence supporting external computation post–carpal arthrodesis is lacking.
- Tenosynovitis of the abductor pollicis longus muscle is a recognized cause of thoracic limb lameness in the dog.

DISCLOSURE

The author has no commercial or financial affiliation/conflicts that would have an impact on the material in this article. The author has nothing to declare.

REFERENCES

1. Johnson KA. Accessory carpal bone fractures in the racing greyhound. Classification and pathology. Vet Surg 1987;16(1):60–4.
2. Johnson KA, Dee JF, Piermattei DL. Screw fixation of accessory carpal bone fractures in racing Greyhounds: 12 cases (1981-1986). J Am Vet Med Assoc 1989; 194(11):1618–25.
3. Neville-Towle JD, Tan CJ, Parr WCH, et al. Three-dimensional kinematics of the canine carpal bones imaged with computed tomography after ex vivo axial limb loading and palmar ligament transection. Vet Surg 2018;47(6):861–71.
4. Andreoni AA, Rytz U, Vannini R, et al. Ground reaction force profiles after partial and pancarpal arthrodesis in dogs. Vet Comp Orthop Traumatol 2010;23(1):1–6.
5. Milgram J, Milshtein T, Meiner Y. The role of the antebrachiocarpal ligaments in the prevention of hyperextension of the antebrachiocarpal joint. Vet Surg 2012; 41(2):191–9.

6. Nakladal B, vom Hagen F, Brunnberg M, et al. Carpal joint injuries in cats - an epidemiological study. Vet Comp Orthop Traumatol 2013;26(5):333–9.
7. Evans H, de Lahunta A. Miller's anatomy of the dog. 4th edition. St. Louis (MO), USA: Saunders/Elsevier; 2013.
8. Milgram J, Slonim E, Kass P, et al. A radiographic study of joint angles in standing dogs. Vet Comp Orthop Traumatol 2004;17:82–90.
9. Allen K, DeCamp CE, Braden TD, et al. Kinematic gait analysis of the trot in healthy mixed breed dogs. Vet Comp Orthop Traumatol 1994;7(04):148–53.
10. Hottinger HA, DeCamp CE, Olivier NB, et al. Noninvasive kinematic analysis of the walk in healthy large-breed dogs. Am J Vet Res 1996;57(3):381–8.
11. Birch E, Leśniak K. Effect of fence height on joint angles of agility dogs. Vet J 2013;198(Suppl):e99–102.
12. Whitelock R. Conditions of the carpus in the dog. Pr 2001;23:2–13.
13. Shetye SS, Malhotra K, Ryan SD, et al. Determination of mechanical properties of canine carpal ligaments. Am J Vet Res 2009;70(8):1026–30.
14. Li A, Bennett D, Gibbs C, et al. Radial carpal bone fractures in 15 dogs. J Small Anim Pract 2000;41(2):74–9.
15. Tomlin JL, Pead MJ, Langley-Hobbs SJ, et al. Radial carpal bone fracture in dogs. J Am Anim Hosp Assoc 2001;37(2):173–8.
16. Gnudi G, Mortellaro CM, Bertoni G, et al. Radial carpal bone fracture in 13 dogs. Vet Comp Orthop Traumatol 2003;16(03):178–83.
17. Johnson K. Canine sports medicine and surgery. In: Bloomberg M, Dee J, Taylor R, editors. Philadelphia: WB Saunders Company; 1998. p. 100–8.
18. Perry K, Fitzpatrick N, Johnson J, et al. Headless self-compressing cannulated screw fixation for treatment of radial carpal bone fracture or fissure in dogs. Vet Comp Orthop Traumatol 2010;23(2):94–101.
19. Gnudi G, Martini FM, Zanichelli S, et al. Incomplete humeral condylar fracture in two English Pointer dogs. Vet Comp Orthop Traumatol 2005;18(4):243–5.
20. Beale BS, Cole G. Minimally invasive osteosynthesis technique for articular fractures. Vet Clin North Am Small Anim Pract 2012;42(5):1051–1068, viii.
21. Johnson K. Piermattei's atlas of surgical approaches to the bones and joints of the dog and cat. 5th edition. Philadelphia (PA): Elsevier - Health Sciences Division; 2004.
22. Palierne S, Delbeke C, Asimus E, et al. A case of dorso-medial luxation of the radial carpal bone in a dog. Vet Comp Orthop Traumatol 2008;21(2):171–6.
23. Miller A, Carmichael S, Anderson T, et al. Luxation of the radial carpal bone in four dogs. J Small Anim Pract 1990;31:148–54.
24. Boudreau B, Hodge S, Alsup J. Surgical update — Fracture of the ulnar carpal bone. Vet Forum 2009;26:30–5.
25. Vedrine B. Comminuted fracture of the ulnar carpal bone in a Labrador retriever dog. Can Vet J 2013;54(11):1067–70.
26. Johnson AL, Piermattei DL, Davis P. Characteristics of accessory carpal bone fractures in 50 racing Greyhounds. Vet Comp Orthop Traumatol 1988;1:104.
27. Pownder SL, Cooley S, Hayashi K, et al. Non-invasive magnetic resonance imaging diagnosis of presumed intermedioradial carpal bone avascular necrosis in the dog. Can Vet J 2016;57(8):879–81.
28. Aiken MJ, Stewart JE, Anderson AA. Avascular necrosis of the canine radial carpal bone: a condition analogous to Preiser's disease? J Small Anim Pract 2013; 54(7):374–6.
29. Harris KP, Langley-Hobbs SJ. Idiopathic ischemic necrosis of an accessory carpal bone in a dog. J Am Vet Med Assoc 2013;243(12):1746–50.

30. Castelli E, Pozzi A, Klisch K, et al. Comparison between high-field 3 Tesla MRI and computed tomography with and without arthrography for visualization of canine carpal ligaments: A cadaveric study. Vet Surg 2019;48(4):546–55.

31. Guilliard MJ, Mayo AK. Sprain of the short radial collateral ligament in a racing greyhound. J Small Anim Pract 2000;41(4):169–71.

32. Nordberg CC, Johnson KA. Magnetic resonance imaging of normal canine carpal ligaments. Vet Radiol Ultrasound 1999;40(2):128–36.

33. Langley-Hobbs SJ, Hamilton MH, Pratt JNJ. Radiographic and clinical features of carpal varus associated with chronic sprain of the lateral collateral ligament complex in 10 dogs. Vet Comp Orthop Traumatol 2007;(20):324–30.

34. Tomlinson JE, Manfredi JM. Evaluation of application of a carpal brace as a treatment for carpal ligament instability in dogs: 14 cases (2008-2011). J Am Vet Med Assoc 2014;244(4):438–43.

35. Beardsley SL, Schrader SC. Treatment of dogs with wounds of the limbs caused by shearing forces: 98 cases (1975-1993). J Am Vet Med Assoc 1995;207(8):1071–5.

36. Benson JA, Boudrieau RJ. Severe carpal and tarsal shearing injuries treated with an immediate arthrodesis in seven dogs. J Am Anim Hosp Assoc 2002;38(4):370–80.

37. Glyde M. Accessory carpal bone disease in agility and working dogs. London: ESVOT; 2016. p. 137–8.

38. Bristow PC, Meeson RL, Thorne RM, et al. Clinical comparison of the hybrid dynamic compression plate and the castless plate for pancarpal arthrodesis in 219 dogs. Vet Surg 2015;44(1):70–7.

39. Johnson KA. Carpal arthrodesis in dogs. Aust Vet J 1980;56:565–73.

40. Keller WG, Chambers JN. Antebrachial metacarpal arthrodesis for fusion of deranged carpal joints in two dogs. J Am Vet Med Assoc 1989;195(10):1382–4.

41. Johnson AL, Houlton JEF, Vannini R, et al. AO principles of fracture management in the dog and cat. Switzerland: Georg Thieme Verlag; 2005.

42. Brown G, Kalff S, Gemmill TJ, et al. Highly comminuted, articular fractures of the distal antebrachium managed by pancarpal arthrodesis in 8 dogs. Vet Surg 2016;45(1):44–51.

43. Worth AJ, Bruce WJ. Long-term assessment of pancarpal arthrodesis performed on working dogs in New Zealand. N Z Vet J 2008;56(2):78–84.

44. Maarschalkerweerd RJ, Hazewinkel HAW, Mey BP, et al. Carpal arthrodesis in dogs, a retrospective study with force plate analysis. Vet Q 1996;18(sup1):22–3.

45. Calvo I, Farrell M, Chase D, et al. Carpal arthrodesis in cats. Long-term functional outcome. Vet Comp Orthop Traumatol 2009;22(6):498–504.

46. Voss K, Geyer H, Montavon P. Antebrachiocarpal luxation in a cat A case report and anatomical study of the medial collateral ligament. Vet Comp Orthop Traumatol 2003;16:266–70.

47. Jerram RM, Walker AM, Worth AJ, et al. Prospective evaluation of pancarpal arthrodesis for carpal injuries in working dogs in New Zealand, using dorsal hybrid plating. N Z Vet J 2009;57(6):331–7.

48. Meeson RL, Goodship AE, Arthurs GI. A biomechanical evaluation of a hybrid dynamic compression plate and a cast L ess arthrodesis plate for pancarpal arthrodesis in dogs. Vet Surg 2012;41(6):738–44.

49. Whitelock RG, Dyce J, Houlton JE. Metacarpal fractures associated with pancarpal arthrodesis in dogs. Vet Surg 1999;28(1):25–30.

50. Diaz-Bertrana C, Darnaculleta F, Durall I, et al. The stepped hybrid plate for carpal panarthrodesis - Part II: a multicentre study of 52 arthrodeses. Vet Comp Orthop Traumatol 2009;22(5):389–97.
51. Lotsikas PJ, Radasch RM. A clinical evaluation of pancarpal arthrodesis in nine dogs using circular external skeletal fixation. Vet Surg 2006;35(5):480–5.
52. Ramirez JM, Macias C. Pancarpal Arthrodesis Without Rigid Coaptation Using the Hybrid Dynamic Compression Plate in Dogs. Vet Surg 2016;45(3):303–8.
53. Clarke SP, Ferguson JF, Miller A. Clinical evaluation of pancarpal arthrodesis using a CastLess plate in 11 dogs. Vet Surg 2009;38(7):852–60.
54. Guerrero TG, Montavon PM. Medial plating for carpal panarthrodesis. Vet Surg 2005;34(2):153–8.
55. Streubel R, Makara M, Guerrero T. Medial radio-carpal arthrodesis in three cats with a 2.0 mm locking maxillofacial plate system. Vet Comp Orthop Traumatol 2011;24(4):294–8.
56. Denny HR, Barr A. Partial carpal and pancarpal arthrodesis in the dog: a review of 50 cases. J Small Anim Pract 1991;32:329–34.
57. Wininger FA, Kapatkin AS, Radin A, et al. Failure mode and bending moment of canine pancarpal arthrodesis constructs stabilized with two different implant systems. Vet Surg 2007;36(8):724–8.
58. Guillou RP, Demianiuk RM, Sinnott MT, et al. In vitro mechanical evaluation of a limited contact dynamic compression plate and hybrid carpal arthrodesis plate for canine pancarpal arthrodesis. Vet Comp Orthop Traumatol 2012;25(2):83–8.
59. Arnott JL, Bailey R, Shields A, et al. An in vitro comparison of a 2.7/3.5 mm hybrid plate alone and combined with crossed K-wires for canine pancarpal arthrodesis. Vet Comp Orthop Traumatol 2008;21(04):307–11.
60. Willer RL, Johnson KA, Turner TM, et al. Partial carpal arthrodesis for third degree carpal sprains. A review of 45 carpi. Vet Surg 1990;19(5):334–40.
61. Haburjak JJ, Lenehan TM, Davidson CD, et al. Treatment of carpometacarpal and middle carpal joint hyperextension injuries with partial carpal arthrodesis using a cross pin technique: 21 cases. Vet Comp Orthop Traumatol 2003;16:105–11.
62. Burton NJ, Miles AW, Pollintine P. Biomechanical comparison of a novel castless arthrodesis plate with T-plate and cross pin techniques for canine partial carpal arthrodesis. Vet Comp Orthop Traumatol 2013;26(3):165–71.
63. Grundmann S, Montavon PM. Stenosing tenosynovitis of the abductor pollicis longus muscle in dogs. Vet Comp Orthop Traumatol 2001;14:95–100.
64. Okamura Y, Okamoto Y, Morita T, et al. Enthesiopathy with an abductor pollicis longus dysfunction in a Rough Collie dog. Aust Vet J 2007;85(8):329–31.
65. Hittmair KM, Groessl V, Mayrhofer E. Radiographic and ultrasonographic diagnosis of stenosing tenosynovitis of the abductor pollicis longus muscle in dogs. Vet Radiol Ultrasound 2012;53(2):135–40.

Physeal Injuries and Angular Limb Deformities

Derek B. Fox, DVM, PhD

KEYWORDS

• Physis • Antebrachium • Angular deformity • Radius • Ulna • Humerus

KEY POINTS

• Because of the normally discordant number, relative activity, and morphology of the physes in the radius and ulna, the antebrachium is more subject to physeal-related developmental abnormalities than other bones within the canine and feline appendicular skeleton.

• Particular and predictable patterns of deformity can result, depending on which physes are dysfunctional.

• Successful correction of deformities requires in-depth understanding of normal physeal activity; patient signalment; and ability to quantify the location, magnitude, and plane of the deformity or deformities.

INTRODUCTION

Physeal injuries are common in the developing dog and cat. Insults to physeal function can result in growth disturbances and malalignment of the forelimb and can be caused by trauma, genetic disorders, nutritional imbalances, or other medical disturbances. Resulting deformities can include limb shortening, angulation, joint incongruity, and subluxation, with subsequent osteoarthritis, joint remodeling, and debilitation. Because of the paired bone configuration and disparity in relative physeal contributions to longitudinal growth between the radial and ulnar physes, the antebrachium is the main source of debilitating angular deformities resulting from physeal disturbance in the forelimb. Angular deformities can be assessed in 3 planes—frontal, sagittal, and transverse—and classified based on their multiplicity and direction. Successful correction of deformities requires in-depth understanding of normal physeal activity; careful consideration of patient signalment; and the ability to quantify the location, magnitude, and plane of the deformity or deformities. The goal of this article is to review normal physeal function, forelimb development, and the ramifications of disturbed physeal activity on forelimb alignment and joint health.

Small Animal Orthopedic Surgery, Department of Veterinary Medicine and Surgery, University of Missouri, Veterinary Health Center, 900 East Campus Drive, Clydesdale Hall, Columbia, MO 65211, USA
E-mail address: foxdb@missouri.edu

Vet Clin Small Anim 51 (2021) 305–322
https://doi.org/10.1016/j.cvsm.2020.11.003
vetsmall.theclinics.com

THE PHYSIS: FORM AND FUNCTION

The purpose of the physis is to elongate the long bones at the level between the epiphyses and metaphyses through the process of endochondral ossification. This is accomplished through the activity of the functional unit of the physis, columns of chondrocytes that proliferate, synthesize extracellular matrix, hypertrophy, mineralize the matrix, signal vascular invasion, and undergo apoptotsis.[1] These functions are intimately regulated intrinsically by growth factor signaling and extrinsically both through hormonal and mechanical influences. The growth plate can be divided into layers both morphologically and functionally. The terminology used to describe the layers can vary among investigators, depending on what microstructural feature or function is described. Functionally, the physis is composed of the following zones: (1) the germinal zone; (2) the columnar zone with upper proliferating area and lower maturation area; (3) the hypertrophic zone with an upper 4/5 possessing nonmineralized matrix and lower 1/5 with mineralized matrix; and (4) the outer metaphysis.[1] The cells within the germinal zone also frequently are referred to as resting cells because they do not proliferate.[2] Whereas these layers provide for longitudinal growth, they do not account for the necessary increasing width of the physis during bone development. The growth plate zones thus are circumscribed by a wedge-shaped area of chondrocyte progenitor cells, known as the perichondral ossification groove of Ranvier, that contributes germinal cells to allow expansion of the bone's width at the physis. Within this groove is the fibrous ring of La Croix, which contains fibers arranged vertically, circumferentially, and obliquely to provide mechanical support in response to compression, tension, and shear loads on the physis.[1,2]

Chondrocyte proliferation within the growth plate is under the primary control of a local negative feedback loop involving 3 signaling molecules synthesized by growth plate chondrocytes: parathyroid hormone–related peptide (PTHrP), Indian hedgehog (Ihh), and transforming growth factor (TGF)-β.[3] The release of Ihh by cells newly undergoing hypertrophic differentiation triggers the release of TGF-β by the perichondrium, which in turn stimulates perichondral and juxta-articular cells to increase synthesis of PTHrP, thus slowing the progression of proliferating cells expressing the PTHrP receptor from advancing into the hypertrophic stage.[4] This feedback loop is greatly modulated by several other systemic and local signaling molecules, including the fibroblast growth factor (FGF) family and its receptors.[4] The specific ramification of genetic mutations of the FGF genes when considering limb development is discussed in greater detail later. In addition, growth hormone produced in the anterior pituitary, and its mediator, insulinlike growth factor, play important roles in physeal chondrocyte proliferation. Chondrocyte maturation and hypertrophy occur in response to the bone morphogenic proteins and their receptors.[5] Once the chondrocytes have terminally differentiated, their purpose is to foster matrix calcification in preparation for osteoblastic bone formation.[6] Subsequent death and removal of the chondrocyte then allow space for infiltrating vasculature and bone marrow stromal cells. Death of terminally differentiated chondrocytes occurs through highly regulated apoptosis or programmed cell death.

During the late embryonic phase of development, the epiphyseal cartilages of the long bones are well vascularized, with vessels frequently crossing the physes.[1] Following birth, the transphyseal vascular bridging vanishes, resulting in physeal vasculature arising from 2 separate sources. Epiphyseal vessels supply cells of the germinating, proliferating, and upper hypertrophic zones through diffusion. Separate metaphyseal vessels permeate to the level of the distal hypertrophic zone. The epiphyseal and metaphyseal vessels normally only anastomose once the physis has closed, marking the onset of skeletal maturity.[7] Premature vascular anastomosis across the physis results in pathologic closure of the growth plate and can result in aberrant long bone development. Disruption of the epiphyseal blood supply is the most devastating injury to the physeal growth plate vasculature. Epiphyseal vessel damage can cause avascular necrosis of both the germinal chondrocytes and secondary ossification center of the epiphysis, resulting in ossification of the growth plate and premature cessation of growth. Injury of the metaphyseal vasculature, however, can result in transitory increases in physeal growth.[1,6] For example, humeral elongation has been reported in dogs incurring distal humeral physeal fractures that have undergone surgical repair.[8]

One hormonal influence of physeal activity that is of particular importance to the veterinary surgeon is that of estrogen. In mammals, low serum levels of estrogen during early sexual maturation result in robust skeletal growth, but high levels during late puberty result in growth plate fusion and cessation of longitudinal bone growth.[9] The mechanisms of action for these opposing effects are not fully understood but appear to depend on maturational stage, serum levels of estrogen, and the presence of functional estrogen receptors in the physis.[10] Investigations regarding the impact of prepubertal gonadectomy in the canine demonstrate that those dogs (both male and female) undergoing spay or castration at or before 7 months of age experience a significant delay in physeal closure and elongation of the radius and ulna compared with control populations of littermates left sexually intact.[11] The specific relevance of this finding when addressing physeal disturbances in the skeletally immature dog is the potential magnification of the severity of an emerging deformity through the performance of gonadectomy before 7 months of age. Gonadectomies in animals with identified deformities attributable to physeal insult should be postponed until the age at which physeal closure is achieved for the specific physis or physes in question. The timing of physeal closure is discussed in more detail in the next section.

BRACHIAL AND ANTEBRACHIAL DEVELOPMENT

The physes at the proximal and distal aspects of the humerus, radius, and ulna drive the majority of development of the forelimb. Understanding each physis' relative contribution to the longitudinal growth of a given bone and its time of closure is critical to guiding decision making when presented with a physeal-related deformity (**Table 1**). Research suggests that approximately 80% of longitudinal growth of the humerus arises from the proximal physis and 20% from the distal physis.[8,12] In 1985, Newton and Nunamaker[13] performed a systematic review of 12 studies aimed at determining the closure times of physes in the dog. They reported average times of closure of the proximal and distal humeral physes in dogs as 375 days and 187 days, respectively.[13] The relatively early closure (approximately 6 months) and lesser contribution (approximately 20%) of overall growth of the distal humeral physis

Table 1					
Physeal closure times and relative contributions to growth of the canine forelimb					
Bone	Humerus		Radius		Ulna
Physis	Proximal	Distal	Proximal	Distal	Distal
Closure time (d)[13]	375	187	258	318	308
Contribution to growth (%)[8,15]	~80	~20	36	64	100

Data from Refs.[8,13,15]

help explain why fractures of this physis typically do not result in humeral shortening after treatment by surgery.[8]

Antebrachial development is considerably more complex than humeral growth and, as a result, is much more prone to insult and resulting deformity. Sources of this complexity arise from the paired bone configuration and the fact that, although elongation of the radius occurs from both proximal and distal physes, 100% of ulnar growth between the elbow and carpus arises from the distal ulnar physis alone. Thus, the singular distal ulnar physis must match the same growth as that divided between 2 radial physes, resulting in a requisite and gradual shifting between the 2 bones during development.[14] With respect to radial development, specifically, percent contributions to overall length from proximal and distal physes are 36% and 64%, respectively.[15] The balance of contribution between the physes is dynamic in that as a puppy matures, the distal physis contributes relatively more over time.[15] The period of most rapid growth of the canine antebrachium is between 10 weeks and 14 weeks of age.[15] Average ages at closure of the proximal and distal radial physes are 258 days and 318 days, respectively, whereas the distal ulna physes closes at a mean age of 308 days.[13] As described previously, closure times of physes are delayed with early gonadectomy.

PHYSEAL PATHOLOGY

Normal physeal activity and bone development can be impaired by a large number of pathologic processes, including trauma, endocrinopathies, genetic skeletal dysplasias, nutritional disorders, infectious pathogens, irradiation, and other concurrent juvenile orthopedic diseases like hypertrophic osteodystrophy. It is beyond the scope of this article to explore each in detail, but the commonality of trauma-induced physeal injuries in the small animal warrants further discussion. Because the physes represent both the sole source of skeletal longitudinal growth as well as the mechanically weakest point of the juvenile skeleton, an understanding of growth plate biomechanics and modes of failure is essential. Physeal fractures are common in the skeletally immature small animal and can result in significant alteration of physiologic growth function. A close relationship exists between the ultrastructural properties of the physeal extracellular matrix and its mechanical behavior. In cadaveric testing, the germinal and proliferating portions of the columnar zones are protected somewhat from excessive external force due to their random organization and higher concentrations of collagen fibers.[16] Experimentally, the hypertrophic zone may represent the weakest region within the growth plate under tensile load due to the lower concentration and more regular organization of collagen and the parallel orientation of chondrocytes.[3] The clinical relevance of these observations depends, however, on the specific anatomic site and complexity of offending forces.

A commonly used classification system of growth plate fractures intended to correlate the characteristics and prognoses of each fracture configuration was proposed by Salter and Harris.[17] Using this classification system, physeal fractures can be categorized into types.

Type I fractures represent a displacement of the epiphysis from the metaphysis as a result of shearing and tensile forces with no associated bone fracture. Type I fractures are more common in younger animals (<6 months of age) and historically were believed to carry more favorable prognoses due to both the larger thickness of the physis at this age and the limitations of the fractures to the hypertrophic zone.[18] Several clinical reports now contradict this, however. A high incidence of damage to the proliferating portion of the columnar physeal zone has been reported in naturally occurring type I fractures in the dog, potentially explaining the common clinical observation of subsequent premature growth cessation in some anatomic locations.[19]

Salter-Harris type II fractures occur along the length of the growth plate but extend into the metaphysis, resulting in a wedge-shaped metaphyseal fragment, which remains attached to the epiphysis. The side on which the metaphyseal fragment occurs is related to the directionality of the impacting force and subsequent bending of the bone. Type III fractures are intra-articular in that an epiphyseal fracture communicates with the fissure extending along the growth plate. With disruption of the articular cartilage and subchondral bone, there exists a higher likelihood for postoperative osteoarthritis. Type IV fractures consist of type III fractures with the addition of a metaphyseal extension of the epiphyseal injury. Like type III fractures, type IV fractures are intra-articular and thus require perfect anatomic reduction to reduce the risk of secondary osteoarthritis. Displaced type IV fractures also must be reduced accurately to minimize the risk of formation of a bone bridge along the fracture line that extends from the joint across the physis and into metaphysis, which can result in subsequent growth retardation.[3]

Type V Salter-Harris fractures classically are described as compression fractures of the growth plate. The offending compression is theorized to result in necrosis of proliferating chondrocytes of the growth plate, resulting in overall growth arrest if the entire physis is affected or angular deformation if only a portion of the physis is involved. The most common location in the canine skeleton to be affected by type V fractures is the distal ulnar physis because of its unique conical shape. Any physis, however, can experience premature cessation subsequent to trauma and, depending on which physis or physes are involved, characteristic constellations of deformity can ensue.

When a physeal fracture is identified and treated, caution should be used in prognosticating how the limb will continue to develop. Numerous other factors that are difficult or impossible to assess have a tremendous impact on the response of the bone as it heals, including the anatomic site involved, the potential for postoperative physiologic compensatory mechanisms to occur, the posttraumatic status of the epiphyseal vasculature, the specific physeal zone affected, and the nature of the insulting forces creating the fracture. The prudent surgeon, however, re-examines the affected patient frequently during development to monitor for the onset of deformity, because, frequently, early intervention is warranted should developing malalignment be observed.

NORMAL FORELIMB ALIGNMENT

A comprehensive understanding of normal limb alignment is critical when assessing a developing deformity, planning corrective surgery, and evaluating postoperative outcomes. Whereas several different methods can be used to assess limb alignment, an objective system with accepted nomenclature called the center of rotation of angulation (CORA) has been adapted from human surgery and applied extensively to small animal veterinary orthopedics. Specifically, several radiographic studies have been completed evaluating the alignment of the normal canine forelimb both as individual segments (brachium and antebrachium) and as the overall limb in toto. Utilizing the CORA methodology, anatomic landmarks for the determination of joint orientation lines of the shoulder, elbow, and carpus in frontal and sagittal planes have been described.[20–22] Both mechanical and anatomic axes have been applied to establish a reference library of joint orientation angles through which the overall alignment of the canine forelimb can be described (**Fig. 1**).[20–24] The precise methodology of determining these lines and axes is reviewed in detail elsewhere.[20,22,24,25] A complete list of joint orientation angles for the canine forelimb can be found in **Table 2**. Important to note regarding the alignment

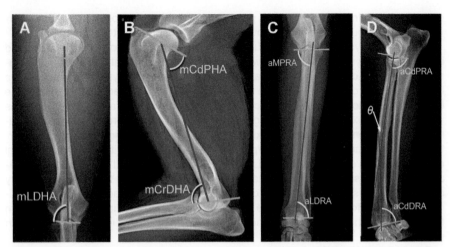

Fig. 1. CORA assessment of normal canine forelimb alignment. (*A*) Humerus frontal plane. (*B*) Humerus sagittal plane. (*C*) Radius and ulna frontal plane. (*D*) Radius and ulna sagittal plane. Green lines, joint orientation lines; red lines, axes; and yellow arcs, joint orientation angles, a, anatomic; A, angle; Cd, caudal; Cr, cranial; D, distal; H, humerus; L, lateral; m, mechanical; M, medial; P, proximal; R, radius; Θ, procurvatum measurement between proximal and distal anatomic axes of the radius in the sagittal plane.

of the canine forelimb in the frontal plane is that the overall limb's mechanical axis (the weight-bearing axis drawn from the center of the humeral head to the center of the metacarpophalangeal joints) lies medial to the center of the elbow, giving rise to a medialized elbow mechanical axis deviation (eMAD) (**Fig. 2**).[23,24] The potential relevance of this finding with respect to medial compartment disease of the elbow is discussed in greater detail in Bruecker and colleagues' article, "Elbow Dysplasia: Medial Compartment Disease and Osteoarthritis," in this issue.

EXAMINATION OF THE PATIENT WITH A FORELIMB DEFORMITY

Assessment of the affected patient begins with obtaining a good history regarding potential traumatic incidences as well as the recent function and activity levels of the

Table 2
Mean joint orientation angles of the canine forelimb (see Fig. 1)

Bone	Humerus[22]		Radius/Ulna[21]		
Plane	Frontal	Sagittal	Frontal	Sagittal	Procurvatum (Θ)
Proximal	NA	mCdPHA = 43°	aMPRA = 83°	aCdPRA = 85°	27°
Distal	mLDHA = 87°	mCrDHA = 72°	aLDRA = 86°	aCdDRA = 77°	

Abbreviations: a, anatomic; A, angle; Cd, caudal; Cr, cranial; D, distal; H, humeral; L, lateral; m, mechanical; M, medial; NA, not applicable; P, proximal; R, radius; procurvatum (Θ), to reflect the angular measurement.

Data from Fasanella FJ, Tomlinson JL, Welihozkiy A et al. Radiographic measurements of the axes and joint angles of the canine radius and ulna. Veterinary Orthopedic Society 37th Annual Conference Abstracts. February 2010;20-27.Breckenridge, CO. https://static1.squarespace.com/static/5571dbd0e4b02ba2bd5bdfdc/t/55f3248fe4b0df1a832c7c0e/1441997967081/VOS-2010-Abstracts-Part-I.pdf. Accessed November 9, 2020 and Wood MC, Fox DB, Tomlinson JL. Determination of the mechanical axis and joint orientation lines in the canine humerus; a radiographic cadaveric study. Vet Surg 2014;43:414-417.

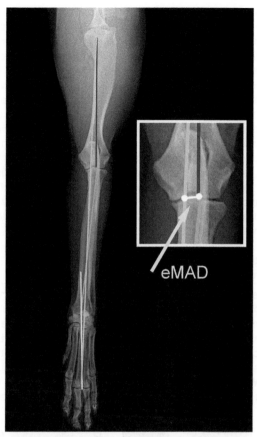

Fig. 2. Overall forelimb alignment for the dog, frontal plane. Red line, humeral mechanical axis; green line, radioulnar mechanical axis; yellow line, metacarpal mechanical axis; and blue line, overall forelimb mechanical axis. (*Inset*) White line, distance between the center of the elbow and the overall limb mechanical axis.

dog. Although some surgical corrections are done prophylactically to help prevent an obvious and severe deformity from having a deleterious impact on the adjacent joints of a developing animal, a decision to intervene is easier for those dogs presenting with a lameness or who are losing quality of life. Next, a thorough orthopedic examination must be completed. This should include watching the animal ambulate on a surface with excellent traction. Lameness is observed for as is how the limb moves during the various phases of the animal's gait. Many specific attributes of forelimb deformities can be predicted prior to radiographic examination simply through careful examination. For example, cranial displacement of the antebrachium with abrupt, sudden carpal flexion during the stance phase is known as buckling[26,27] and can indicate the presence of excessive radial procurvatum. The range of motion of the shoulder, elbow, and carpus should be determined as well as if any pain is elicited on palpation. Special attention should be paid to how the joints palpate at the endpoints of their respective ranges of motion in each plane. In the sagittal plane, both carpus and elbow should be hyperflexed and hyperextended. Elbow incongruity, common with certain types of antebrachial deformity, frequently results in significant pain on elbow hyperextension.

Hyperextension of the carpus may reveal excessive motion in this direction and thus suggest that laxity of the antebrachial flexors is present, not uncommon as a secondary soft tissue compensatory change when excessive radioulnar procurvatum is present. Such a finding is important to note prior to surgical correction of any bone deformity because intentional under-correction may be necessary to avoid the creation of an iatrogenic palmigrade stance. Conversely, pain on carpal hyperflexion may suggest significant carpal bone malformation, which also can be a source of valgus deformation.[28] Equally important is to palpate each joint out of the plane of primary motion. For example, the mediolateral stability of the carpus is critical to evaluate to determine if frontal plane malalignment of the radius and ulna has resulted in stretching and laxity of the collateral support of the joint, because this finding would dramatically alter the prognosis after correction. Finally, the torsional alignment of the antebrachium can be assessed by placing the dog on its back, flexing both elbow and carpus 90°, and assessing the alignment of the metacarpals with respect to the antebrachium and brachium. Malalignment in this view can indicate whether internal or external torsion is present (**Fig. 3**).

PATTERNS OF FORELIMB DEFORMITY
Deformities of Chondrodystrophism

It is well established that aberrational activity of any of the physes that give rise to longitudinal growth of the radius, ulna, and humerus can result in maldevelopment and alteration of normal alignment of the forelimb. As described previously, there are several different etiopathogeneses that can lead to physeal disturbance. One of the more common is chondrodystrophy, a type of skeletal dysplasia that results in disproportionate dwarfism. The term, *chondrodystrophy*, first was introduced by Hansen[29] to describe dogs with premature degeneration of the intervertebral disks and characteristic shortening and malalignment of the long bones of the appendicular skeleton.

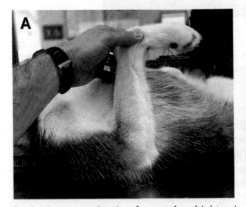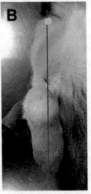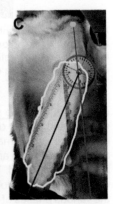

Fig. 3. Gross examination for antebrachial torsion. (*A*) Dorsal recumbent positioning of the dog with the forelimb placed in 90°–90° flexion at the elbow and carpus. The forelimb is examined from above, looking down the axis of the antebrachium. *Yellow line* outlines the contour of the manus. (*B*) Normal forelimb alignment. Blue dot demarks the greater tubercle of the humerus. Red line highlights straight alignment between humerus, elbow, carpus, and metacarpals. (*C*) Examination of a forelimb with external antebrachial torsion. Blue dot demarks the greater tubercle of the humerus. Red line highlights humeral axis. Blue line highlights axis of metacarpals. A goniometer centered on the carpus is used to measure angular difference between metacarpal axis and humeral axis (approximately 30°) demonstrating external torsion.

Two genetic mutations now have been associated with canine chondrodystrophy, consisting of copied sections of the canine FGF4 retrogene inserted into 2 aberrant locations of chromosomes 12 and 18.[30,31] Whereas the mutations can occur independently, those breeds with the most extreme limb maldevelopment inherit both in high frequency and include the basset hound, Welsh corgi, and dachshund.[30] Whereas the hallmark of forelimb changes associated with chondrodystrophism historically has been limb shortening, coincident angular deformities also can be present and may be severe. To be clear, a majority of chondrodystrophic dogs do not exhibit untoward effects as a result of their distinct and characteristic conformation. A study aimed at classifying antebrachial deformities in a mixed population of dogs determined, however, that chondrodystrophic dogs typically had more complex patterns of malalignment with a higher likelihood of possessing concurrent joint osteoarthritis and remodeling.[32] Specifically, those chondrodystrophic dogs that present with a forelimb lameness attributable to antebrachial angulation typically possess partially compensated biapical frontal plane radial deformities (proximal radial varus and distal valgus) with concurrent excessive procurvatum and external torsion (**Fig. 4**).[20,32] Fortunately, humeral changes related to chondrodystrophism appear to be limited to shortening and thickening of the bone with subtle changes in the sagittal plane, which are not believed to hold clinical relevance.[33]

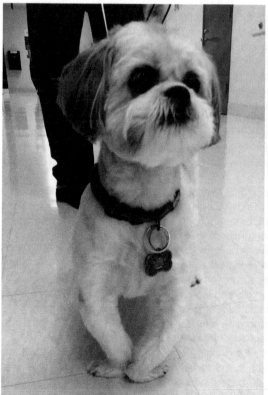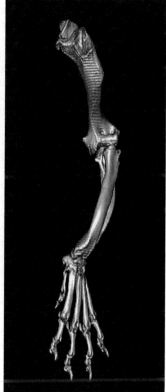

Fig. 4. Chondrodystrophic dog demonstrating excessive bilateral biapical partially compensated torsion-angulation antebrachial deformities as viewed grossly (*left*) and on computed tomographic surface reconstruction (*right*).

Discerning whether a chondrodystrophic dog with partially compensated biapical deformities requires surgical correction can be challenging. Corrective surgery is invasive and never should be completed for cosmetics but rather reserved for those dogs whose quality of life is negatively affected by the deformity in question. Although specific guidance regarding correction techniques of biapical antebrachial deformities is beyond the scope of this article, different strategies exist, and readers are referred to those references that discuss them. Although some research suggests good outcomes can be achieved through addressing such deformities through the performance of single osteotomies,[34] the relatively large residual translation with this technique suggests that double-level corrective osteotomies based on each radial CORA may result in a more geometrically accurate correction.[20,25,27,34] No prospective clinical trial comparing the outcome of the 2 approaches, however, has been completed to date. The concurrent incidence of humeroulnar incongruity that can exist as a component of biapical deformities of chondrodystrophism is discussed in the next section.

Premature Closure of the Distal Ulnar Physis

Of all reported forelimb deformities that arise secondary to physeal insult, the most common is the premature closure of the distal ulnar physis.[35] As described previously, all ulnar growth distal to the elbow occurs at the distal growth plate, and this growth must match that of both the proximal and distal radial physes. Thus, even subtle alterations in the activity of the distal ulnar physis can have potentially serious ramifications on antebrachial development. The distal ulnar physis also is unique in that its morphology is quite different from both radial physes. Figuratively, the distal ulnar physis can be described as a cone within a cone, versus both radial physes that are more akin to stacked plates. This morphology is believed to make the distal ulnar physis more stable in resisting fracture separation and yet more susceptible to compression from forces arising from a larger variety of directions. Consequently, both compressive and shearing forces can result in Salter-Harris type V fractures of the distal ulnar physis whereas such shearing forces likely would separate the distal radial physis. Thus, initial injury to the distal ulnar physis may go unnoticed by owners or be observed only as a transient lameness not requiring immediate medical attention.

Because of the caudolateral positional relationship of the distal ulna with respect to the radius, premature closure of the distal ulnar physis results in a predictable set of sequelae with respect to the development of the antebrachium: shortening, excessive procurvatum, valgus, and external torsion (**Fig. 5**). In 12% of cases, shortening of the ulna also can result in loss of humeroulnar congruity with gross remodeling of the anconeal process and elongation of the ulnar trochlear notch (**Fig. 6**).[35] Pain associated with humeroulnar incongruity also can be the chief complaint of some chondrodystrophic dogs presenting with a forelimb lameness. Such cases can be challenging to treat because there are 2 potential sources of lameness: the malalignment of the antebrachium and the joint incongruity. Studies have demonstrated that in limbs with a partially compensated biapical deformity of the antebrachium secondary to chondrodystrophism, concurrent elbow pathology is evident in 83%.[32] In another study, 53% of dogs presenting with humeroulnar incongruity requiring surgical treatment were chondrodystrophic, with basset hounds overrepresented.[36]

Treatment strategies of premature closure of the distal ulnar physis depend on the nature of the deformity present, patient signalment, severity of angulation, and client capabilities. Humeroulnar incongruity subsequent to ulnar shortening is readily treated by ulnar elongation. This can be achieved either through acute or gradual correction

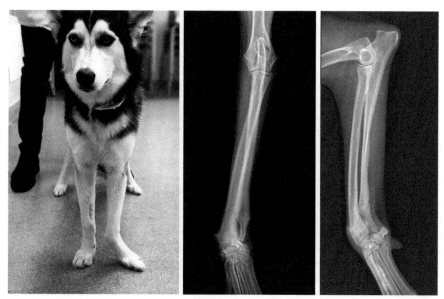

Fig. 5. A 1-year-old husky presenting with antebrachial angulation secondary to premature closure of the distal ulnar physis (same dog seen in **Fig. 3**) exhibiting distal antebrachial valgus, external torsion, and procurvatum on gross examination and orthogonal radiographs. (*left panel*) Gross appearance of valgus deformity with external torsion. (*middle panel*) Frontal plane radiograph of the affected antebrachium demonstrating valgus and torsion of the distal radius. (*Right*) Sagittal plane radiograph demonstrating excessive procurvatum and torsion of the distal radius.

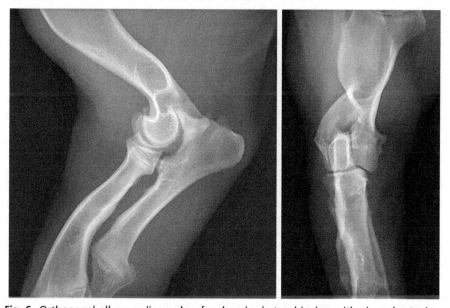

Fig. 6. Orthogonal elbow radiographs of a chondrodystrophic dog with ulnar shortening, humeroulnar incongruity, and elongation of the ulnar trochlear notch. (*Left panel*) Sagittal plane radiographs of the affected elbow. (*Right panel*) Frontal plane radiographs of the affected elbow.

with rigid fixation[37] or, more commonly, via dynamic proximal ulnar ostectomy (DPUO).[36] The advantages of the latter are a less invasive and less expensive approach. The DPUO utilizes the pull of the triceps muscle group to distract the proximal ulna into congruency with the humerus. Execution of DPUO alone also is a reasonable first step in the staged treatment of a chondrodystrophic dog with biapical radial deformities and concurrent humeroulnar incongruity, especially if the malalignment is not deemed to be that severe. Many dogs improve significantly after normalizing their elbow congruity and may not require additional corrective surgery.

When premature distal ulnar physeal closure is the source of antebrachial angulation, more invasive treatments are required to normalize alignment and thereby improve comfort and function. Although distal ulnar physectomy or ostectomies may mitigate worsening of the radial angulation in a skeletally immature animal, they do not appear to allow consistent autocorrection of the radius to normalcy. Thus, more aggressive surgical intervention aimed at restoring normal alignment of the antebrachium frequently is required. In growing dogs, this is achieved most successfully with gradual correction with Ilizarov-style external fixation and the principles of distraction osteogenesis to simultaneously elongate and align the radius and ulna.[38] Once skeletal growth has stopped, either gradual or acute correction with either internal fixation or external fixation can be utilized successfully. Most antebrachial angular deformities that occur secondary to premature closure of the distal ulnar physis are uniapical and occur distally, in the proximity of the distal radial and ulnar physes.[32] As described previously, a majority of these deformities exhibit distal radial valgus, excessive procurvatum, and external torsion, thus representing deformity discernible in all 3 planes: frontal, sagittal, and transverse. Accurate correction requires calculating the obliquity of the plane of the deformity between frontal and sagittal planes.[25,38] Furthermore, the torsional component of the deformity can result in artifact when calculating the angular magnitude of the CORA and must be accounted for via special segmental radiographic views or imaging modalities like computed tomography.[27,34,39] Three-dimensional printing and rapid prototyping also have demonstrated utility in helping to plan the correction of complex torsion-angulation radioulnar deformities.[26,27,40]

Successful correction of uniapical, oblique-plane radioulnar torsion-angulation deformities has been achieved through several different methods, including Ilizarov-style fixators,[38] hybrid fixators,[37] and internal fixation with bone plates.[41] Osteotomy types vary by technique and method of fixation but usually involve either closing or opening wedges. Recent reports, however, describe the adaptation of a type of osteotomy utilized in human medicine to specifically address torsion-angulation deformities in the canine radius, called the oblique plane inclined osteotomy.[41,42]

Premature Closure of the Distal Radial Physis

As described previously, the distal radial physis contributes to the majority of radial growth and remains open longer than the proximal physis. As with other physes, the distal radial physis can undergo premature closure secondary to insult and may be affected symmetrically or asymmetrically either medially or laterally. Asymmetric closure of the lateral aspect appears to be the most common presentation.[43] On physical examination, the limb can appear grossly similar to that affected by premature closure of the distal ulnar physis, with an apparent valgus deformity of the distal radius, carpus, and manus and antebrachial shortening with compensatory elbow hyperextension.[44] Characteristic radiographic changes, however, distinguish this condition (**Fig. 7**).[43–45] The lateral aspect of the distal radial physis appears narrowed, with lateral deviation of the distal radial epiphysis and valgus malalignment of the carpus

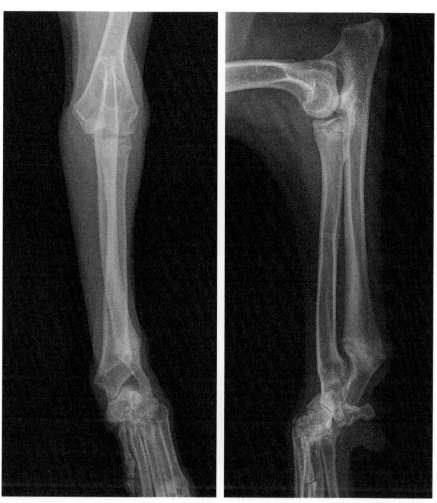

Fig. 7. Orthogonal radiographs of the antebrachium of a 6-month-old Labrador retriever with asymmetric premature closure of the lateral aspect of the distal radial physis. Note radial shortening, widening of the humeroradial joint space with loss of humeroulnar congruity, valgus deviation of the distal radial epiphysis, wedge-shaped opening, subluxation of the radiocarpal joint on the frontal plane, and cranial subluxation of the radiocarpal joint on the sagittal plane and ulnar recurvatum. (*Left panel*) Frontal plane radiographs of the affected elbow. (*Right panel*) Sagittal plane radiographs of the affected elbow.

and manus. Although not consistently seen, a wedge-like opening and loss of joint congruence of the radiocarpal joint may be apparent on frontal plane radiographs, with cranial subluxation of the carpus on sagittal plane views. Because the radius is the retarding force on antebrachial development with this condition, the ulna may exhibit recurvatum. Finally, the radius may be shortened at the level of the elbow, resulting in a widening of the humeroradial joint space with humeroulnar subluxation. Asymmetric closure of the medial aspect of the physis resulting in varus deformity also can occur but is seen less commonly (**Fig. 8**). Lastly, symmetric closure of the distal radial physis has been described. This condition may result in similar elbow incongruency proximally and can cause a varus deformity of the carpus and manus distally as

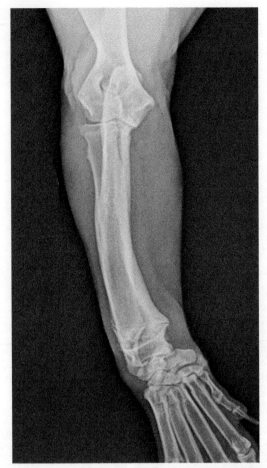

Fig. 8. Frontal plane radiograph of a 10-month-old mixed breed dog with asymmetric premature closure of the medial aspect of the distal radial physis and resulting distal antebrachial varus.

the ulna outgrows the radius, thus pushing the distal extremity medially.[46,47] Surgical correction of premature closure of the distal radial physis must be tailored to the type of closure present (symmetric vs asymmetric or lateral vs medial) as well as the location and magnitude of the deformity. Correction can be achieved via different techniques but is recommended to occur at an early age and prioritizes (1) optimizing elbow joint congruency via elongation of the radius or shortening of the ulna, (2) correcting malalignment of the distal extremity, and (3) restoring length of the antebrachium.[43–48]

Premature Closure of the Proximal Radial Physis

The proximal radial physis also can undergo premature closure, far less frequently, however, than the distal physis. This likely is due to the fact that the load across the elbow is distributed fairly evenly between the radial head and coronoid processes. Thus, the proximal radial physis is more protected from sudden overloading and preferential physeal compression. Still, trauma, infection, or inflammatory conditions can result in retardation of the activity of the proximal physis. Resulting pathology is evident in the form of radial shortening, increasing humeroradial joint space, and loss of humeroulnar congruence in the absence of antebrachial angulation. This condition can be distinguished from symmetric distal physeal closure by the narrowed and closed appearance of the proximal radial physis in the presence of a distal radial physis that is normal. Treatment of this condition differs depending on the age of the patient but constitutes guided radial elongation in an actively growing dog and either radial elongation or ulnar shortening in a mature animal.

CLINICS CARE POINTS

- Gonadectomies in animals with emerging physeal-related deformities should be postponed until the physes of the affected limb have closed.
- Distal humeral condylar fractures possess a low risk of subsequent deformities owing to the earlier closure time and lesser contribution of growth of the distal physis.
- The canine antebrachium elongates most rapidly between 10 and 14 weeks of age.
- Forelimb "buckling" during ambulation can indicate excessive antebrachial procurvatum.
- Antebrachial torsion must be evaluated through gross examination pre-operatively as surgical correction is largely based on visual appearance.
- Most chondrodystrophic dogs presenting for deformity of the radius and ulna will possess partially compensated biapical deformities of the antebrachium with associated osteoarthritis of the elbow and carpus.
- Premature closure of the distal ulnar physis causes elbow incongruity in at least 12% of cases and should always be evaluated.
- Radial deformities that exhibit deformity in the frontal and sagittal plane are considered oblique-plane deformities.
- When present, torsion will artifactually affect the accurate radiographic measurement of the angular component of a deformity and must be accounted for.
- Premature closure of the lateral distal radial physis may grossly appear similar to premature closure of the distal ulnar physis, but requires diagnostic distinction for appropriate corrective measures.

DISCLOSURE

The author has no commercial or financial interests associated with any of the information provided in this article.

REFERENCES

1. Farriol F, Shapiro F. Bone development: interaction of molecular components and biophysical forces. Clin Orthop Relat Res 2005;432:14–33.
2. Iannotti JP. Growth plate physiology and pathology. Orthop Clin North Am 1990; 21:1–17.
3. Ianotti JP, Goldstein S, Kuhn J, et al. The formation and growth of skeletal tissues. In: Buckwalter JA, Einhorn TA, Simon SR, editors. Orthopaedic basic science, biology and biomechanics of the musculoskeletal system. 2nd edition. Rosemont (II): American Academy of Orthopaedic Surgeons; 2000. p. 77–109.

4. Kronenberg HM, Lee K, Lanske B, et al. Parathyroid hormone-related protein and Indian hedgehog control the pace of cartilage differentiation. J Endocrinol 1997; 154:S39–45.

5. Volk SW, Leboy PS. Regulating the regulators of chondrocyte hypertrophy. J Bone Miner Res 1999;14:483486.

6. Ballock RT, O'Keefe RJ. The biology of the growth plate. J Bone Joint Surg Am 2003;85A:715–26.

7. Shapiro F. Epiphyseal and physeal cartilage vascularization: a light microscope and trtiated thymidine autoradiographic study of cartilage canals in newborn and young postnatal rabbit. Anat Rec 1998;252:140–8.

8. Lefebvre JGNG, Robertson TR, Baines SJ, et al. Assessment of humeral length in dogs after repair of Salter–Harris type IV fracture of the lateral part of the humeral condyle. Vet Surg 2008;37:545–51.

9. Juul A. The effects of oestrogens on linear bone growth. Hum Reprod Update 2001;7:303–13.

10. Börjesson AE, Lagerquist MK, Windahl SH, et al. The role of estrogen receptor α in the regulation of bone and growth plate cartilage. Cell Mol Life Sci 2013;70: 4023–37.

11. Salmeri KR, Bloomberg MS, Scruggs SL, et al. Gonadectomy in immature dogs: effects on skeletal, physical, and behavioral development. J Am Vet Med Assoc 1991;198:1193–203.

12. Pritchett JW. Growth plate activity in the upper extremity. Clin Orthop Relat Res 1991;268:235–42.

13. Newton CD. Canine and feline epiphyseal plate closure and appearance of ossification centers, Appendix C. In: Newton CD, Nunamaker DM, editors. Textbook of small animal orthopedics. Philadelphia (PA): JB Lippincott; 1985. p. 1108–13.

14. Carrig CB. Growth abnormalities of the canine radius and ulna. Vet Clin North Am 1983;13:91–115.

15. Conzemius MG, Smith GK, Brighton CT, et al. Analysis of physeal growth in dogs, using biplanar radiography. Am J Vet Res 1994;55:22–7.

16. Fujii T, Takai S, Arai Y, et al. Microstructural properties of the distal growth plate of the rabbit radius and ulna: biomechanical, biochemical, and morphological studies. J Orthop Res 2000;18:87–93.

17. Salter RB, Harris WR. Injuries involving the epiphyseal plate. J Bone Joint Surg Am 1963;45:587–622.

18. Braden TD. Histophysiology of the growth plate and growth plate injuries. In: Bojrab MJ, Sneak DD, Bloomberg MS, editors. Disease mechanisms in small animal surgery. 2nd edition. Malvern (PA): Lea & Febiger; 1993. p. 1027–39.

19. Johnson JM, Johnson AL, Eurell JA. Histologic appearance of naturally occurring canine physeal fractures. Vet Surg 1994;23:81–6.

20. Fox DB, Tomlinson JL, Cook JL, et al. Principles of uniapical and biapical radial deformity correction using dome osteotomies and the center of rotation of angulation methodology in dogs. Vet Surg 2006;35:67–77.

21. Fasanella FJ, Tomlinson JL, Welihozkiy A, et al. Radiographic measurements of the axes and joint angles of the canine radius and ulna. Veterinary Orthopedic Society 37th Annual Conference Abstracts. February 2010;20-27.Breckenridge, CO.   Available   at: https://static1.squarespace.com/static/ 5571dbd0e4b02ba2bd5bdfdc/t/55f3248fe4b0df1a832c7c0e/1441997967081/ VOS-2010-Abstracts-Part-I.pdf. Accessed November 9, 2020.

22. Wood MC, Fox DB, Tomlinson JL. Determination of the mechanical axis and joint orientation lines in the canine humerus; a radiographic cadaveric study. Vet Surg 2014;43:414–7.
23. Saviori CM, Fox DB, Tomlinson JL. Determination of thoracic limb mechanical axes in the dog: a cadaveric radiographic study in the frontal plane. Steamboat (CO): Abstract. Veterinary Orthopedic Society; 2009.
24. Goodrich ZJ, Norby B, Eichelberger BM, et al. Evaluation of standing versus recumbent frontal plane radiography. Vet Surg 2014;43:791–803.
25. Fox DB, Tomlinson JL. Principles of angular limb deformity correction. In: Johnston SA, Tobias KM, editors. Veterinary surgery, small animal (vol 1). 2nd edition. St. Louis (MO): Elsevier; 2018. p. 762–74.
26. Crosse KR, Worth AJ. Computer-assisted surgical correction of an antebrachial deformity in a dog. s 2010;23:354–61.
27. Kwan TW, Marcellin-Little DJ, Harrysson OLA. Correction of biapical radial deformities by use of bi-level hinged circular external fixation and distraction osteogenesis in 13 dogs. Vet Surg 2014;43:316–29.
28. Comerford EJ, Doran IC, Owen MR. Carpal derangement and associated carpal valgus in a dog. Vet Comp Orthop Traumatol 2006;19:113–6.
29. Hansen HJ. A pathologic-anatomical interpretation of disc degeneration in dog, with special reference to the so-called enchondrosis intervertebralis. Acta Orthop Scand Suppl 1952;11:1–117.
30. Brown EA, Dickinson PJ, Mansour T, et al. FGF4 retrogene on CFA12 is responsible for chondrodystrophy and intervertebral disk disease in dogs. Proc Natl Acad Sci U S A 2017;114:11476–81.
31. Parker HG, VonHoldt BM, Quignon P, et al. An expressed FGF4 retrogene is associated with breed-defining chondrodysplasia in domestic dogs. Science 2009; 325:995–8.
32. Knapp JL, Tomlinson JL, Fox DB. Classification of angular limb deformities affecting the canine radius and ulna using the center of rotation of angulation method. Vet Surg 2016;45:295–302.
33. Smith EJ, Marcellin-Little DJ, Harrysson OL, et al. Influence of chondrodystrophy and brachycephaly on geometry of the humerus in dogs. Vet Comp Orthop Traumatol 2016;29:220–6.
34. Fitzpatrick, Nikolaou C, Farrell M, et al. The double-arch modified type-1b external skeletal fixator: Technique description and functional outcome for surgical management of canine antebrachial limb deformities. Vet Comp Orthop Traumatol 2011;5:374–82.
35. Ramadan RO, Vaughan LC. Premature closure of the distal ulnar growth plate in dogs: a review of 58 cases. J Small Anim Pract 1978;19:647–67.
36. Gilson SD, Piermattei DL, Schwarz PD. Treatment of humeroulnar subluxation with a dynamic proximal ulnar osteotomy: a review of 13 cases. Vet Surg 1989;18: 114–22.
37. Sereda CW, Lewis DD, Radasch RM, et al. Descriptive report of antebrachial growth deformity correction in 17 dogs from 1999 to 207 using hybrid linear-circular external fixator constructs. Can Vet J 2009;50:723–32.
38. Marcellin-Little DJ, Ferretti A, Roe SC, et al. Hinged Ilizarov fixation for correction of antebrachial deformities. Vet Surg 1998;27:231–45.
39. Piras LA, Peirone B, Fox DB. Effects of antebrachial torsion on the measurement of angulation in the frontal plane: a cadaveric radiographic analysis. Vet Comp Orthop Traumatol 2012;25:89–94.

40. Dismukes DI, Fox DB, Tomlinson JL. Use of radiographic measures and three-dimensional computed tomographic imaging in the surgical correction of an antebrachial deformity in a dog. J Am Vet Med Assoc 2008;232:68–73.

41. Frankllin SP, Dover RK, Andrade N, et al. Correction of antebrachial angulation-rotation deformities in dogs with oblique plane inclined osteotomies. Vet Surg 2017;46:1078–85.

42. Kim SY, Snowdon KA, DeCamp CE. Single olique osteotomy for correction of antebrachial angular and torsional deformities in a dog. J Am Vet Med Assoc 2017; 251:333–9.

43. Newton CD. Principles and techniques of osteotomy. In: Newton CD, Nunamaker DM, editors. Textbook of small animal orthopedics. Philadelphia (PA): JB Lippincott; 1985. p. 529–44.

44. Preston CA. Distraction osteogenesis to treat premature distal radial growth plate closure in a dog. Aust Vet J 2000;78:387–91.

45. Passman D, Wolff EF. Premature closure of the distal radial growth plate in dog. J Am Vet Med Assoc 1975;167:391–3.

46. Newton CD, Nunamaker DM, Dickinson CR. Surgical management of radial physeal growth disturbances in dogs. J Am Vet Med Assoc 1975;167:1011–8.

47. Olson NC, Carrig CB, Brinker WO. Asynchronous growth of the canine radius and ulna: Effects of retardation of longitudinal growth of the radius. Am J Vet Res 1979;40:351–5.

48. Barr ARS, Denny HR. The management of elbow instability caused by premature closure of the distal radial growth plate in dogs. J Small Anim Pract 1985;26: 427–35.

The Shoulder Joint and Common Abnormalities

Rebecca Stokes, DVM[a], David Dycus, DVM, MS, CCRP[b],*

KEYWORDS

- Medial shoulder syndrome • Supraspinatus tendinopathy • Bicipital tendinopathy
- Arthroscopy • Osteochondrosis • Osteochondritis dissecans
- Infraspinatus contracture • Shoulder luxation

KEY POINTS

- The shoulder is a complex joint composed mostly of static and dynamic capsuloligamentous support structures.
- Thorough orthopedic and neurologic examination, radiographs, advanced imaging techniques (musculoskeletal ultrasound, computed tomography, and magnetic resonance imaging), and/or arthroscopy are used to obtain accurate diagnosis.
- Osteochondrosis/osteochondritis dissecans is an important developmental disease commonly affecting the caudal humeral head.
- Canine bicipital and supraspinatus tendinopathies show similarities to humans; however, accurate diagnosis and clinical significance are difficult to determine.
- Medial shoulder syndrome is one of the most common shoulder pathologies occurring in greater frequency than luxation.

INTRODUCTION

The shoulder is a diarthrodial joint capable of immense range of motion because it is composed primarily of capsuloligamentous supporting structures but mainly functions in flexion and extension.[1] Additionally, the shoulder is capable of abduction, adduction, and internal and external rotation. Both passive (static) and active (dynamic) mechanisms provide stability and counteract forces that otherwise would destabilize the joint.[2] Passive mechanisms require no muscle activity and allow a wide range of joint motion. Passive stabilizers include the limited joint volume, adhesion/cohesion mechanisms, concavity compression, and capsuloligamentous restraints (medial glenohumeral ligament [MGL], lateral glenohumeral ligament [LGL], joint capsule [JC], labrum, and origin of the biceps tendon).[3,4] Active stabilizers require coordinated muscle contraction and include the cuff muscles (supraspinatus, infraspinatus, teres

[a] Department of Small Animal Clinical Sciences, College of Veterinary Medicine, Iowa State University, Vet Med, 1800 Christensen Drive, Ames, IA 50011, USA; [b] Department of Orthopedic Surgery, Nexus Veterinary Bone & Joint Center, Baltimore, MD 21224, USA
* Corresponding author.
E-mail address: dldycus@gmail.com

Vet Clin Small Anim 51 (2021) 323–341
https://doi.org/10.1016/j.cvsm.2020.11.002
0195-5616/21/© 2020 Elsevier Inc. All rights reserved.

minor, and subscapularis)[5,6] and, to a lesser extent, biceps brachii, long head of the triceps brachii, deltoideus, and teres major muscles.[7]

Shoulder pathology plays an important role in canine forelimb lameness. Historically, shoulder discomfort was generalized into large categories; however, imaging technique advances have allowed for emergence and greater understanding of various disorders. In addition to shoulder palpation, thorough investigation of the elbow and neurologic evaluation are necessary with forelimb lameness because elbow pathology, spinal abnormalities, and peripheral nerve sheath tumors are important differentials.[5] This article gives an updated review of common canine shoulder pathologies, including osteochondrosis, bicipital and supraspinatus tendinopathies, infraspinatus contracture, medial shoulder syndrome (MSS), and luxation.

OSTEOCHONDROSIS/OSTEOCHONDRITIS DISSECANS

Osteochondrosis (OC) is a developmental disease resulting from incomplete endochondral ossification. When progression leads to disruption of the articular surface and flap formation, osteochondritis dissecans (OCD) results (**Fig. 1**).[8,9] OC/OCD commonly affects young, large, and giant breed dogs and occurs bilaterally in 27% to 68% of dogs.[10,11] Although it overwhelmingly is a disease of canines, a single report of feline shoulder OCD has been documented.[12] The caudocentral and caudomedial humeral head are common sites affected[13] (see **Fig. 1**), with less favorable outcomes associated with caudocentral lesions.[14]

Clinical signs often occur at 4 months to 8 months of age.[8] Later presentations likely are secondary to osteoarthritis from a lesion missed in the immature dog. Mild to moderate lameness, worse upon rising and after activity, are described. Examination often

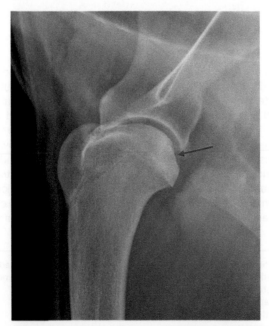

Fig. 1. Lateral shoulder radiograph revealing caudal humeral head OCD lesion. Note the subchondral defect (*arrow*) with flattening of the caudal humeral head and surrounding sclerosis.

reveals discomfort on deep shoulder flexion because this places direct pressure on the caudal humeral head.[8] Radiographs may appear normal or reveal a caudal humeral head subchondral defect (see **Fig. 1**).[15] When no defect is observed but high clinical suspicion exists, musculoskeletal ultrasound, arthrography, computed tomography (CT), and/or magnetic resonance imaging (MRI) may aid in diagnosis.[16,17] Conservative management is recommended only for those less than 6 months of age with mild lameness and no radiographic abnormalities. Surgery otherwise is standard of care and involves flap removal, surrounding unadhered cartilage excision, and encouraging local fibrocartilage formation through arthrotomy or arthroscopy (**Fig. 2**).[9,14] Larger defects or refractory cases can be addressed with osteochondral autografts[18] or synthetic plug implantation.[19] Activity restriction and rehabilitation are integral to a successful outcome.[20] Overall, return to normal or near normal function generally is good following surgery.[11]

BICIPITAL TENDINOPATHY

Bicipital tendinopathy (historically termed, tenosynovitis) once was thought to be a common pathologic finding. Advances in diagnostic capabilities through arthroscopy (**Fig. 3**), musculoskeletal ultrasound (**Fig. 4**), CT, and MRI, however, have led to identification of other soft tissue pathologies not previously recognized.[21,22] Bicipital tendinopathy affects middle-aged to older, medium to large breed dogs, often resulting in chronic, progressive lameness worse after exercise.[8,23,24] The pathogenesis largely is unknown but can be classified as primary or secondary tendinopathies.[25] Primary bicipital tendinopathy is thought to occur secondary to chronic microtrauma.[23,25] The biceps tendon origin is relatively hypovascular, which may predispose it to mechanical failure.[2,25] Secondary bicipital tendinopathy occurs as a result of trauma, impingement via joint mice or enlarged supraspinatus, and/or intraarticular pathology.[24]

Chronic intermittent or progressive weight-bearing lameness, which initially may be noticeable only upon rising or following activity and may or may not be responsive to

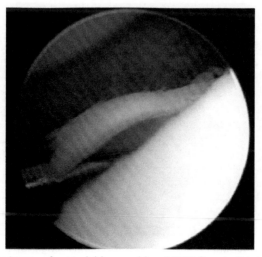

Fig. 2. Arthroscopic image of a caudal humeral head OCD flap. In this image, cranial is to the right. A hypodermic needle can be seen lifting the flap up.

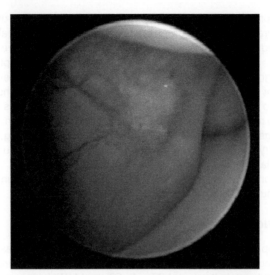

Fig. 3. Arthroscopic image of a normal biceps. The origin of the biceps from the supraglenoid tubercle is noted in the top of the image.

anti-inflammatories, is common. Diagnosis is obtained through examination abnormalities (discomfort on direct shoulder palpation, positive biceps stretch test, and so forth) and diagnostic imaging (radiographs, musculoskeletal ultrasound, MRI, and/or arthroscopy).[5,24,25] Tension upon shoulder flexion and discomfort during biceps stretch test (**Fig. 5**) may be present. Importantly, in contrast, those with a biceps tear have loss of end-feel. Radiographs largely are normal; however, tendon calcification may be present in chronic cases (**Fig. 6**). Given their close anatomic relationship, it may be difficult to distinguish calcification within the biceps versus supraspinatus. Skyline radiographic views are used to help identify calcification within the

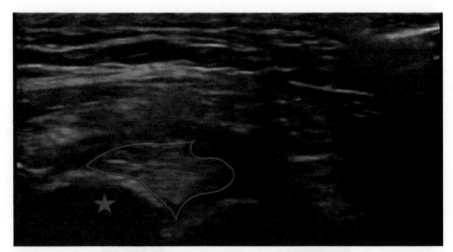

Fig. 4. Musculoskeletal ultrasound image of the normal origin of the biceps (*outlined*) arising from the supraglenoid tubercle (*star*). (*Courtesy of* D. Canapp, DVM, Annapolis Junction, MD.)

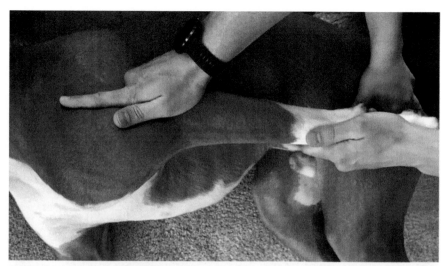

Fig. 5. Biceps stretch test is performed by full flexion of the shoulder and extension of the elbow. The dogs head is to the left.

intertubercular groove.[23] Ultrasound changes consistent with biceps tendinopathy include a sonolucent line around the tendon on the transverse view (**Fig. 7**), enlarged hypoechoic tendon with fiber pattern disruption, and/or bicipital groove irregularities.

Treatment is largely conservative with exercise restriction and formal rehabilitation to facilitate healing and improve tissue flexibility. For moderate or refractory cases, intra-articular therapies (corticosteroids, plasma products, and other biologics) are considered.[20,23,26–29] Should a patient not respond to any intervention, other pathologies should be ruled out prior to recommending surgery. Surgery consists of biceps release (tenotomy) (**Fig. 8**) or tenodesis.[25]

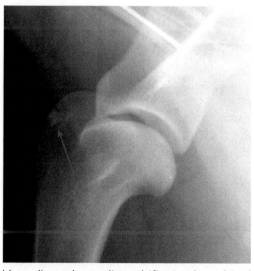

Fig. 6. Lateral shoulder radiograph revealing calcification (*arrow*) in the region of the biceps/supraspinatus.

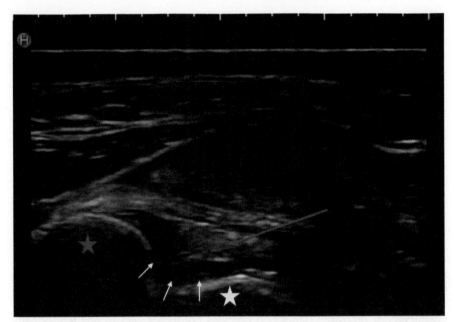

Fig. 7. Musculoskeletal ultrasound of biceps tendinopathy. The biceps (*red arrow*)has a hy-poechoic fiber patter at its origin on the supraglenoid tubercle (*red star*). In addition, there is fluid (*yellow arrows*) surrounding the biceps tendon. The yellow star is the bicipital groove for reference. (*Courtesy of* D. Canapp, DVM, Annapolis Junction, MD.)

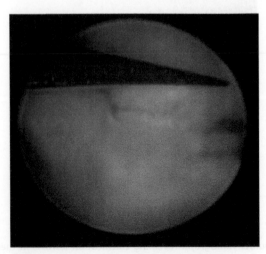

Fig. 8. Arthroscopic biceps tenotomy using arthroscopic scissors.

SUPRASPINATUS TENDINOPATHY

Supraspinatus tendinopathies are documented in humans and to lesser extent in canines with similarities that include the proposed pathogenesis (hypovascularity), clinical evaluation, potential effects on the biceps, and management strategies.[26,30–32] Supraspinatus tendinopathies also can have mineralization.[33] With pathogenesis largely unknown, several theories exist, including hypoxia, degenerative changes due to overuse or concurrent pathology, and metabolic disorders.[26,30] Although distinct areas of hypovascularity or avascularity are documented (similar to humans), the significance is unknown but may lead to fibrocartilaginous transformation.[30] Myxomatous degeneration and/or cartilaginous metaplasia are common histopathologic changes.[33] Similarly, the clinical implication of mineralization is unclear[26,31,33–35] and concurrent disease often is present.[36]

Supraspinatus tendinopathies occur in medium to large breeds, with Labrador retrievers and rottweilers overrepresented.[26,34] History and examination may be similar to biceps tendinopathy. Lameness may be unilateral even with bilateral disease.[33] Supraspinatus tendinopathies resulting from compression of the biceps often are more affected.[37] Examination may include discomfort and tension on shoulder flexion and/or direct supraspinatus insertion palpation.[38]

Similarly, radiographs largely are normal.[33] Ultrasound is a noninvasive tool for confirming supraspinatus tendinopathy and further investigating other periarticular structures (**Figs. 9** and **10**).[32] It can be helpful particularly in differentiating active inflammation within or surrounding the supraspinatus tendon from static mineralization.[32,34,36] Common ultrasound changes include increased tendon size, irregular fiber pattern, nonhomogeneous echogenicity, and/or calcifications (**Fig. 11**).[36] Mistieri and colleagues[32] proposed that MRI is more helpful for investigating concurrent biceps tendon impingement. Care should be used, however, because MRI supraspinatus

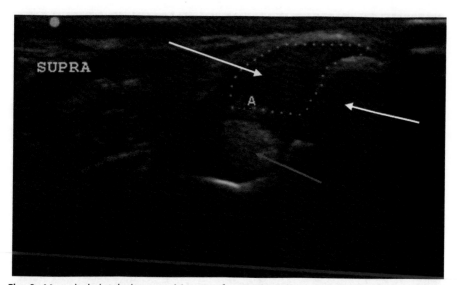

Fig. 9. Musculoskeletal ultrasound image of normal supraspinatus tendon (*yellow arrow*) and biceps tendon (*red arrow*). The white arrow is the greater tubercle of the humerus where the supraspinatus tendon inserts. (*Courtesy of* D. Canapp, DVM, Annapolis Junction, MD.)

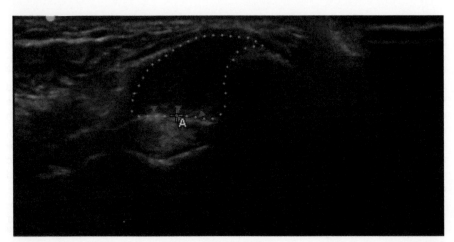

Fig. 10. Musculoskeletal ultrasound image of supraspinatus tendinopathy (*outlined by dots*). The enlarged supraspinatus is compressing the biceps (*arrowheads*) contributing to secondary tendinopathy. (*Courtesy of* D. Canapp, DVM, Annapolis Junction, MD.)

description reveals a normal trilaminar appearance on sagittal and transverse images and should not be mistaken as evidence of a tendinopathy.[39]

Management largely is conservative with exercise restriction, formal rehabilitation, and/or intralesional injections considered. Two studies reported ultrasound appearance and gait analysis improvement after ultrasound-guided injections of adipose-derived progenitor cells and platelet-rich plasma (PRP) or bone marrow aspirate

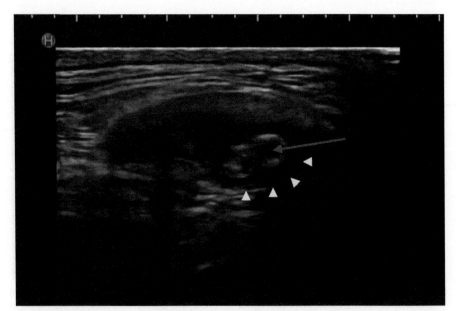

Fig. 11. Musculoskeletal ultrasound of calcified supraspinatus tendinopathy (*arrow*). An anechoic halo (*arrowheads*) surrounds the calcification.

concentrate and PRP.[40,41] Another study found subjective improvement with a single PRP injection in 10 dogs.[42] Additional success with extracorporeal shock wave therapy has been observed.[43] Surgical treatment is controversial, with varying success rates,[31,33,34] and consists of mineralization removal and/or tendon debulking to relieve pressure on the biceps.[26,33,34] Mineralization may recur but may not lead to clinical disease.[34]

INFRASPINATUS CONTRACTURE

The infraspinatus' main function is abduction and rotation of the humerus and to a lesser extent flexion and extension of the joint.[44] The infraspinatus traverses the shoulder laterally, acting as a dynamic stabilizer.[44] Infraspinatus contracture is an uncommon condition overall but is associated with active, medium to large breed dogs, specifically working, hunting, and sporting dogs.[8] Most are affected unilaterally; however, bilateral cases have been documented.[45–47] Although the etiology is unknown, based on histopathology and electromyography testing, it is thought to be a primary muscle disorder resulting from repetitive microtrauma during vigorous exercise rather than an acute trauma or neuropathy.[8,45,48]

History often reveals abrupt forelimb lameness, shoulder discomfort, and/or swelling of the infraspinatus musculature after strenuous activity.[49] Within 2 weeks to 6 weeks, the lameness and discomfort resolve. Fibrosis and contracture, however, result in a nonpainful, characteristic circumducted gait abnormality.[8,44,45,48–50] Range of motion often is limited in pronation and abduction. The affected limb is positioned with the elbow adducted and paw abducted (**Fig. 12**).

Diagnosis is made through history, gait evaluation, and examination. If there is uncertainty, imaging can be completed. Radiographs often are unremarkable; however, calcification may be present.[46,51] Musculoskeletal ultrasound is more useful, especially when additional supraspinatus pathology is suspected.[46,52] Although less common, supraspinatus contracture has been reported and is important to differentiate.[8,49]

Because most cases are found in the contracted phase, the treatment of choice is infraspinatus tenotomy.[8] Following transection, immediate tissue release with characteristic popping sound and full shoulder range of motion should be appreciated.[8] Tenotomy carries a good prognosis for return to full function, including sport and work.[49] Early rehabilitation postoperatively, however, is critical for successful outcome.[20,49]

MEDIAL SHOULDER SYNDROME

The MGL, LGL, and JC comprise the static stabilizers because they do not respond to changes in joint position. The dynamic stabilizers contract and relax in response to changes in joint position and are composed of the periarticular cuff muscles, as described previously.[1,5,7,53,54]

MSS is an important cause of canine forelimb lameness, occurring with much greater frequency than luxations.[5] MSS is defined by abnormal motion or translation of the humeral head within the glenoid fossa.[5,55] Pathology commonly occurs medially (80% of cases)[56]; however, lateral instability and multidirectional instability have been reported.[5,57–60] Pathology occurs when 1 or more stabilizer is affected, the MGL being most common (**Fig. 13**).[57,58] It is unknown, however, which stabilizers and what severity produce clinical signs.[61]

Although MSS is becoming recognized more commonly, diagnosis is difficult to obtain and often achieved through careful examination and diagnostic imaging. MSS occurs in middle-aged, medium to large breeds. Acute, traumatic events have

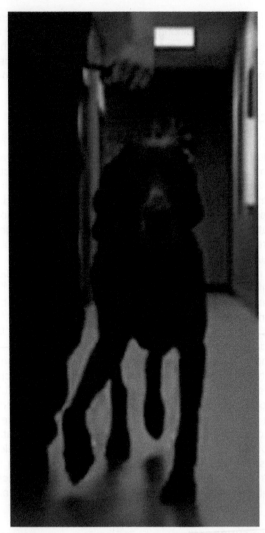

Fig. 12. Characteristic gait of an infraspinatus contracture patient. Note the external rotation of the humerus with elbow adduction and paw abduction during swing phase.

been documented but chronic overuse injuries are suspected of playing a larger role.[5,57,58,62] Chronic forelimb lameness, ranging from subtle and intermittent to severe and continuous (depending on the severity and structures affected), often is described.

Although nonspecific, muscle atrophy and/or pain on manipulation of the shoulder may be appreciated.[5] Various palpation techniques to confirm medial pathology have been postulated. The drawer test was described first; however, it can be technically challenging for unexperienced evaluators, and sedation is required.[5] Additionally, a hyperabduction test was described by Cook and colleagues.[57] This test technically is easier and a good alternative to the drawer test; however, interpretation should be made cautiously between breeds and individuals.

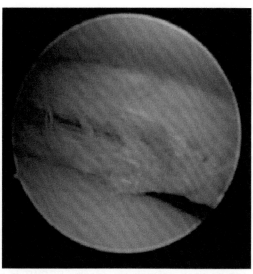

Fig. 13. Arthroscopic image of midbody MGL fraying. For reference, cranial is to the left.

Studies investigating the accuracy and repeatability of the hyperabduction test are conflicting.[7,57,59,62,63] Initially, dogs with medial shoulder pathology had higher abduction angles (>50°) compared with normal shoulder joints; however, arthroscopic shoulder evaluation was not used to define normal/abnormal.[57] Later studies showed similar results of larger abduction angle in affected dogs[57,62]; however, hyperabduction was observed with medial and lateral instability.[62] Additionally, sedation and muscle atrophy can affect measurements.[7] Divitt and colleagues[59] found that both techniques had minimal effects on arthroscopic medial compartment changes. Negative hyperabduction test, however, was 7 times more likely to occur in those without medial compartment changes. Given this, it can be concluded that it is relatively sensitive but lacks specificity.[59] An important aspect when performing the abduction test is the maintenance of shoulder extension. Because joint laxity increases with flexion, inability to maintain extension could elevate the angle falsely.[64] Comparison of contralateral limb angle may be helpful in unilateral disease.[57,63,64] A recent report noted the abduction test has poor interobserver variability, with increasing accuracy achieved by more experienced observers.[64]

Radiographs are performed to rule out boney abnormalities and assess degenerative joint disease (DJD), a majority showing no abnormalities. In the absence of OCD lesion, all shoulder joints with DJD should be investigated for MSS.[5,56] Stress radiography can be helpful; however, results may be similar to hyperabduction tests.[63] Although musculoskeletal ultrasound cannot identify direct pathology to the MGL, LGL, and subscapularis, it may be useful in investigating periarticular pathology.[21,57,62] In contrast, MRI can identify the MGL and subscapularis tendons; however, disease severity often is underestimated compared with arthroscopy.[21] Arthroscopy commonly is used because it allows direct visualization of the intraarticular components (see **Fig. 13**) and dynamic evaluation via probing and range of motion.[5]

MSS management is a topic of debate. To date, no literature supports superiority of surgery over conservative management. For those moderately to severely affected or with medial or multidirectional instability, however, surgery is recommended.[60,65]

Common techniques include open tendon transposition, open subscapularis imbrication, open or arthroscopic-assisted prosthetic repair, and radiofrequency-induced thermal capsulorrhaphy (RITC) (**Fig. 14**) or arthroscopic thermal capsulorrhaphy.[56,58,65–68]

Tendon transpositions were among the first described for medial stabilization and involve transposition of the biceps brachii tendon of origin or supraspinatus tendon (less common).[6,66,67] Their major drawback is the alteration of joint biomechanics leading to temporary or permanent functional gait abnormality and osteoarthritis.[6,66,67] For cases of intact tendons and mild laxity, subscapularis imbrication alone may be effective.[68] Alternatively, prosthetic repair techniques have shown promise in restoring a more biomechanically similar joint. One study described improved clinical results and minimal gait abnormalities in 9/10 dogs that underwent prosthetic MGL repair using bone tunnels, suture anchors, and monofilament suture.[69] Additionally, an arthroscopic assisted approach using a prosthetic ligament was described in 39 cases of varying severity.[70] Overall complication rate was 15% with no catastrophic complications and 77% return to normal function.[70]

Management of milder pathology largely is conservative with exercise restriction and formal rehabilitation. Some individuals utilize a hobbles vest to prevent shoulder abduction. Intra-articular biologics (platelet products) and extracorporal shock wave therapy (ECSWT) can be used adjunctively. Ideally, ECSWT is utilized initially and again 4 weeks to 6 weeks later.[71] The use and effectiveness of RITC are controversial and adopted from human medicine. With RITC, thermal energy is applied to lax ligaments and JC, causing collagen bundle shrinkage and tightening.[58,72] Although immediate tightening is observed, strict activity restriction and owner compliance are essential because these tissues lose their mechanical properties 2 weeks to 4 weeks after treatment.[58,72,73] Therefore, a non–weight-bearing sling (velpeau) or hobbles to prevent abduction is crucial. Afterward, a strengthening and conditioning program should be implemented to allow controlled stimulus while fibroblast infiltration and proliferation restore mechanical properties and improve muscle mass.[58,72] Subjectively, improved function is expected at 12 weeks to 16 weeks, with optimal improvement 5 months to 6 months following treatment. Initial reports showed 93% good and 79% excellent clinical improvement.[58] More recently, an 80% success rate was

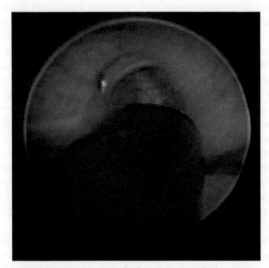

Fig. 14. Arthroscopic MGL RITC using a radiofrequency probe.

described but was not significantly better than nonsurgical management.[60] Contraindications for RITC include lateral, multidirectional, or bilateral instability, overt DJD, complete MGL tears, and neurologic dysfunction.[58] Although RITC has shown some success, based on the data, it cannot be considered superior to other surgical options. Therefore, RITC should be reserved for patients without overt instability that have failed conservative management whereas reconstruction is recommended if gross instability exists.[20]

SHOULDER LUXATION

Shoulder luxation is uncommon, can be congenital or traumatic, and may be acute or chronic in nature. A majority occur medially or laterally, with cranial and caudal luxation occurring with much less frequency. Congenital luxation typically occurs in toy and small breeds, whereas traumatic luxation is common in larger breed dogs.[8,66,74–76] A weight-bearing or non–weight-bearing lameness may be present, depending on the underlying cause, severity, and chronicity. With traumatic luxations, notable localized swelling, bruising, and discomfort may be present. With both, a palpable difference in the distance from the acromion to the greater tubercle may be noted. With medial luxation, the elbow tends to be flexed and adducted with the distal limb abducted and supinated. Lateral luxation shows a similar appearance; however, the distal limb is adducted.[8] Diagnosis is obtained using orthogonal radiographs and help rule out concurrent fractures.

Traumatic Luxation

Although traumatic luxation often occurs medially, large breeds also develop lateral luxation.[66] Prompt diagnosis, reduction, and stabilization are key to a successful outcome regardless of whether conservative management (manual reduction and coaptation) or surgical intervention is pursued. In the acute phase, luxations are relatively easy to manually reduce under general anesthesia, but residual instability may be present due to damage of the supporting structures.[66] Following reduction, coaptation is warranted for continued stabilization wherein a velpo sling is indicated for medial luxation whereas a spica splint is applied for lateral luxations.[76] Following at least 2 weeks of coaptation, continued activity restriction and rehabilitation is indicated for an additional 2 weeks to 6 weeks.[8,20] Those relatively stable after reduction tend to have successful outcomes. Surgery is indicated with unsuccessful manual reduction, failed closed reduction, gross instability after closed reduction, and/or chronic luxation.[8,66,75]

Surgical stabilization typically involves reconstruction or augmentation of the JC and glenohumeral ligamants.[66] Current described techniques include medial or lateral biceps brachii tendon transposition for medial, lateral, and cranial luxations; supraspinatus tendon transposition for medial luxation; and suture augmentation techniques.[66,67,70,76–80] Suture augmentation is preferred because tendon transpositions have a higher tendency of temporary or permanent joint incongruence and subsequent DJD.[6,66,67] With concurrent (peri)articular fractures, surgery also must include fracture reduction and rigid fixation.[81] In a single canine with severe shoulder instability and contralateral elbow luxation, ligament reconstruction and temporary transarticular bridging locking plate was successful.[82] Additionally, augmented repair with a woven poly-L-lactide device has shown experimental promise.[83] Transarticular pinning and lateral capsular reefing are historical techniques and no longer recommended.[66] Salvage procedures include excisional arthroplasty (glenoid and humeral head resection resulting in pseudojoint) and arthrodesis. These procedures may be indicated with excessive DJD, failed previous stabilization attempts, chronic luxations, and/or when adequate stabilization cannot be accomplished.[8,66,67,76,84]

Full functional recovery is achievable, with those addressed in the acute phase (with conservative management or surgery) generally carrying a good prognosis.[76] Conversely, those undergoing excisional arthroplasty or arthrodesis experience a functional gait abnormality and decreased range of motion.[8,66,75,84]

Congenital Luxation

Congenital luxation occurs in toy and small breeds between 3 months and 10 months of age[66,85] and typically is unilateral; however, bilateral cases are documented. Although much less common, some luxations occur in adults with minor trauma. Luxation almost always is medial.[66,85] Closed reduction often is not successful given the inherent glenoid and/or humeral head abnormalities. Therefore, surgical stabilization with the previously described techniques often are warranted. Additionally, affected animals should undergo sterilization because it may be heritable.[66]

SUMMARY

Shoulder pathologies are a common cause of canine forelimb lameness. Obtaining early and exact diagnosis is critical. Due to the shoulder's complex anatomy and biomechanics, orthopedic and neurologic examination, radiographs, advanced imaging (musculoskeletal ultrasound, CT, and MRI), and/or arthroscopy often are used. In the immature dog, OC/OCD is considered a top differential for forelimb lameness with shoulder discomfort. In the mature dog, diagnostics are used to differentiate biceps and/or supraspinatus tendinopathy and MSS. For mild cases, conservative management with exercise restriction and guided rehabilitation plan[20] should be implemented. Intra-articular and ultrasound-guided injections are considered for mild, nonresponsive cases. Surgery is reserved for moderate to severe or refractory cases. Prompt luxation reduction is key to a successful outcome. Prognosis is good for conservatively managed, acute, traumatic luxation with mild disruption and prompt reduction. Surgery is indicated, however, for severe disruption and chronic or congenital luxation.

CLINICS CARE POINTS

- In young, large to giant breed dogs with shoulder discomfort, a high clinical suspicion for shoulder OC/OCD should exist.
- During biceps stretch test, biceps tendinopathy elicits discomfort and moderate tension whereas biceps tears have a loss of end-feel.
- Biceps and/or supraspinatus tendon mineralization should be interpreted with caution because it does not always correlate with an active problem.
- Infraspinatus contracture elicits characteristic circumducting gait and examination abnormalities (elbow adduction, paw abduction, limited shoulder abduction, and pronation).
- During hyperabduction test, maintaining shoulder extension and comparing contralateral angles increase accuracy.
- Prompt luxation reduction and stabilization are crucial for a successful outcome.

DISCLOSURE

The authors certify that they have no affiliations with or involvement in any organization or entity with any financial interest or nonfinancial interest in the subject matter or materials discussed in this article.

REFERENCES

1. Evans HE. Arthrology. In: Miller's anatomy of the dog. 3rd edition. Philadelphia: Saunders Company; 1993. p. 233–6.
2. Rochat MC. Ch 50: The Shoulder. In: Johnston SA, Tobia KM, editors. Veterinary surgery: small animal. 2nd edition. St Louis (MO): Elsevier Health Sciences; 2017. p. 800–20.
3. Sager M, Herten M, Dreiner L, et al. Histological variations of the glenoid labrum in dogs. Anat Histol Embryol 2013;42(6):438–47.
4. Schwarz T, Johnson VS, Voute L, et al. Bone scintigraphy in the investigation of occult lameness in the dog. J Small Anim Pract 2004;45(5):232–7.
5. Bardet JF. Diagnosis of shoulder instability in dogs and cats: a retrospective study. J Am Anim Hosp Assoc 1998;34(1):42–54.
6. Vasseur PB, Moore D, Brown SA. Stability of the canine shoulder joint: an in vitro analysis. Am J Vet Res 1982;43(2):352–5.
7. Gray MJ, Lambrechts NE, Maritz NG, et al. A biomechanical investigation of the static stabilizers of the glenohumeral joint in the dog. Vet Comp Orthop Traumatol 2005;18(02):55–61.
8. Piermattei D, Flo G, DeCamp C. The shoulder joint. In: Handbook of small animal orthopedics and fracture repair. 4th edition. St Louis (MO): Saunders/Elsevier; 1998. p. 264–96.
9. Johnston SA. Osteochondritis dissecans of the humeral head. Vet Clin Small Anim Pract 1998;28(1):33–49.
10. Berzon JL. Osteochondritis dissecans in the dog: diagnosis and therapy. J Am Vet Med Assoc 1979;175(8):796–9.
11. Biezynski J, Skrzypczak P, Piatek A, et al. Assessments of treatment of Osteochondrosis dissecans (OCD) of shoulder joint in dogs-the result of two years of experience. Pol J Vet Sci 2012;15(2):285–90.
12. Peterson CJ. Osteochondritis dissecans of the humeral head of a cat. N Z Vet J 1984;32(7):115–6.
13. Xia Y, Moody JB, Alhadlaq H, et al. Characteristics of topographical heterogeneity of articular cartilage over the joint surface of a humeral head. Osteoarthritis Cartilage 2002;10(5):370–80.
14. Olivieri M, Ciliberto E, Hulse DA, et al. Arthroscopic treatment of osteochondritis dissecans of the shoulder in 126 dogs. Vet Comp Orthop Traumatol 2007;20(01): 65–91.
15. Kippenes H, Johnston G. Diagnostic imaging of osteochondrosis. Vet Clin Small Anim Pract 1998;28(1):137–60.
16. Wall CR, Cook CR, Cook JL. Diagnostic sensitivity of radiography, ultrasonography, and magnetic resonance imaging for detecting shoulder osteochondrosis/osteochondritis dissecans in dogs. Vet Radiol Ultrasound 2015;56(1):3–11.
17. Vandevelde B, Van Ryssen B, Saunders JH, et al. Comparison of the ultrasonographic appearance of osteochondrosis lesions in the canine shoulder with radiography, arthrography, and arthroscopy. Vet Radiol Ultrasound 2006;47(2): 174–84.
18. Fitzpatrick N, Van Terheijden C, Yeadon R, et al. Osteochondral autograft transfer for treatment of osteochondritis dissecans of the caudocentral humeral head in dogs. Vet Surg 2010;39(8):925–35.
19. Egan P, Murphy S, Jovanovik J, et al. Treatment of osteochondrosis dissecans of the canine stifle using synthetic osteochondral resurfacing. Vet Comp Orthop Traumatol 2018;31(02):144–52.

20. Marcellin-Little DJ, Levine D, Canapp SO Jr. The canine shoulder: selected disorders and their management with physical therapy. Clin Tech Small Anim Pract 2007;22(4):171–82.
21. Murphy SE, Ballegeer EA, Forrest LJ, et al. Magnetic resonance imaging findings in dogs with confirmed shoulder pathology. Vet Surg 2008;37(7):631–8.
22. Bardet JF. Lesions of the biceps tendon diagnosis and classification. Vet Comp Orthop Traumatol 1999;12(04):188–95.
23. Stobie D, Wallace L, Lipowitz A, et al. Chronic bicipital tenosynovitis in dogs: 29 cases (1985-1992). J Am Vet Med Assoc 1995;207(2):201–7.
24. Lincoln J, Potter K. Tenosynovitis of the biceps branchii tendon in dogs. J Am Anim Hosp Assoc 1984;20(3):382–5.
25. Gilley RS, Wallace LJ, Hayden DW. Clinical and pathologic analyses of bicipital tenosynovitis in dogs. Am J Vet Res 2002;63(3):402–7.
26. Muir P, Johnson KA. Supraspinatus and biceps brachii tendinopathy in dogs. J Small Anim Pract 1994;35(5):239–43.
27. Bruce WJ, Burbidge HM, Bray JP, et al. Bicipital tendinitis and tenosynovitis in the dog: a study of 15 cases. N Z Vet J 2000;48(2):44–52.
28. Ibrahim V, Groah S, Libin A, et al. Use of platelet rich plasma for the treatment of bicipital tendinopathy in spinal cord injury: a pilot study. Top Spinal Cord Inj Rehabil 2012;18(1):77–8.
29. Barker SL, Bell SN, Connell D, et al. Ultrasound-guided platelet-rich plasma injection for distal biceps tendinopathy. Shoulder Elbow 2015;7(2):110–4.
30. Kujat R. The microangiographic pattern of the rotator cuff of the dog. Arch Orthop Trauma Surg 1990;109(2):68–71.
31. Flo GL, Middleton D. Mineralization of the supraspinatus tendon in dogs. J Am Vet Med Assoc 1990;197(1):95–7.
32. Mistieri ML, Wigger A, Canola JC, et al. Ultrasonographic evaluation of canine supraspinatus calcifying tendinosis. J Am Anim Hosp Assoc 2012;48(6):405–10.
33. Pilar Lafuente M, Fransson BA, Lincoln JD, et al. Surgical treatment of mineralized and nonmineralized supraspinatus tendinopathy in twenty-four dogs. Vet Surg 2009;38(3):380–7.
34. Laitinen OM, Flo GL. Mineralization of the supraspinatus tendon in dogs: a long-term follow-up. J Am Anim Hosp Assoc 2000;36(3):262–7.
35. Muir P, Johnson KA, Cooley AJ, et al. Force-plate analysis of gait before and after surgical excision of calcified lesions of the supraspinatus tendon in two dogs. Vet Rec 1996;139(6):137–9.
36. Canapp SO, Canapp DA, Carr BJ, et al. Supraspinatus tendinopathy in 327 dogs: a retrospective study. Vet Evid 2016;1(3).
37. Kriegleder H. Mineralization of the supraspinatus tendon: clinical observations in seven dogs. Vet Comp Orthop Traumatol 1995;8(02):91–7.
38. Muir P, Goldsmid SE, Rothwell TL, et al. Calcifying tendinopathy of the biceps brachii in a dog. J Am Vet Med Assoc 1992;201(11):1747–9.
39. Pownder SL, Caserto BG, Hayashi K, et al. Magnetic resonance imaging and histologic features of the supraspinatus tendon in nonlame dogs. Am J Vet Res 2018;79(8):836–44.
40. Canapp SO Jr, Canapp DA, Ibrahim V, et al. The use of adipose-derived progenitor cells and platelet-rich plasma combination for the treatment of supraspinatus tendinopathy in 55 dogs: a retrospective study. Front Vet Sci 2016;3:61.
41. McDougall RA, Canapp SO, Canapp DA. Ultrasonographic Findings in 41 Dogs Treated with Bone Marrow aspirate concentrate and Platelet-rich Plasma for a supraspinatus Tendinopathy: a retrospective study. Front Vet Sci 2018;5:98.

42. Ho LK, Baltzer WI, Nemanic S, et al. Single ultrasound-guided platelet-rich plasma injection for treatment of supraspinatus tendinopathy in dogs. Can Vet J 2015;56(8):845.

43. Danova NA, Muir P. Extracorporeal shock wave therapy for supraspinatus calcifying tendinopathy in two dogs. Vet Rec 2003;152:208–9.

44. Carberry CA, Gilmore DR. Infraspinatus muscle contracture associated with trauma in a dog. J Am Vet Med Assoc 1986;188(5):533–4.

45. Pettit GD, Chatburn CC, Hegreberg GA, et al. Studies on the pathophysiology of infraspinatus muscle contracture in the dog. Vet Surg 1978;7(1):8–11.

46. Franch J, Bertran J, Remolins G, et al. Simultaneous bilateral contracture of the infraspinatus muscle. Vet Comp Orthop Traumatol 2009;22(03):249–52.

47. Bennett D, Campbell JR. Unusual soft tissue orthopaedic problems in the dog. J Small Anim Pract 1979;20(1):27–39.

48. Devor M, Sørby R. Fibrotic contracture of the canine infraspinatus muscle. Vet Comp Orthop Traumatol 2006;19(02):117–21.

49. Bennett RA. Contracture of the Infraspinatus Muscle in Dogs – A Review of 12 Cases. J Am Anim Hosp Assoc 1986;22(4):481–7.

50. Dillon EA, Anderson LJ, Jones BR. Infraspinatus muscle contracture in a working dog. N Z Vet J 1989;37(1):32–4.

51. McKee WM, Macias C, May C, et al. Ossification of the infraspinatus tendon-bursa in 13 dogs. Vet Rec 2007;161(25):846–52.

52. Orellana-James NG, Ginja MM, Regueiro M, et al. Sub-acute and chronic MRI findings in bilateral canine fibrotic contracture of the infraspinatus muscle. J Small Anim Pract 2013;54(8):428–31.

53. Karduna AR, Williams GR, Iannotti JP, et al. Kinematics of the glenohumeral joint: influences of muscle forces, ligamentous constraints, and articular geometry. J Orthop Res 1996;14(6):986–93.

54. Talcott KW, Vasseur PB. Luxation of the scapulohumeral joint. In: Slatter DH, editor. Textbook of small animal surgery. 3rd edition. Philadelphia: W.B. Saunders; 2003. p. 1897–904.

55. Sidaway BK, McLaughlin RM, Elder SH, et al. Role of the tendons of the biceps brachii and infraspinatus muscles and the medial glenohumeral ligament in the maintenance of passive shoulder joint stability in dogs. Am J Vet Res 2004;65(9):1216–22.

56. Bardet JF. Shoulder diseases in dogs. Vet Med 2002;97(12):909–18.

57. Cook JL, Renfro DC, Tomlinson JL, et al. Measurement of angles of abduction for diagnosis of shoulder instability in dogs using goniometry and digital image analysis. Vet Surg 2005;34(5):463–8.

58. Cook JL, Tomlinson JL, Fox DB, et al. Treatment of dogs diagnosed with medial shoulder instability using radiofrequency-induced thermal capsulorrhaphy. Vet Surg 2005;34(5):469–75.

59. Devitt CM, Neely MR, Vanvechten BJ. Relationship of physical examination test of shoulder instability to arthroscopic findings in dogs. Vet Surg 2007;36(7):661–8.

60. Franklin SP, Devitt CM, Ogawa J, et al. Outcomes associated with treatments for medial, lateral, and multidirectional shoulder instability in dogs. Vet Surg 2013;42(4):361–4.

61. Fujita Y, Yamaguchi S, Agnello KA, et al. Effects of transection of the cranial arm of the medial glenohumeral ligament on shoulder stability in adult Beagles. Vet Comp Orthop Traumatol 2013;26(02):94–9.

62. Cogar SM, Cook CR, Curry SL, et al. Prospective evaluation of techniques for differentiating shoulder pathology as a source of forelimb lameness in medium and large breed dogs. Vet Surg 2008;37(2):132–41.

63. Livet V, Harel M, Taroni M, et al. Stress radiography for the diagnosis of medial glenohumeral ligament rupture in canine shoulders. Vet Comp Orthop Traumatol 2019;32(06):433–9.

64. Jones SC, Howard J, Bertran J, et al. Measurement of shoulder abduction angles in dogs: an ex vivo study of accuracy and repeatability. Vet Comp Orthop Traumatol 2019;32(06):427–32.

65. Pucheu B, Duhautois B. Surgical treatment of shoulder instability. Vet Comp Orthop Traumatol 2008;21(04):368–74.

66. Bone DL. Chronic luxations. Vet Clin North Am Small Anim Pract 1987;17(4): 923–42.

67. Craig E, Hohn RB, Anderson WD. Surgical stabilization of traumatic medial shoulder dislocation [dogs]. J Am Anim Hosp Assoc 1980;16(1):93–102.

68. Pettitt RA, Clements DN, Guilliard MJ. Stabilisation of medial shoulder instability by imbrication of the subscapularis muscle tendon of insertion. J Small Anim Pract 2007;48(11):626–31.

69. Fitch RB, Breshears L, Staatz A, et al. Clinical evaluation of prosthetic medial glenohumeral ligament repair in the dog (ten cases). Vet Comp Orthop Traumatol 2001;14(04):222–8.

70. O'Donnell EM, Canapp SO Jr, Cook JL, et al. Treatment of medial shoulder joint instability in dogs by extracapsular stabilization with a prosthetic ligament: 39 cases (2008–2013). J Am Vet Med Assoc 2017;251(9):1042–52.

71. Durant A, Millis D. Applications of extracorporeal shockwave in small animal rehabilitation. In: Canine rehabilitation and physical therapy. Philadelphia: WB Saunders; 2014. p. 381–92.

72. Hayashi K, Markel MD. Thermal capsulorrhaphy treatment of shoulder instability: basic science. Clin Orthop Relat Res 2001;390:59–72.

73. O'neill T, Innes JF. Treatment of shoulder instability caused by medial glenohumeral ligament rupture with thermal capsulorrhaphy. J Small Anim Pract 2004; 45(10):521–4.

74. Hohn RB, Rosen H, Bohning JR, et al. Surgical stabilization of recurrent shoulder luxation. Vet Clin North Am 1971;1(3):537–48.

75. McKee M, Macias C. Orthopaedic conditions of the shoulder in the dog. In Pract 2004;26(3):118–29.

76. Puglisi TA. Canine humeral joint instability -Part I. Comp Contin Educ Pract Vet 1986;8:593–601.

77. DeAngelis M, Schwartz A. Surgical correction of cranial dislocation of the scapulohumeral joint in a dog. J Am Vet Med Assoc 1970;156(4):435.

78. Leighton RL, Kagan KG. Surgical repair of lateral shoulder luxation. Mod Vet Pract 1976;57(9):702.

79. Leighton RL, Kagan KG. Repair of medial shoulder luxation in dogs. Mod Vet Pract 1976;57(8):604.

80. Wolff EF. Transposition of the biceps brachii tendon to repair luxation of the canine shoulder joint (review of a procedure). Vet Med Small Anim Clin 1974; 69(1):51.

81. Huck JL, Bergh MS. Traumatic craniolateral shoulder luxation and fracture of the lesser tubercle of the humerus in a dog. Vet Comp Orthop Traumatol 2011;24(06): 474–7.

82. Post C, Guerrero T, Voss K, et al. Temporary transarticular stabilization with a locking plate for medial shoulder luxation in a dog. Vet Comp Orthop Traumatol 2008;21(02):166–70.
83. Derwin KA, Codsi MJ, Milks RA, et al. Rotator cuff repair augmentation in a canine model with use of a woven poly-L-lactide device. J Bone Joint Surg Am Vol 2009; 91(5):1159.
84. Montasell X, Dupuis J, Huneault L, et al. Short-and Long-term outcomes after shoulder excision arthroplasty in 7 small breed dogs. Can Vet J 2018;59(3):277.
85. Vaughan LC, Jones DG. Congenital dislocation of the shoulder joint in the dog. J Small Anim Pract 1969;10(1):1–3.

Common Neoplastic Diseases Affecting the Forelimb

Janis Lapsley, DVM, Laura E. Selmic, MPH, ACVS, DACVS-SA, DECVS*

KEYWORDS

- Canine • Feline • Cats • Dogs • Tumor • Neoplasia • Extremity

KEY POINTS

- When neoplasia affects the forelimb, companion animals may present with lameness, new occurrence of swelling, or a mass.
- Fine needle aspiration or a biopsy of masses to obtain a diagnosis before treatment is critical for neoplasia affecting extremities.
- The planning of surgical treatment of limb tumors is essential to maximize the chance of complete excision.

INTRODUCTION

Lameness, new occurrence of a swelling, or a mass are the most common reasons for presentation in companion animals when neoplasia affects the limbs. Although neoplasia may not be the first differential diagnosis that comes to mind when evaluating animals presenting for an evaluation for lameness, it is important to consider neoplasia as a differential diagnosis when working through the patient assessment, orthopedic examination, and investigation. A rapid and accurate diagnosis of the etiology of lameness, swelling, or mass can help to decrease patient suffering and allow treatment options to be presented at an earlier stage of the disease, allowing for increased treatment options and/or an improved prognosis.

PATIENT ASSESSMENT

Patient signalment may help to identify disease susceptibilities, because some breeds commonly present for specific neoplastic conditions of the limbs (**Table 1**). Most malignancies affect middle-aged to older dogs, but younger animals may still be affected. Osteosarcoma has been reported in dogs as young as 6 months old.[1]

Department of Veterinary Clinical Sciences, College of Veterinary Medicine, The Ohio State University, 601 Vernon L Tharp Street, Columbus, OH 43210, USA
* Corresponding author. Surgical Oncology.
E-mail address: Selmic.1@osu.edu

Vet Clin Small Anim 51 (2021) 343–356
https://doi.org/10.1016/j.cvsm.2020.11.004
vetsmall.theclinics.com
0195-5616/21/© 2020 Elsevier Inc. All rights reserved.

Table 1
Breeds commonly presented for specific neoplastic processes affecting the limbs

Tissue	Tumor Types	Overrepresented Breeds
Skin and subcutaneous	Mast cell tumor[1,2]	Boxer Labrador retriever Golden retriever Bulldog Boston terrier Fox terrier Weimaraner Cocker spaniel Rhodesian ridgeback Dachshund American cattle dog
Digit	Malignant melanoma[3,4] Squamous cell carcinoma[4,5]	Scottish terrier Rottweiler Dachshund Flat coat retriever Standard poodle Black Labrador Giant schnauzer Gordon setter Rottweiler
Joint/periarticular	Periarticular histiocytic sarcoma[6]	Bernese mountain dog Flat coat retriever Rottweiler
Bone	Osteosarcoma[7–11]	Saint Bernard Great Dane Irish Setter Doberman Pinscher Rottweiler German Shepherd Golden Retriever

The patient history can help to ascertain the natural history of the lameness, swelling, or mass and may give clues for a neoplastic cause. Often, lameness owing to neoplastic causes may have an insidious onset and be persistent or progressively worsening. Lameness may show limited or a lack of improvement to analgesics. There may be a severe deterioration associated with a pathologic fracture if the bone is weakened by neoplasia.

When evaluating patients for the assessment of a new swelling or mass, it is essential to characterize what structure the mass may be arising from (ie, dermis, subcutis, muscle, joint, or bone). A body map helps to document the location and measurements of masses and allows comparison with earlier physical examination findings. With older dogs, it is not uncommon to see multiple masses present. Dogs with mast cell tumors (MCT), thyroid carcinoma, or malignant melanoma were more commonly found to have concurrent malignancies.[12] An orthopedic examination may identify bone or joint swelling or pain on deep bone palpation that may not be evident with a more general physical examination. These findings are important for recommendations regarding diagnostics.

DIAGNOSTIC APPROACH
Assessing the Local Lesion

For a mass arising in soft tissues, fine needle aspiration (FNA) is crucial to obtain a diagnosis before surgical removal to plan surgical margins accurately. The limb is an area where complete surgical resection at the first surgery is desired because there is minimal additional tissue for further surgeries in the event of residual microscopic disease or local tumor recurrence. An incisional biopsy may be needed if cytology is nondiagnostic or additional information regarding the grade or histopathologic diagnosis may change treatment. The location of the biopsy should be immediately overlying the mass, because the biopsy tract will need to be able to be removed or treated later owing to contamination.

For a soft tissue mass involving the digit, a bony swelling, or swelling or mass close to or around a joint, orthogonal radiographs of the area will assess for underlying bone proliferation or lysis. If bone lysis is present in cases with digital masses, this entity may help with the presumptive diagnosis of digital neoplasia, because bone lysis is more likely to be caused by malignancies.[13] An FNA can be a helpful diagnostic tool for assessing digital and bony lesions. When adequately cellular, an FNA can help to rule out other differential diagnoses like osteomyelitis and may yield a definitive diagnosis. Other diagnostics such as urine fungal antigen tests are indicated in dogs in endemic fungal areas or with a travel history to these areas to rule out fungal disease. If cytology is nondiagnostic, then a bone biopsy or incisional biopsy may be required.

Assessing the Extent of Regional or Distant Metastasis

Further assessment for any regional or distant spread should be performed for most malignancies before proceeding with treatment, because the extent of the tumor spread may change treatment options and decisions. Often assessments of lymphatic spread are restricted to lymph nodes that are easily palpable to perform FNA. There are significant limitations of this approach; the locoregional lymph node predicted by anatomic proximity to the tumor may differ from the primary draining node for the tumor lymphatic basin, and FNA has been shown to only be sensitive for the detection of nodal metastasis in 68% to 75% of cases depending on the tumor type.[14,15]

Sentinel lymph nodes (SLNs) are defined as the first lymph nodes that receive direct lymphatic drainage from a tumor. The SLN concept is based on the existence of an orderly and predictable pattern of lymphatic drainage and metastasis to a specific lymph node in a regional lymphatic basin before drainage into other regional nodes.[16] SLN mapping techniques to guide SLN biopsy are an important consideration in patient workup because the SLN status may help to predict patient outcomes and guide therapy recommendations. SLN mapping is rapidly becoming incorporated into veterinary medicine, and multiple techniques exist for mapping.[16] The standard of care in humans involves a peritumoral injection of radioactive markers followed by scintigraphy and the intraoperative use of gamma cameras combined with vital dye for direct visualization of lymphatic pathways.[16,17] More readily accessible techniques using computed tomography (CT) lymphography, radiographic studies, and peritumoral vital dyes have recently been well-described in veterinary patients for multiple tumor types.

Evaluation of the thoracic cavity for the presence of metastatic disease or other abnormalities can be performed using 3-view thoracic radiographs or CT scans. A CT scan is more sensitive for detecting metastatic pulmonary lesions, especially when lesions are less than 7 mm.[18] The accurate diagnosis of a pulmonary metastasis is critical for appropriate patient staging and may dramatically influence prognosis and treatment recommendations for some patients. Abdominal imaging is generally performed using ultrasound examination or a CT scan; visceral organ changes on a CT scan and ultrasound examination may be subtle or nonspecific. Even if normal on imaging, routine FNA of these organs is warranted in diseases where visceral metastasis is associated with a shorter survival and a poorer prognosis. The reported sensitivity of ultrasound examination in detecting mast cell infiltration of the spleen and liver was 43% and 0%, respectively, compared with FNA cytology in one study of high-grade MCT.[19]

SPECIFIC TUMORS

In this section, we discuss the biologic behavior of malignant tumor types that can affect the limbs and explain the staging tests as well as the treatment options.

Digital Tumors

Most dogs and cats with digit tumors present owing to a digital mass with or without lameness. The disease tends to occur in older dogs (median age, 10 years).[13] There are several differential diagnoses for digital masses that should be considered (**Table 2**). The most common tumor seen in dogs is squamous cell carcinoma (SCC), which can occur concurrently in multiple digits in some dogs.[4,13] A malignant melanoma arising from the subungual tissues or the haired skin is the second most common tumor.[4,13] In cats, the most common tumors are carcinomas (SCC or adenocarcinoma), but sarcomas (fibrosarcoma, osteosarcoma, and hemangiosarcoma [HSA]) have also been reported.[5] The involvement of multiple digits has been documented in cats with adenocarcinoma.[5,20] In 64 cats with digital carcinomas, 87.5% of lesions represented metastasis from primary lung tumors, which is referred to as feline lung–digit syndrome.[20] Malignant melanoma has also been reported in 5 cats.[21]

The most common digital tumors in companion animals can metastasize; a minimum database of regional lymph node FNA (axillary and superficial cervical) and thoracic radiographs are recommended. The diagnosis or suspicion of some malignancies may necessitate a complete assessment, including abdominal ultrasound examination and other diagnostic tests. In a study in dogs with digital SCC, metastases were detected at diagnosis in 8.8% to 13.0% of dogs and subsequently in 17.0% to

Table 2	
Differential diagnoses to consider for patients presenting with a digital mass	
Benign or Non-neoplastic	**Malignant Neoplastic**
Previous trauma	SCC
Osteomyelitis	Malignant melanoma
Pyogranulomatous inflammation	STS
Epidermal inclusion cyst	MCT
Benign adnexal tumors	Osteosarcoma
Histiocytomas	Adenocarcinoma
Hemangiomas	Malignant adnexal tumors
Basal cell tumors	Round cell tumor (plasmacytoma, lymphoma)
Infiltrating lipomas	HSA
Fibromas	
Papillomas	
Cysts	

26.1% of dogs after surgery.[4,13] In dogs with malignant melanoma, 28% to 32% had a metastasis at presentation with a further 17% developing metastasis subsequently.[13] In cats, the metastatic potential of primary digital malignancies is not well-known. Of 8 cats with primary SCC of the digit in one study, only 1 had a metastasis to the draining lymph node at the time of amputation, and none of the 3 cats that had thoracic radiographs had metastases suspected on follow-up.[20] For feline digital melanoma cases, only the rate of subsequent metastasis is known; 3 of the 5 cases developed metastases to a lymph node, lung, and bone.[21]

Surgery has been the predominant treatment evaluated for digital tumors. Digital amputation at the metacarpophalangeal joint may constitute a wide excision for small tumors, but partial foot amputation or limb amputation may need to be considered for larger tumors. The prognosis reported with surgery for dogs with SCC of the digit is 1- and 2-year survival rates of 50% to 83% and 18% to 62%, respectively.[4,13,22] Dogs with SCC arising from the subungual epithelium may have a better prognosis than SCC arising from other digital structures (1- and 2-year survival rates of 95% and 74%, respectively).[13] Cats have been reported to have shorter survival with digital SCC, ranging from 73 days to 2 years, with a median survival of 12.5 weeks.[5,20] Dogs with digital malignant melanoma have had reported 1- and 2-year survival rates of 42% to 57% and 13% to 36%, respectively, reflecting the tumor's high metastatic rate.[3,4,13,22,23] In a recent study evaluating the outcome in dogs with haired skin melanoma, 16 cases were overlying digits and had an overall survival time of 1363 days, which was not statistically different from other sites.[24] The role of adjuvant therapies, including radiation therapy and chemotherapy, has not been established. Given the highly metastatic nature of this digital melanoma, adjuvant therapies are commonly offered in clinical practice, including nonsteroidal anti-inflammatory drugs, carboplatin chemotherapy, and melanoma vaccine. In a recent study evaluating the effect of carboplatin after surgery in dogs with melanoma, the median overall survival time for all dogs with digital melanoma was 1350 days. There was no difference in survival between dogs receiving carboplatin after surgery and those that did not.[25] Another recent study reported the response in dogs that received a xenogeneic tyrosinase vaccine for the treatment of melanoma.[26] Fifty-eight dogs with digital melanoma were included in this study with 57 receiving surgical excision, 3 dogs receiving adjuvant chemotherapy, and 2 dogs receiving radiation therapy. Sixteen of the dogs (27%) had metastases at diagnosis. Treatment results yielded 1- and 2-year survival rates of 63% and 32%, respectively. In this study, metastases at diagnosis were associated with a worse outcome.[26] Little is known about the prognostic factors for digital tumors given that these entities are uncommon, and few studies have assessed treatment outcome.

Skin and Subcutaneous Tumors

Mast cell tumors

MCTs are the most common cutaneous neoplasm in dogs representing up to 21% of all canine skin tumors.[27–29] There is currently no reported age or gender predisposition.[2] An increased incidence is recognized in several breeds (see **Table 1**), of these breeds, dogs of bulldog ancestry generally have low-grade tumors whereas the Shar Pei breed generally has more biologically aggressive MCTs.[28]

MCTs typically arise in the dermis or subcutaneous tissues and are generally solitary lesions ranging in appearance from raised, hairless, erythematous masses to diffuse nodular swellings or rashes with 25% to 40% occurring on the limbs.[1,28,30] Multiple lesions are noted in 11% to 14% of dogs.[31] Well-differentiated tumors are often slow-growing, small, solitary lesions present for several months. In contrast, undifferentiated MCT often grow or change in size quickly, are ulcerated, and can cause significant inflammation and edema of the surrounding tissues. Subcutaneous MCTs are soft and fleshy, with indistinct borders, and are commonly misdiagnosed as lipomas.

The diagnosis is typically straightforward with cytology. Previous reports have identified several major prognostic factors, including tumor grade, mitotic index, regional lymph node metastasis, tumor diameter greater than 3 cm, body site location of tumor, and metastasis to more than 2 sites.[32] Although cytology is useful for diagnosing MCTs and a new cytologic grading system has been proposed,[33] a histopathologic analysis is required for tumor grading. The histologic grade is considered the most reliable prognostic factor and is based on cellular differentiation and the mitotic index. The original Patnaik grading system was found to have considerable disagreement between pathologists and failed to identify a subset of well-differentiated or intermediately differentiated tumors that would behave aggressively.[1] The Kiupel grading system was developed to differentiate tumors as low grade or high grade based on the mitotic index, presence of multinucleated cells, bizarre nuclei, and karyomegaly in an attempt to increase intraobserver agreement and better predict tumor behavior.[34] The Patnaik and Kiupel systems are commonly reported together, although multiple studies have demonstrated the superiority of the Kiupel system with regard to predicting MCT associated mortality and metastasis.[30]

Preoperative or postoperative staging is performed on a patient-dependent basis and can include regional lymph node aspiration, abdominal ultrasound examination, and liver and splenic FNA. For dogs of breeds predisposed to low-grade tumors with a low metastatic rate, full staging is rarely necessary. A multilevel staging system has been proposed to help address the needs of different subsets of MCT populations.[35]

The current treatment standards for MCT include surgical excision with wide, proportional, or metric 2cm margins with locoregional lymph node aspirate or biopsy.[1] Long-term survival after complete excision of well-differentiated and intermediate-grade tumors is expected in 80% to 90% and 75% of dogs, respectively.[31,36] The reported 1-year survival rate for poorly differentiated tumors is low. For poorly differentiated or incompletely excised MCTs, additional therapy such as adjuvant radiation therapy and chemotherapy should be considered.

Soft Tissue Sarcomas

Soft tissue sarcomas (STS) are a group of mesenchymal tumors that account for approximately 15% of skin tumors in dogs.[37] These tumors are mostly solitary, found in in middle-aged or older animals, and have been associated with radiation, trauma, foreign bodies, orthopedic implants, and *Spirocerca lupi*.[37] These tumors represent a heterogenous group originating from mesenchymal tissues such as the muscular, adipose, neurovascular, fascial, and fibrous tissues. These tumors generally behave in a locally expansile invasive manner, but have a low to moderate metastatic rate after surgical excision. Some tumors are excluded from this group owing to individual biologic behavior or histologic appearance. These tumors include histiocytic sarcoma, synovial cell sarcoma (SCS), HSA, lymphangiosarcoma, rhabdomyosarcoma, oral fibrosarcoma, gastrointestinal stromal tumors, and some peripheral nerve sheath tumors.

The diagnosis of STS can be challenging with FNA, with a reported cytologic accuracy of between 63% to 97% with fewer false-negative results when the cytology was evaluated by a boarded clinical pathologist.[37] A nondiagnostic cytology can still be valuable because it assists in excluding other readily exfoliating tumors (eg, round cell tumors) and can support a suspected STS diagnosis. Biopsy of these tumors can be warranted to obtain a diagnosis and help to determine an appropriate treatment plan. The biopsy-reported grade is not always reliable; in one study, an incorrect histologic grade was found in 41% of cases when the biopsy was compared with definitive surgical samples (29% underestimating grade, 12% overestimating grade).[38] This error likely occurs owing to the heterogeneity of the tumor and the grade being based on differentiation, mitosis, and necrosis. Additional preoperative staging should include thoracic and abdominal imaging, evaluation of the regional lymph node, and sometimes regional imaging of the STS. Because the lungs are the most common site of metastasis,[37] 3-view thoracic radiographs or a CT scan should be performed before definitive treatment.

Excisional biopsy or unplanned incomplete resection of these tumors commonly occurs in practice but is not recommended. STS is generally a surgical disease with wide excision (3-cm lateral and 1 fascial plan deep margins) recommended. Wide excision can be challenging for distal limb STS because there is an overall lack of skin for tension-free closure and a defined deep fascial plane in these areas. Marginal excision of suspected low-grade tumors of the distal limbs may be acceptable because these tumors have been shown to have low recurrence (10.8%) and metastatic (0%) rates, with a median disease-free interval of 697.8 days and a median survival of 703.5 days.[39] Higher grade tumors in these areas can be treated with wide excision followed by reconstruction with tissue flaps or grafts or allowed to heal by secondary intention or radical resection via limb amputation.

Postoperative therapy is recommended for incompletely excised or recurrent tumors, which can include additional surgery, radiation therapy, chemotherapy, or electrochemotherapy. Optimal radiation plans have not been defined for STS in dogs, but a greater cumulative dose seems to provide better local tumor control.[37] The reported median time to local recurrence with radiation therapy after incomplete tumor resection is between 412 and 789 days, with overall median survival time of 2270 days.[37] The use of chemotherapy in patients with STS remains controversial because no significant survival benefit has been reliably shown. Metronomic (low-dose continuous) chemotherapy may have some benefit in preventing tumor recurrence via inhibiting tumor growth by antiangiogenic and immunomodulatory effects.[40] Electrochemotherapy has recently become of interest for the treatment of STS in dogs. This therapy uses electrical stimulation of the tissues after local administration of chemotherapeutic agents, which causes an increased uptake of the agent through cell membranes allowing for the delivery of higher local doses of chemotherapy. Multiple studies have shown promising results with median disease-free intervals of 243 to 857 days when electrochemotherapy was used postoperatively in incompletely excised tumors.[41,42] The overall prognosis for extremity STS is generally good, especially if complete excision is performed.

Joint and Periarticular Tumors

Common periarticular tumors are histiocytic sarcoma (PAHS), SCS, synovial myxoma/myxosarcoma, and malignant fibrous histiocytoma (previously called undifferentiated pleomorphic sarcoma). Patients are typically middle-aged large breed dogs that present with lameness associated with a periarticular soft tissue mass. Radiographically, a soft tissue mass is apparent with bony proliferative or destructive changes seen spanning the affected joint. The involvement of more than 1 bone surrounding an affected joint helps to differentiate these lesions from a primary bone tumor. These tumors can be difficult to differentiate from one another, often requiring the use of immunohistochemical staining, including CD18, vimentin, and cytokeratin.[43]

Histiocytic sarcoma arises from dendritic antigen-presenting cells and can occur in many locations, including the lung, liver, spleen, stomach, pancreas, skin, skeletal muscle, central nervous system, and bone.[6] PAHS is the most commonly reported periarticular tumor in dogs[43] and has been reported to occur around large appendicular joints, such as the stifle, elbow, and shoulder.[44] PAHS has been reported to occur with an increased frequency at sites of prior joint disease.[45] Before definitive surgery, a biopsy may be helpful for definitive classification of the tumor type and owner decision making. PAHS is typically vimentin positive, CD18 positive, and cytokeratin negative. Owing to the proximity of the tumor to articular and neurovascular structures, preservation of the limb is generally impossible, and surgical excision via limb amputation is recommended. For dogs where limb amputation is not feasible, radiation therapy should be considered. A recent review evaluated survival outcomes in dogs treated with surgery or radiation therapy in combination with adjuvant systemic chemotherapy.[44] The overall median time to progression was 336 days for operated dogs and 217 days for irradiated dogs, with a median overall survival of 398 days for operated dogs and 240 days for irradiated dogs. Of irradiated dogs, 91.2% experienced a clinical improvement in their lameness during treatment. In this study, regional lymph node metastasis was found via cytology in 71.4% of cases with a distant metastasis present in 24.5%. Regional lymph node and distant metastases were associated with an increased risk of overall disease progression. The median survival time with limb amputation alone is reported at 161 days, with an increased median survival of up to 568 days reported with multimodal therapy.[6]

SCS presents similarly to PAHS. SCS is differentiated via immunohistochemical staining with these tumors being vimentin positive, cytokeratin positive, and CD18 negative. Two histologic forms exist (monophasic or biphasic) based on the presence or absence of an epithelioid component with the monophasic form being most common.[46] The median survival time for SCS after amputation depends on the tumor grade and is reported to be between 455 and 976 days with a metastatic rate of 8% to 32%.[47]

Synovial myxomas are similar to SCS and PAHS in appearance and presentation, with the major difference being their histologic appearance. Histologically, they contain multiple myxoid islands with widely spaced stellate cells. Grossly, they are gelatinous, producing a viscous fluid when incised. They stain positive for vimentin, variably positive for CD18, and negative for cytokeratin. These tumors generally occur in the stifle or digits and are treated with amputation or local resection via synovectomy. Survival times of more than 2 years have been reported, even with incomplete resection.[48]

Bone Tumors

Most dogs with bone tumors present owing to lameness. Any large or giant breed dog with metaphyseal swelling should raise concern for the possibility of primary bone tumor, especially in middle-aged to older dogs.[7,11] After localization of lameness and lesion, orthogonal radiographs help to assess for an underlying bone lesion. The radiographic appearance of bone tumors can be variable, from bone lysis to bone proliferation or osteoblastic activity to a mix of these. None of the findings are specific for primary bone tumors, so differential diagnoses for these aggressive bone lesions should be considered (**Table 3**).

Other diagnostics such as bone FNA and bone biopsy may be performed to differentiate between these diagnoses. Bone cytology has been shown to have high accuracy (83%) compared with bone biopsy and histopathology (82%) and can be performed blind or with ultrasound guidance.[49,50]

Table 3
Differential diagnoses for aggressive bone lesions

Benign or Non-neoplastic	Malignant Neoplastic
Previous trauma/fracture	Primary bone tumors Osteosarcoma Chondrosarcoma Fibrosarcoma HSA
Bacterial or fungal osteomyelitis	Secondary bone tumors Multiple myeloma Lymphoma Urogenital carcinoma
Bone cyst	

Osteosarcoma is the most common primary bone tumor in the dog (≤85% of all bone malignancies).[8–10] Osteosarcoma predominantly occurs in the metaphyses of long bones and is a highly metastatic tumor, with fewer than 10% of dogs presenting with pulmonary metastases but more than 90% of dogs having microscopic metastasis. Staging is indicated to assess for advanced disease. Lymph node metastasis is rare (4.4%), but lymph node FNA can be performed to check for spread.[51] Thoracic imaging is indicated to assess for pulmonary metastasis. CT scanning has been shown to have an increased sensitivity to detect pulmonary metastasis in canine patients with osteosarcoma in several studies.[52–54] Bone metastasis may be assessed with bone radiographs or whole body CT scans, although these modalities are thought to be less sensitive than bone scintigraphy. The prevalence of concurrent bone metastasis at diagnosis is variable (1.4%–28% dogs).[55–57] An abdominal ultrasound examination can be performed for screening for visceral metastases, but these entities are rare (0%–2.5% dogs at diagnosis).[58,59]

The treatment options for primary bone tumors are commonly presented as palliative intent (which provide symptomatic relief) or definitive or curative intent (which aim to kill or remove the primary lesion and treat microscopic metastasis).[47] Palliative-intent options include analgesics, bisphosphonates, coarse fractionated radiation therapy, and amputation. Definitive-intent options include local tumor therapies of amputation or stereotactic radiation therapy or limb-sparing surgery combined with cytotoxic chemotherapy. Multiple chemotherapeutic agents and combinations have been used, including single-agent carboplatin or cisplatin, single-agent doxorubicin, and doxorubicin and carboplatin or cisplatin combined or alternating. There have been recent clinical trials evaluating new therapeutic approaches, including immunotherapy.[60] The outcome is variable and depends on the treatment approach used, as well as the tumor histopathology. Amputation alone for appendicular osteosarcoma results in a shorter survival time than amputation with cytotoxic chemotherapy.[61,62] Additionally, a recent meta-analysis showed that the serum alkaline phosphatase and proximal humeral osteosarcoma were negative prognostic indicators in canine appendicular osteosarcoma.[62]

Other Tumors

Subcutaneous and intramuscular hemangiosarcoma
HSA is a tumor of vascular origin; subcutaneous and intramuscular primary HSA are uncommonly reported in the veterinary literature. A retrospective study, including 71 dogs with intramuscular or subcutaneous HAS, found an overall survival time of

172 days.[63] The presence of lameness, anemia, evidence of metastatic disease at presentation, larger tumors, and incomplete resections were associated with shorter survival times in this population. For dogs with subcutaneous or intramuscular tumors without evidence of metastasis at initial staging where adequate local tumor control was achieved and who received adjuvant doxorubicin, the overall survival time is reported to be between 246 and 1189 days.[63,64] Shorter median survival times of 272.5 days have been reported for intramuscular versus subcutaneous HSA[64]; however, the patient population was small. Subcutaneous and intramuscular HSA seem to carry a similarly poor prognosis; the visceral form has a reported 1-year survival rate of 24%.[63] Although considered rare, HSA can also occur as metastatic lesions, and thus a full evaluation of any patient with a muscular lesion is important. A recent study retrospectively evaluated dogs with primary HSA who had undergone a full-body CT scan during staging.[65] This study found the presence of skeletal muscle metastasis in 15 of 61 dogs (24.6%) evaluated, with 75.4% of dogs also having metastatic lesions to other sites. The most common clinical sign noted in dogs with muscular metastasis of HSA was lameness. HSA also occurs in the dermis, typically on the ventrum of light-colored thin-haired dogs with solar exposure and has a markedly better prognosis.

SUMMARY

Multiple neoplasms are reported to affect the limbs of dogs and cats. A full diagnostic workup, including a cytologic or histologic diagnosis of the primary mass, evaluation of regional lymph nodes, local tumor imaging, and thoracic and abdominal imaging, is typically recommended before surgical intervention. The stage and grade of disease are often prognostic for patient outcome and are specific to each neoplastic disease.

CLINIC CARE POINTS

- Obtaining a diagnosis before treatment is critical for neoplasia affecting the extremities.
- Fine needle aspiration is often a good starting point to rule out non-neoplastic processes and definitively diagnose some tumors.
- Incisional biopsy may be helpful if cytology is nondiagnostic before treatment. This will give information about tumor type to help guide owners toward definitive treatment and advise on the prognosis.
- If a malignant neoplasm of the extremity is diagnosed, staging tests are indicated to screen for more advanced disease before treatment.

DISCLOSURE

The authors have no conflicts of interest or funding to disclose.

REFERENCES

1. London CA, Thamm DH. Mast cell tumors. In: Vail DM, Thamm DH, Liptak JM, editors. Withrow & MacEwen's small animal clinical oncology. 6th edition. St Louis: Elsevier; 2020. p. 382–93.
2. Kiupel M. Mast cell tumors. In: Meuten DJ, editor. Tumors in domestic animals. Ames (IA): 2017. p. 176–93.

3. Schultheiss PC. Histologic features and clinical outcomes of melanomas of lip, haired skin, and nail bed locations of dogs. J Vet Diagn Invest 2006;18:422–5.

4. Wobeser BK, Kidney BA, Powers BE, et al. Diagnoses and clinical outcomes associated with surgically amputated canine digits submitted to multiple veterinary diagnostic laboratories. Vet Pathol 2007;44:355–61.

5. Wobeser BK, Kidney BA, Powers BE, et al. Diagnoses and clinical outcomes associated with surgically amputated feline digits submitted to multiple veterinary diagnostic laboratories. Vet Pathol 2007;44:362–5.

6. Clifford C, Graig A, Skorupski KA, et al. Miscellaneous tumors. In: Vail DM, Thamm DH, Liptak JM, editors. Withrow & MacEwen's small animal clinical oncology. St Louis: Elsevier; 2020. p. 794–7.

7. Misdorp W, Hart AA. Some prognostic and epidemiologic factors in canine osteosarcoma. J Natl Cancer Inst 1979;62:537–45.

8. Brodey R, Riser W. Canine osteosarcoma. A clinicopathologic study of 194 cases. Clin Orthop Relat Res 1969;62:54–64.

9. Brodey RS, McGrath JT, Reynolds H. A clinical and radiological study of canine bone neoplasms. I. J Am Vet Med Assoc 1959;134:53–71.

10. Dorfman SK, Hurvitz AI, Patnaik AK. Primary and secondary bone tumours in the dog. J Small Anim Pract 1977;18:313–26.

11. Brodey RS, Abt DA. Results of surgical treatment in 65 dogs with osteosarcoma. J Am Vet Med Assoc 1976;168:1032–5.

12. Rebhun RB, Thamm DH. Multiple distinct malignancies in dogs: 53 cases. J Am Anim Hosp Assoc 2010;46:20–30.

13. Marino DJ, Matthiesen DT, Stefanacci JD, et al. Evaluation of dogs with digit masses: 117 cases (1981-1991). J Am Vet Med Assoc 1995;207:726–8.

14. Fournier Q, Cazzini P, Bavcar S, et al. Investigation of the utility of lymph node fine-needle aspiration cytology for the staging of malignant solid tumors in dogs. Vet Clin Pathol 2018;47:489–500.

15. Ku CK, Kass PH, Christopher MM. Cytologic-histologic concordance in the diagnosis of neoplasia in canine and feline lymph nodes: a retrospective study of 367 cases. Vet Comp Oncol 2017;15:1206–17.

16. Beer P, Pozzi A, Rohrer Bley C, et al. The role of sentinel lymph node mapping in small animal veterinary medicine: a comparison with current approaches in human medicine. Vet Comp Oncol 2018;16:178–87.

17. Tuohy JL, Milgram J, Worley DR, et al. A review of sentinel lymph node evaluation and the need for its incorporation into veterinary oncology. Vet Comp Oncol 2009; 7:81–91.

18. Nemanic S, London CA, Wisner ER. Comparison of thoracic radiographs and single breath-hold helical CT for detection of pulmonary nodules in dogs with metastatic neoplasia. J Vet Intern Med 2006;20:508–15.

19. Book AP, Fidel J, Wills T, et al. Correlation of ultrasound findings, liver and spleen cytology, and prognosis in the clinical staging of high metastatic risk canine mast cell tumors. Vet Radiol Ultrasound 2011;52:548–54.

20. van der Linde-Sipman JS, van den Ingh TS. Primary and metastatic carcinomas in the digits of cats. Vet Q 2000;22:141–5.

21. Luna LD, Higginbotham ML, Henry CJ, et al. Feline non-ocular melanoma: a retrospective study of 23 cases (1991-1999). J Feline Med Surg 2000;2:173–81.

22. Henry CJ, Brewer WG, Whitley EM, et al. Canine digital tumors: a veterinary cooperative oncology group retrospective study of 64 dogs. J Vet Intern Med 2005;19: 720–4.

23. Aronsohn MG, Carpenter JL. Distal extremity melanocytic nevi and malignant melanoma in dogs. J Am Anim Hosp Assoc 1990;26:605–12.

24. Laver T, Feldhaeusser BR, Robat CS, et al. Post-surgical outcome and prognostic factors in canine malignant melanomas of the haired skin: 87 cases (2003-2015). Can Vet J 2018;59:981–7.

25. Brockley LK, Cooper MA, Bennett PF. Malignant melanoma in 63 dogs (2001-2011): the effect of carboplatin chemotherapy on survival. N Z Vet J 2013;61:25–31.

26. Manley CA, Leibman NF, Wolchok JD, et al. Xenogeneic murine tyrosinase DNA vaccine for malignant melanoma of the digit of dogs. J Vet Intern Med 2011;25:94–9.

27. Sledge DG, Webster J, Kiupel M. Canine cutaneous mast cell tumors: a combined clinical and pathologic approach to diagnosis, prognosis, and treatment selection. Vet J 2016;215:43–54.

28. Govier SM. Principles of treatment for mast cell tumors. Clin Tech Small Anim Pract 2003;18:103–6.

29. Shoop SJ, Marlow S, Church DB, et al. Prevalence and risk factors for mast cell tumours in dogs in England. Canine Genet Epidemiol 2015;2:1.

30. Kiupel M, Camus M. Diagnosis and prognosis of canine cutaneous mast cell tumors. Vet Clin North Am Small Anim Pract 2019;49:819–36.

31. Mullins MN, Dernell WS, Withrow SJ, et al. Evaluation of prognostic factors associated with outcome in dogs with multiple cutaneous mast cell tumors treated with surgery with and without adjuvant treatment: 54 cases (1998-2004). J Am Vet Med Assoc 2006;228:91–5.

32. Ferrari R, Marconato L, Buracco P, et al. The impact of extirpation of non-palpable/normal-sized regional lymph nodes on staging of canine cutaneous mast cell tumours: a multicentric retrospective study. Vet Comp Oncol 2018;16:505–10.

33. Camus MS, Priest HL, Koehler JW, et al. Cytologic criteria for mast cell tumor grading in dogs with evaluation of clinical outcome. Vet Pathol 2016;53:1117–23.

34. Kiupel M, Webster JD, Bailey KL, et al. Proposal of a 2-tier histologic grading system for canine cutaneous mast cell tumors to more accurately predict biological behavior. Vet Pathol 2011;48:147–55.

35. Horta RS, Lavalle GE, Monteiro LN, et al. Assessment of canine mast cell tumor mortality risk based on clinical, histologic, immunohistochemical, and molecular features. Vet Pathol 2018;55:212–23.

36. Murphy S, Sparkes AH, Smith KC, et al. Relationships between the histological grade of cutaneous mast cell tumours in dogs, their survival and the efficacy of surgical resection. Vet Rec 2004;154:743–6.

37. Liptak JM, Christensen NI. Soft tissue sarcomas. In: Vail DM, Thamm DH, Liptak JM, editors. Withrow & MacEwen's small animal clinical oncology. 6th edition. St Louis: Elsevier; 2020.

38. Perry JA, Culp WT, Dailey DD, et al. Diagnostic accuracy of pre-treatment biopsy for grading soft tissue sarcomas in dogs. Vet Comp Oncol 2014;12:106–13.

39. Stefanello D, Morello E, Roccabianca P, et al. Marginal excision of low-grade spindle cell sarcoma of canine extremities: 35 dogs (1996-2006). Vet Surg 2008;37:461–5.

40. Bray JP. Soft tissue sarcoma in the dog - part 1: a current review. J Small Anim Pract 2016;57:510–9.

41. Spugnini EP, Vincenzi B, Amadio B, et al. Adjuvant electrochemotherapy with bleomycin and cisplatin combination for canine soft tissue sarcomas: a study of 30 cases. Open Vet J 2019;9:88–93.

42. Torrigiani F, Pierini A, Lowe R, et al. Soft tissue sarcoma in dogs: a treatment review and a novel approach using electrochemotherapy in a case series. Vet Comp Oncol 2019;17:234–41.

43. Craig LE, Julian ME, Ferracone JD. The diagnosis and prognosis of synovial tumors in dogs: 35 cases. Vet Pathol 2002;39:66–73.

44. Marconato L, Sabattini S, Buchholz J, et al. Outcome comparison between radiation therapy and surgery as primary treatment for dogs with periarticular histiocytic sarcoma: an Italian society of veterinary oncology study. Vet Comp Oncol 2020;18(4):778–86.

45. Manor EK, Craig LE, Sun X, et al. Prior joint disease is associated with increased risk of periarticular histiocytic sarcoma in dogs. Vet Comp Oncol 2018;16:E83–8.

46. Monti P, Barnes D, Adrian AM, et al. Synovial cell sarcoma in a dog: a misnomer-cytologic and histologic findings and review of the literature. Vet Clin Pathol 2018; 47:181–5.

47. Ehrhart NP, Christensen NI, Fan T. Tumors of the skeletal system. In: Vail DM, Thamm DH, Liptak JM, editors. Withrow & MacEwen's small animal clinical oncology. St Louis: Elsevier; 2020. p. 553.

48. Craig LE, Krimer PM, Cooley AJ. Canine synovial myxoma: 39 cases. Vet Pathol 2010;47:931–6.

49. Samii VF, Nyland TG, Werner LL, et al. Ultrasound-guided fine-needle aspiration biopsy of bone lesions: a preliminary report. Vet Radiol Ultrasound 1999;40:82–6.

50. Sabattini S, Renzi A, Buracco P, et al. Comparative assessment of the accuracy of cytological and histologic biopsies in the diagnosis of canine bone lesions. J Vet Intern Med 2017;31:864–71.

51. Hillers KR, Dernell WS, Lafferty MH, et al. Incidence and prognostic importance of lymph node metastases in dogs with appendicular osteosarcoma: 228 cases (1986-2003). J Am Vet Med Assoc 2005;226:1364–7.

52. Talbott JL, Boston SE, Milner RJ, et al. Retrospective evaluation of whole body computed tomography for tumor staging in dogs with primary appendicular osteosarcoma. Vet Surg 2017;46:75–80.

53. Oblak ML, Boston SE, Woods JP, et al. Comparison of concurrent imaging modalities for staging of dogs with appendicular primary bone tumours. Vet Comp Oncol 2013;13(1):28–39.

54. Oblak ML, Boston SE, Higginson G, et al. The impact of pamidronate and chemotherapy on survival times in dogs with appendicular primary bone tumors treated with palliative radiation therapy. Vet Surg 2012;41:430–5.

55. Berg J, Lamb CR, O'Callaghan MW. Bone scintigraphy in the initial evaluation of dogs with primary bone tumors. J Am Vet Med Assoc 1990;196:917–20.

56. Hahn KA, Hurd C, Cantwell HD. Single-phase methylene diphosphate bone scintigraphy in the diagnostic evaluation of dogs with osteosarcoma. J Am Vet Med Assoc 1990;196:1483–6.

57. Parchman MB, Flanders JA, Erb HN, et al. Nuclear medical bone imaging and targeted radiography for evaluation of skeletal neoplasms in 23 dogs. Vet Surg 1989;18:454–8.

58. Sacornrattana O, Dervisis NG, McNiel EA. Abdominal ultrasonographic findings at diagnosis of osteosarcoma in dogs and association with treatment outcome. Vet Comp Oncol 2013;11:199–207.

59. Wallace M, Selmic L, Withrow SJ. Diagnostic utility of abdominal ultrasonography for routine staging at diagnosis of skeletal OSA in dogs. J Am Anim Hosp Assoc 2013;49:243–5.
60. Poon AC, Matsuyama A, Mutsaers AJ. Recent and current clinical trials in canine appendicular osteosarcoma. Can Vet J 2020;61:301–8.
61. Spodnick GJ, Berg J, Rand WM, et al. Prognosis for dogs with appendicular osteosarcoma treated by amputation alone: 162 cases (1978-1988). J Am Vet Med Assoc 1992;200:995–9.
62. Schmidt AF, Groenwold RH, Amsellem P, et al. Which dogs with appendicular osteosarcoma benefit most from chemotherapy after surgery? Results from an individual patient data meta-analysis. Prev Vet Med 2016;125:116–25.
63. Shiu KB, Flory AB, Anderson CL, et al. Predictors of outcome in dogs with subcutaneous or intramuscular hemangiosarcoma. J Am Vet Med Assoc 2011;238:472–9.
64. Bulakowski EJ, Philibert JC, Siegel S, et al. Evaluation of outcome associated with subcutaneous and intramuscular hemangiosarcoma treated with adjuvant doxorubicin in dogs: 21 cases (2001-2006). J Am Vet Med Assoc 2008;233:122–8.
65. Carloni A, Terragni R, Morselli-Labate AM, et al. Prevalence, distribution, and clinical characteristics of hemangiosarcoma-associated skeletal muscle metastases in 61 dogs: a whole body computed tomographic study. J Vet Intern Med 2019;33:812–9.

Neurologic Causes of Thoracic Limb Lameness

Sharon C. Kerwin, DVM, MS[a], Amanda R. Taylor, DVM[b,c],*

KEYWORDS

- Lameness • Thoracic limb • Intervertebral disc disease
- Cervical spondylomyelopathy • Brachial plexus • Root signature
- Nerve sheath tumor

KEY POINTS

- Intervertebral disc extrusion to one side (lateralized) and nerve sheath tumors are the neurologic causes of thoracic limb lameness that are seen most commonly.
- Dogs with neurologic causes of lameness often have detectable abnormalities on neurologic examination.
- Advanced imaging is necessary to determine the underlying cause of neurologic thoracic limb lameness.

INTRODUCTION

Thoracic limb lameness can be a challenging clinical sign to investigate. Although orthopedic disease is by far the most common reason for lameness, there are important neurologic diseases to consider and rule out when an orthopedic cause is not identified. Not uncommonly, a patient may have both orthopedic and neurologic disease.

Common neurologic diseases that cause thoracic limb lameness include those that affect the spinal cord, nerve roots, nerves, and muscles. If an orthopedic examination does not identify an area of concern, neurologic examination should be performed. Diseases that can cause lameness include cervical intervertebral disc extrusion, diseases of the brachial plexus (avulsion, neoplasia, and neuritis), cervical spondylomyelopathy (CSM), and myopathies (polymyositis). When the nerve roots are diseased due to compression or destruction, resulting lameness is called a root signature.

[a] Department of Small Animal Clinical Sciences, College of Veterinary Medicine & Biomedical Sciences, Texas A&M University, TAMU 4474, College Station, TX 77843-4474, USA; [b] MedVet Dayton, 2714 Springboro West, Moraine, OH 45439, USA; [c] BluePearl North Hills, PA, USA
* Corresponding author. MedVet Dayton, 2714 Springboro West, Moraine, OH 45439.
E-mail addresses: amanda.taylordvm@medvet.com; amanda.taylor@bluepearlvet.com

Vet Clin Small Anim 51 (2021) 357–364
https://doi.org/10.1016/j.cvsm.2020.12.003
0195-5616/21/© 2020 Elsevier Inc. All rights reserved.

CERVICAL INTERVERTEBRAL DISC DISEASE

Cervical intervertebral disc extrusion that is lateralized, or herniated to one side, resulting in disc material lodged within the intervertebral foramen or compressing nerve roots as they arise from the spinal cord, can cause thoracic limb lameness. Clinical suspicion of this disease should be raised in consideration of multiple factors, including the history, signalment, and neurologic examination. The history often is an acute onset of lameness and the client also may report the dog crying out with exertion or sudden movement. Low head carriage and reluctance to lift the head or turn the neck also may be described by the client. Signalment is an important consideration, because a disc extrusion is more likely in chondrodystrophic breeds and young to middle-aged dogs. For example, a 3-year-old dachshund (miniature or standard) with an acute onset of lameness in the thoracic limb should have this differential high on the list because this breed does not have a high prevalence of orthopedic disease of the elbow. In contrast, a 3-year-old Labrador retriever with thoracic limb lameness likely has orthopedic disease of the elbow, such as elbow dysplasia with secondary osteoarthritis.

Neurologic examination can include multiple abnormalities that are identified with cervical intervertebral disc disease but may be normal in many cases of foraminal disc extrusion.[1] Gait evaluation may identify scuffing of the involved thoracic limb and associated proprioceptive ataxia of the pelvic limbs or all limbs. Head carriage may be neutral or low/angled toward the ground. When standing, the affected thoracic limb may be knuckled over so that the dorsal aspect of the foot rests on the ground, or the limb may be held abducted or flexed with reluctance to bear weight. The postural reactions, or proprioceptive positioning, should be delayed in the affected thoracic limb (including knuckling and hopping tests) and also may be delayed in other limbs, depending on the degree of associated spinal cord injury. Reflexes often are affected, with a decrease in the degree of strength displayed in the withdrawal reflex and incomplete flexion of the shoulder, elbow, or carpal joints. Lateralized disc extrusions typically do not affect the cutaneous trunci or cause Horner syndrome, an important differentiation from other diseases reviewed. Dogs often display cervical hyperesthesia, or pain and vocalization, on palpation of the affected area as well as resistance to range of motion of the cervical spine.

Once clinical suspicion for a lateralized extrusion is raised, advanced diagnostics are necessary to confirm a diagnosis. The imaging modality of choice is magnetic resonance imaging (MRI). Abnormalities identified on MRI include an extradural compression of the nerve root and possibly spinal cord with intervertebral disc material overlying the affected intervertebral disc space (Fig. 1). Mineralized, degenerative intervertebral disc material also can be identified on computed tomography (CT); however, this imaging modality is considered a good diagnostic test only when MRI is not available. A myelogram is not recommended because lateralized material in a foramen may not alter the column of contrast material in the cervical spinal canal. The comparison of MRI to CT and myelography for suspect disc herniation recently has been reviewed in the literature; MRI is the most accurate modality for determining disc herniation site and side.[2]

Treatment is directed toward relieving the compression directly with surgery; traditional medical management to include rest, analgesics, and anti-inflammatory medications; or perineural steroid injection combined with rest for foraminal extrusions.[3] If the disc extrusion is accessible via ventral slot, in the authors' experience, surgical decompression may provide faster and more durable relief than medical management if the patient is a surgical candidate. Cervical hemilaminectomy has been successful in

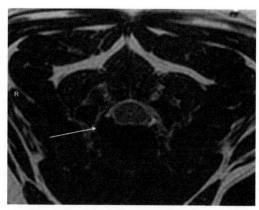

Fig. 1. Transverse T2-weighted MRI of the cervical spinal cord at the level of an interverte-bral disc space. The arrow identifies hypointense extruded intervertebral disc material within the intravertebral foramen compressing the nerve root.

cases of lateralized herniation as well, although this approach can be more challenging.[4]

DISEASES OF THE BRACHIAL PLEXUS

An intricate network of nerves provides innervation to the thoracic limb. These nerves reside in a group called the brachial plexus, which encompasses the spinal nerves from C6 through T2.[5] Nerves of the brachial plexus are susceptible to injury in trauma where the thoracic limb is caught and pulled, known as brachial plexus avulsion. Neoplasia also can develop within the myelin covering the nerve, which is called a nerve sheath tumor. Inflammation of the nerves secondary to infection or autoimmune disease results in neuritis. Although there are other miscellaneous conditions that could affect the nerves, this article focuses on the 3 differentials, discussed previously, because they are encountered most frequently.

Brachial plexus avulsion encompasses degrees of injury depending on the trauma endured. Clinical history includes obvious trauma, such as being hit by a car, being kicked by a horse, human abuse, or falling from a height. Patients with traumatic injury can be of any signalment. Evaluation for concurrent injuries, such as pneumothorax, fractures of the limbs or vertebral column, and others, should be considered. On exam-ination, the dog or cat is unable to extend the carpal and, in some cases, elbow joints to bear weight. The limb may be carried by holding the elbow flexed or may be advanced by flexing the elbow and flipping the paw forward with motion. Postural reactions are decreased to absent in the affected limb, whereas the other limbs are normal. Reflexes in the affected limb are decreased to absent, depending on the degree of injury.

There are 2 possible concurrent abnormalities that are an indication that the brachial plexus has been severely affected. The first is the absence of movement of the cuta-neous trunci on the side ipsilateral to the injured limb when the cutaneous trunci reflex is tested. Cutaneous trunci muscles receive motor innervation from the lateral thoracic nerve, which arises from the eighth cervical and first thoracic nerve roots.[5] Sensation is not affected by this injury; therefore, a pinch of the skin a few centimeters lateral to the dorsal midline at the level of the caudal lumbar vertebral column still results in an ascending signal that causes the cutaneous trunci reflex to be positive on the side opposite the injury.

Sympathetic innervation of the pupil, which is responsible for dilation, has a complex pathway that travels from the hypothalamus, through the brainstem, into the cervical spinal cord, and then out the intervertebral foramen between the first and fourth thoracic vertebrae in the ramus communicans.[6] At this level, the innervation is susceptible to injury concurrent with brachial plexus injury. Injury to the sympathetic innervation results in some or all signs seen with Horner syndrome in the eye ipsilateral to the injured limb including miosis, elevation of the third eyelid, ptosis, and enophthalmos.

Severity of injury can range from neuropraxia, where the nerve is mildly injured but remains intact; to axonotmesis, where the nerve fibers are severed or torn to varying degrees but the myelin sheath around the nerve remains intact; or to neurotmesis, where the axons and the myelin sheath are torn or transected. The first 2° of injury are recoverable, but it is important to keep in mind that should axons have to regrow, they do so at a rate of 1 mm per day, so in an animal with a limb that is a length of 12 in length, recovery could take 8 months.

Regarding diagnostics for this type of injury, cervical vertebral column radiographs are recommended to rule out a fracture. MRI can document the severity of the injury in some cases; however, most cases are not worked up to this degree because the findings are unlikely to change recommendations and outcome. Treatment is directed toward physical rehabilitation to strengthen the limb and encourage nerve signaling. In cases where the injury is severe and permanent loss of function occurs, it may be necessary to amputate the limb.

Peripheral Nerve Sheath Tumor

Peripheral nerve sheath tumors are neoplasms of the Schwann cells or other perineural supporting tissues around peripheral nerves, primarily in dogs. Although they do occur in cats, they tend to affect the distal limb (digits and carpus) and can cause lameness as they expand in the soft tissues.[7] They often affect the brachial plexus and typically cause a vague, progressive forelimb lameness, often of months' duration, that mimics orthopedic disease, but radiographic imaging of the limb is unrewarding. Careful palpation of the axillary region may reveal a palpable mass in up to 30% of cases, often with notable pain on manipulation of the mass in approximately half of the cases, with palpable masses or pain on manipulation of the cervical spine.[8] Many of these cases tend to present late in their course and once the neoplasm has invaded the cervical vertebral canal. Ipsilateral pelvic limb deficits may be noted on neurologic examination, in addition to muscle atrophy, decreased withdrawal, and sometimes decreased proprioception in the affected forelimb. As seen with a brachial plexus injury, there may be concurrent Horner syndrome and loss of the cutaneous trunci reflex on the same side as the nerve sheath tumor. A definitive diagnosis cannot be made (apart from surgical exploration of the affected brachial plexus with biopsy) without advanced imaging, preferably with MRI (**Fig. 2**).[9] Prognosis is guarded to grave depending on whether or not the neoplasia has progressed into the canal. Treatment consists of excision of the tumor, which can be as extensive as amputation of the affected limb and nerves in combination with a cervical hemilaminectomy and radiation therapy.

Neuritis

Although peripheral nerve sheath tumors are the most common cause of spinal nerve enlargement in dogs, non-neoplastic neuritis also should be considered. Hypertrophic ganglioneuritis has been reported in dogs[10,11] and cats.[12,13] Idiopathic bilateral C2 hypertrophic ganglioneuritis, diagnosed using MRI, has been reported in a case series of 12 dogs, including 9 Staffordshire bull terriers.[11] Eight of these dogs also had clinical

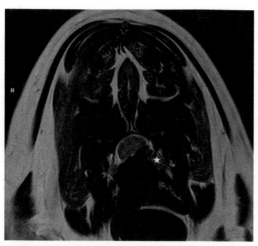

Fig. 2. Transverse T2-weighted MRI of the cervical spinal cord at the level of the C6-7 intervertebral foramen. There is a large mass associated with the left C7 nerve root, identified with a star, consistent with a nerve sheath tumor. The mass is causing compression of the spinal cord, shifting the cord dorsolaterally.

signs consistent with a C1-C5 neurolocalization, and spinal cord compression was a feature in some dogs. Nerve root enlargement was best seen on transverse images at the level of the C1-C2 intervertebral foramen, causing mild to moderate distortion of the spinal cord, and typically contrast enhancement. These cases may begin with a forelimb lameness, progressing to paresis either unilaterally or bilaterally and eventually to weakness and ataxia. Some dogs responded well to immunosuppressive doses of prednisone.[11] Ganglioneuritis also has been reported secondary to disc extrusion in a dog, presumably from local inflammation caused by extruded disc material.[14] Foreign body migration into the brachial plexus also has been reported in the dog, causing a forelimb lameness and neck pain.[15] Infectious neuritis due to mycobacterium has been reported in the cat.[16]

CERVICAL SPONDYLOMYELOPATHY

CSM, or Wobbler syndrome, is a term that refers both to dogs with static compression of the spinal cord and surrounding structures secondary to stenosis of the spinal canal with associated proliferation of the supporting structures (articulations and ligaments) and to dogs with associated disc protrusion. A review of the full pathophysiology of this disease is beyond the scope of this article and has been well reviewed previously.[17] Rather, this article focuses on how CSM can cause lameness.

Large breed and giant breed dogs affected by static CSM, including breeds, such as the Great Dane and mastiff, develop lameness as a sign of their disease state when the foramina become stenotic. The foramina may be narrowed by osseous proliferation of the facets, proliferation of articular surface with fibrotic tissue, or a combination of both processes. As a result, the nerve root becomes compressed along the course of exit from the spinal canal (**Fig. 3**). Dogs with disc-associated CSM, such as the Doberman pinscher, may develop lameness secondary to narrowing of the foramina during dynamic movement in the face of canal narrowing or secondary to disc protrusion to one side (**Fig. 4**).

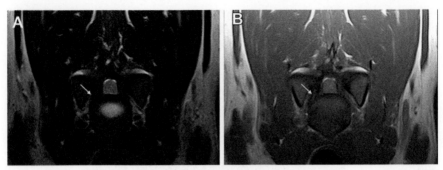

Fig. 3. MRI of a dog with static CSM. Transverse (*A*) T2-weighted and (*B*) T1-weighted MRIs of the cervical spinal cord at the level of the C5-6 intervertebral foramen. The spinal canal is rectangular in shape secondary to osseous stenosis, resulting in loss of the normal fat and fluid signal surrounding the spinal cord. The arrows identify narrowing of the right intervertebral foramina, resulting in compression of the C6 nerve root.

Regarding diagnostics, MRI is the modality of choice to identify the cause of spinal cord disease and whether or not there are changes within the spinal cord parenchyma.[18] Where MRI is unavailable, CT and myelography can achieve a diagnosis. Dynamic imaging, where traction is applied to the cervical region or the neck is flexed and extended, has been reported but no standard established.[19–21]

In either type of CSM, in addition to lameness, there should be other indications of spinal cord disease, in particular, reluctance to raise the head, proprioceptive deficits, and proprioceptive ataxia. Treatment of this disease is controversial and no consensus has been reached on which medical or surgical approach is best for either disease. In the authors' experience, however, mildly affected dogs that are ambulatory are managed with analgesics, anti-inflammatories, chest harness walks, and physical rehabilitation temporarily or lifelong, depending on the response. Dogs that do not improve or worsen with medical management can be considered candidates for surgical treatment. Surgical treatment is sought with the goal of improving comfort and

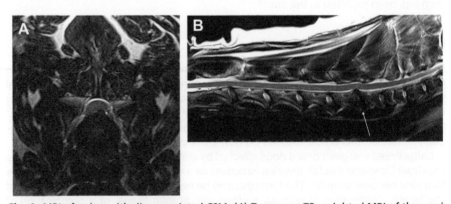

Fig. 4. MRI of a dog with disc-associated CSM. (*A*) Transverse T2-weighted MRI of the cervical spinal cord at the level of the C5-6 intervertebral disc. There is a disc protrusion present, with a left lateral bulge, identified by the asterisk, which is compressing the left C6 nerve root. (*B*) Sagittal T2-weighted MRI of the same dog, with the arrow identifying the C5-6 intervertebral disc space. The dorsal protrusion of the disc and resulting spinal cord compression can be identified above the arrow.

preventing progression of disease. The type of surgical approach generally sought is a ventral decompression with or without stabilization for disc-associated CSM and a dorsal approach for dogs with osseous CSM. Prognosis is guarded with this disease because there typically are multiple sites of stenosis, and further disc protrusions or proliferation of fibrosis can continue to occur.

SUMMARY

There are several neurologic diseases that can result in lameness. The key to identifying them as different from orthopedic cases is to perform a thorough examination to determine if there are neurologic deficits. Because the nerve root typically is affected, the reflexes in the limb are affected. The diagnostic modality of choice for these cases, generally, is MRI, keeping in mind that an expanded field of view, rather than simply focusing on the spine, is key to imaging the brachial plexus in addition to the spinal cord. Treatment of many of these diseases can be challenging, because a compressed or diseased nerve root can result in significant discomfort, and analgesia is a key component of the management of these cases. For intervertebral disc disease and CSM, when signs become progressive, severe, or do not improve, further steps in treatment, such as surgery, are considered.

CLINICS CARE POINTS

- Neurologic diseases that result in lameness likely cause abnormalities in reflexes and proprioception in the limb affected.
- An MRI of the cervical intumescence and brachial plexus provides the most complete investigation of possible neurologic causes of lameness.
- Medical management of neurologic disease with oral analgesics and rest is warranted when signs are mild and early in progression.
- Advanced treatment, such as surgery, may be necessary in cases that continue to progress in the face of good medical management.

DISCLOSURE

The authors of this article have no commercial or financial conflicts of interest.

REFERENCES

1. Bersan E, McConnell F, Trevail R, et al. Cervical intervertebral foraminal disc extrusion in dogs: clinical presentation, MRI characteristics and outcome after medical management. Vet Rec 2015;176(23):597.
2. Robertson I, Thrall DE. Imaging dogs with suspected disc herniation: pros and cons of myelography, computed tomography, and magnetic resonance. Vet Radiol Ultrasound 2011;52(Suppl 1):S81–4.
3. Giambuzzi S, Pancotto T, Ruth J. Perineural injection for treatment of root-signature signs associated with lateralized disk material in five dogs (2009-2013). Front Vet Sci 2016;3:1.
4. Schmied O, Golini L, Steffen F. Effectiveness of cervical hemilaminectomy in canine Hansen Type I and Type II disc disease: a retrospective study. J Am Anim Hosp Assoc 2011;47(5):342–50.

5. Hermanson JW, de Lahunta A, Evans HE. Miller and Evans' anatomy of the dog. 5th edition. Elsevier; 2020.

6. Uemura E. Visual system. In: Fundamentals of canine neuroanatomy and neurophysiology. Wiley; 2015.

7. Schulman FY, Johnson TO, Facemire PR, et al. Feline peripheral nerve sheath tumors: histologic, immunohistochemical, and clinicopathologic correlation (59 tumors in 53 cats). Vet Pathol 2009;46(6):1166–80.

8. Brehm DM, Vite CH, Steinberg HS, et al. A retrospective evaluation of 51 cases of peripheral nerve sheath tumors in the dog. J Am Anim Hosp Assoc 1995;31: 349–59.

9. Kraft S, Ehrhart EJ, Gall D, et al. Magnetic resonance imaging characteristics of peripheral nerve sheath tumors of the canine brachial plexus in 18 dogs. Vet Radiol Ultrasound 2007;48(1):1–7.

10. Rodenas S, Summers BA, Saveraid T, et al. Chronic hypertrophic ganglioneuritis mimicking spinal nerve neoplasia: clinical, imaging, pathologic findings, and outcome after surgical treatment. Vet Surg 2013;42(1):91–8.

11. Joslyn S, Driver C, McConnell F, et al. Magnetic resonance imaging of suspected idiopathic bilateral C2 hypertrophic ganglioneuritis in dogs. J Small Anim Pract 2015;56(3):184–9.

12. Garosi L, de Lahunta A, Summers B, et al. Bilateral, hypertrophic neuritis of the brachial plexus in a cat: magnetic resonance imaging and pathological findings. J Feline Med Surg 2006;8(1):63–8.

13. Kobatake Y, Sakai H, Nishida H, et al. Hypertrophic neuritis causing tetraparesis in a cat. J Vet Med Sci 2018;80(8):1277–80.

14. Mouradian-Darby AE, Young BD, Griffin JFt, et al. Lymphocytic ganglioneuritis secondary to intervertebral disc extrusion in a dog. J Small Anim Pract 2014; 55(9):471–4.

15. Walmsley G, Scurrell E, Summers B, et al. Foreign body induced neuritis masquerading as a canine brachial plexus nerve sheath tumour. Vet Comp Orthop Traumatol 2009;22(5):427–9.

16. Paulsen DB, Kern MR, Weigand CM. Mycobacterial neuritis in a cat. J Am Vet Med Assoc 2000;216(10):1589–91, 1569.

17. da Costa RC. Cervical spondylomyelopathy (wobbler syndrome) in dogs. Vet Clin North Am Small Anim Pract 2010;40(5):881–913.

18. da Costa RC, Parent J, Dobson H, et al. Comparison of magnetic resonance imaging and myelography in 18 Doberman pinscher dogs with cervical spondylomyelopathy. Vet Radiol Ultrasound 2006;47(6):523–31.

19. Penderis J, Dennis R. Use of traction during magnetic resonance imaging of caudal cervical spondylomyelopathy ("wobbler syndrome") in the dog. Vet Radiol Ultrasound 2004;45(3):216–9.

20. Provencher M, Habing A, Moore SA, et al. Evaluation of osseous-associated cervical spondylomyelopathy in dogs using kinematic magnetic resonance imaging. Vet Radiol Ultrasound 2017;58(4):411–21.

21. Ramos RM, da Costa RC, Oliveira AL, et al. Effects of flexion and extension on the diameter of the caudal cervical vertebral canal in dogs. Vet Surg 2015;44(4): 459–66.

Juvenile Disease Processes Affecting the Forelimb in Canines

Nina R. Kieves, DVM

KEYWORDS

- Canine • Forelimb • Juvenile diseases • Panosteitis • HOD
- Retained cartilaginous core

KEY POINTS

- Several diseases affect the juvenile forelimb in dogs; these disease most commonly include hypertrophic osteodystrophy, panosteitis, and retained cartilaginous cores.
- In many cases of hypertrophic osteodystrophy and panosteitis, the outcome is good in the long term.
- Severe cases of hypertrophic osteodystrophy may require hospitalization and supportive care, and can be fatal.
- Panosteitis is self-limiting, but dogs can have several cases of recurrence particularly before the age of 2 years.
- Many cases of retained cartilaginous are asymptomatic, but they can retard growth of the distal ulnar physis leading to angular limb deformity that may require corrective osteotomy.

HYPERTROPHIC OSTEODYSTROPHY

Hypertrophic osteodystrophy (HOD) is a developmental orthopedic disease that affects large and giant breed dogs, primarily during times of rapid growth (2–8 months of age, most present between the ages of 3 and 4 months). It has also been referred to as infantile scurvy, juvenile scurvy, skeletal scurvy, metaphyseal osteopathy, Moller Barlow's disease, osteodystrophy II, and more recently metaphyseal osteopathy.[1] The underlying etiology is not known. Males are over-represented, being 2.3 times more likely to develop HOD than females.[2] Although any breed can develop HOD, Boxers, Chesapeake Bay Retrievers, German Shepherd dogs, Great Danes, Golden Retrievers, Irish Setters, Labrador Retrievers, and Weimaraners are over-represented,[2–6] with Great Danes and Weimaraners making up the majority of cases.[7] However, any breed can develop HOD.

Small Animal Orthopedic Surgery, The Ohio State University, 601 Vernon L Tharp Street, Columbus, OH 43210, USA
E-mail address: kieves.1@osu.edu

Vet Clin Small Anim 51 (2021) 365–382
https://doi.org/10.1016/j.cvsm.2020.12.004

Previous exploration into the etiology of HOD has investigated the role of infection (including canine distemper virus, and *Escherichia coli*), vaccinations, inflammation, hypovitaminosis C, excess vitamins and minerals, vascular anomalies, and genetics.[2–5] Ultimately, many of these etiologies have been ruled out, or deemed unlikely to be the cause of HOD.[5,8,9] Heritability in some breeds has been suggested for breeds at increased risk of developing HOD.[2,7,8,10]

Experimentally, Bohning and colleagues[11] were able to reproduce lesions similar to HOD by feeding dogs a free choice high calorie diet high in protein and calcium. However, many dogs that present with HOD do not have a history of excessive vitamin and mineral supplementation, and conversely, dogs on high levels of supplementation do not always develop HOD.

Infectious causes have been extensively assessed for their contribution to the development of HOD,[10,12,13] with canine distemper virus being found in bone cells of the metaphyseal region in experimental models.[12,13] One case report, found a dog to have positive blood cultures for *E coli*,[14] although predominately no infectious agents have been found to be associated with the disease.[2,15]

An autoimmune or a hyperinflammatory etiology has also been proposed for the development of HOD. Most recently, a study evaluated the serum levels of inflammatory markers in 26 dogs with HOD and 102 control dogs.[16] The dogs with HOD had significantly increased serum levels of innate immunity cytokines including IL-1-beta, IL-18, IL-6, and tumor necrosis factor among others compared with control dogs.[16] Additionally, dogs that developed HOD had elevated values of these markers both during active disease and after they had recovered, suggesting a possible mechanism of autoinflammatory disease similar to some human disorders in children in these dogs.[16]

Clinical Presentation

Most frequently, dogs present with a grossly observable swelling of the distal metaphysis of the radius, ulna, and tibia, although the proximal metaphysis may be affected in some cases (**Fig. 1**). This finding can be mistaken for joint swelling, but adequate palpation and orthopedic examination should distinguish the two entities. Typically, the dog is affected bilaterally. In addition to the swelling, dogs often have some degree of systemic involvement with pyrexia, anorexia, pain with resultant reluctance to move,[17] and possibly a history of diarrhea.[1] There is severe pain with palpation of the metaphyseal region of the long bones, and dogs are typically reluctant to ambulate. A secondary angular limb deformity may develop as a sequela to disruption of the growth plate, causing cranial bowing of the radius with a concurrent valgus deformity of the carpus

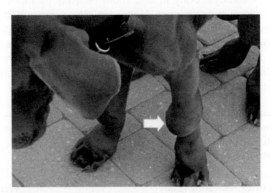

Fig. 1. Typical thickening of the distal antebrachium seen with dogs presenting with HOD.

or cause varus deformity of the tibia (**Figs. 2** and **3**).[17] This deformity is secondary to excessive bone formation in the metaphyseal region with bridging of the physis, or synostosis between the radius and the ulna,[3,7] but is uncommon.

Diagnosis

A definitive diagnosis is made on survey radiographs, with changes becoming apparent 24 to 48 hours after the onset of clinical signs.[18] Initially, a thin, radiolucent line is seen in the metaphysis parallel to the epiphyseal plate, referred to as a pseudophyseal line (**Figs. 4** and **5**). This line is often seen best in the radius. Histologically, this line corresponds with the diseased area with infiltration of neutrophils and mononuclear cells with evidence of hemorrhage, osteoclastic resorption, fibrosis, and necrosis of the trabeculae.[8] As HOD progresses, an extraperiosteal cuff of calcification will develop along the metaphysis. This calcification corresponds with subperiosteal hemorrhage that elevates the periosteum (**Figs. 6** and **7**). The lucent line initially seen will disappear, to be replaced by an increased radiodensity. The extraperiosteal thickening often will regress with age; however, the metaphysis can remain permanently thickened. If a dog develops a relapse of the disease, a new radiolucent line will appear between the physis and the radiodense region.[5]

The differential diagnosis for HOD include hypertrophic osteopathy, secondary nutritional hyperparathyroidism, retained cartilaginous cores, trauma, and septic polyarthritis. Radiographs should be informative to definitively make the diagnosis of HOD.

Treatment

Most dogs will respond well to supportive care of rest, coupled with pain management with a nonsteroidal anti-inflammatory drug (NSAID). Symptoms will typically subside after 1 week or so, but can recur every few weeks until growth has ended. One study found no difference in outcome between no treatment, treatment with antibiotics alone, treatment with antibiotics plus corticosteroids, and treatment with antibiotics plus corticosteroids plus vitamin C.[1] More severe cases will require aggressive supportive care, with intravenous opioids for pain management, antacids, possibly feeding tube placement to provide nutritional support, and either an NSAID or a corticosteroid. It has been reported in the literature that Weimaraners in particular may respond better to corticosteroid treatment compared with NSAID therapy.[10,18] Safra and colleagues[18] found that 100% of Weimaraners treated with a tapering dose of corticosteroids (prednisone) had clinical remission of symptoms within 8 to 48 hours of treatment compared with only 45.5% of those treated with an NSAID. Those dogs that did not enter remission with a 1-week duration of treatment with an NSAID were washed out for 24 to 48 hours and started on prednisone. These dogs all subsequently went on to achieve clinical remission, suggesting that corticosteroids may be a superior treatment compared with NSAIDs for Weimaraners in particular.

Although the clinical signs typically resolve within 7 to 10 days, radiographic resolution may take several months. If a relapse occurs, a new radiolucent line and periosteal reaction will appear.[9] The prognosis is good to excellent for most cases; however, severe refractory cases can be fatal.

Summary

HOD typically affects young large and giant breed dogs. The diagnosis is made based on survey radiographs. Although most dogs recover with supportive care, it can affect the growth plates permanently leading, to angular limb deformities that may require correction. In rare cases, dogs remain refractory to pain management and humane euthanasia may be indicated.

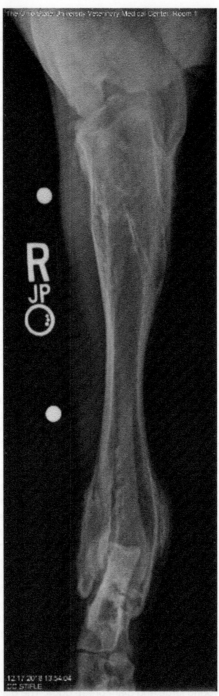

Fig. 2. This dog presented for evaluation of an angular limb deformity secondary to HOD. There is proximal and distal tibial and fibular metaphyseal expansion with surrounding irregular periosteal proliferation and soft tissue thickening, malformation of the tibial plateau, and abnormal stifle conformation; this includes varus deformity of the distal femur and valgus deformity of the proximal tibiae.

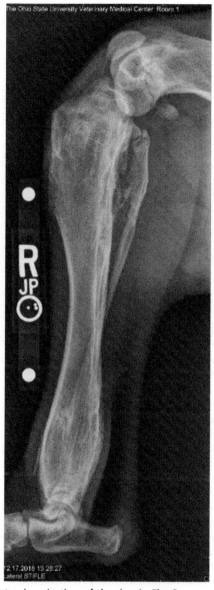

Fig. 3. Corresponding lateral projection of the dog in **Fig. 2**.

PANOSTEITIS

Panosteitis is an inflammatory disease that affects the adipose tissue of the bone marrow of the long bones. It is considered a developmental disease and is typically self-limiting. Dogs are typically affected between 2 and 12 months of age; however, it has been reported in dogs as young as 2 months and as old as 15 years of age.[11,19] The majority of the cases, 82%, that present are less than 18 months of age.[11] Panosteitis also been referred to as enostosis, eosinophilic panosteitis, juvenile osteomyelitis, fibrous osteodystrophy, and shifting leg lameness.

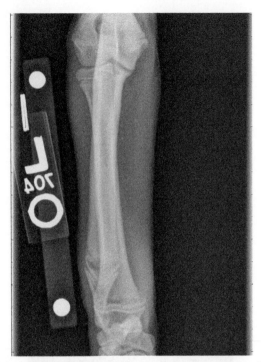

Fig. 4. Craniocaudal projection of a dog with HOD of the distal antebrachium. A thin, radio-lucent line is seen in the metaphysis parallel to the epiphyseal plate, referred to as a pseu-dophyseal line.

Large and giant breed dogs are more commonly affected, but small breeds can develop the disease. It is most commonly reported in German Shepherd dogs (McLaughlin[20]), with Basset hounds being the second highest at risk breed[19]; however, numerous other breeds are considered to be predisposed to developing panosteitis including Afghans, Airedale Terriers, Bernese Mountain Dogs, Cocker Spaniels, Doberman Pinschers, Irish Setters, German Shorthair Pointers, Golden Retrievers, Great Danes, Labrador Retrievers, Mastiffs, Newfoundlands, Rottweilers, Saint Bernards, Shar Peis, and mixed breed dogs. Males are affected 4 times more frequently than females.[6,11,21]

No definitive etiology has been identified as the cause of panosteitis. Historically allergies, autoimmune disease, endocrine dysfunction, hemophilia, metabolic disease, parasitism, and vascular anomalies have been considered.[17,19] To date, no bacterial infectious agents have been isolated from dogs with panosteitis.[22] And although a viral cause has been postulated, it has not been proven.[19]

Histologically, the adipose and hematopoietic tissue of the long bones are temporarily replaced by fibrous tissue. There is a loss of normal adipose tissue with fibrous proliferation and intramembranous ossification with osteoclastic removal of the trabeculae. More severe cases will also have changes to the periosteum and cortex.[3,20]

The initial changes are seen as empty spaces in the adipose bone marrow, with vascular proliferation and local bone formation that is centered around the nutrient foramen. This process causes congestion of the vasculature, increasing the intraosseous pressure from normal 6 to 24 mm Hg up to 25 to 54 mm Hg. This increased pressure leads to additional local bone formation and secondary periosteal bone growth with enlargement of the Haversian system.[8,21] The areas of this local bone formation

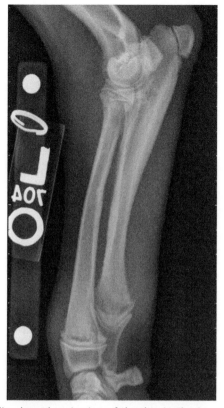

Fig. 5. The corresponding lateral projection of the dog in **Fig. 3**.

coalesce and connect to the endosteum. Ultimately, this new bone is remodeled into hematopoietic bone marrow, and finally normal adipose bone marrow as the disease regresses.[8] At no time is there evidence of acute or chronic inflammation.

Clinical Presentation

Dogs may present with mild lameness to severe lameness with an inability to walk, but most exhibit a mild to moderate lameness. In some cases, the lameness may be reported at a puppy visit as a resolved shifting leg lameness because resolution can be rapid in some cases. There is no history of trauma. Although some reports of concurrent systemic illness such as fever and systemic eosinophilia, along with inappetence and muscle atrophy have been made,[23] others dispute these systemic signs as being disease related.[11] Although any limb can be affected, the forelimb is affected 4 times more frequently than the hindlimb.[8] Which bone—the ulna or humerus—is most commonly affected varies with reports.[11,24] In 1 series of cases, the ulna was most commonly affected (42%), followed by the radius (25%), humerus (14%), femur (11%), and tibia (8%).[24] Another reported cases most frequently in the humerus (68%), and femur (68%), followed by the ulna (54%), radius (27%) and tibia (24%).[11] Although it is uncommon for the same bone to be affected more than once (1%), the same limb is often affected multiple times with recurrence.[11]

Pain is elicited with palpation of the affected bones. The clinician must be careful to palpate deeply, moving aside musculature gently to truly assess for bone pain rather

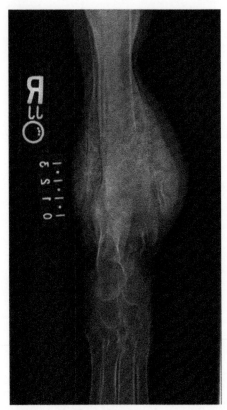

Fig. 6. Craniocaudal projection of a distal tibia in a dog with a more severe presentation of HOD. There is severe, irregularly marginated new bone formation surrounding the proximal and distal tibial and fibular metaphyses, extending to the mid diaphyses. The soft tissues surrounding the metaphyses are circumferentially thickened. The osseous structures of the right pes are lucent. There is smoothly marginated periosteal perforation surrounding the mid tibial and fibular diaphyses.

than interpreting discomfort from pushing on musculature. It is imperative to complete a full physical examination because more than 1 limb may be affected at once; 49% of cases have more than 1 limb affected at some point in the course of the disease, and 53% of cases having multiple bones involved.[11]

In addition to numerous limbs being affected at once, other developmental orthopedic diseases occur frequently in many of the breeds that are predisposed to panosteitis, so the clinician must assess for these as well. Concurrent disease was reported in 26% of cases in 1 report,[11] and in many cases, it is the concurrent disease that is the primary cause of lameness rather than the panosteitis. Of particular note for consideration is elbow dysplasia in German Shepherd dogs (and other large breed dogs), as well as hip dysplasia. If the panosteitis is not the primary cause of the dog's lameness, this factor must be accounted for in a treatment plan.

Diagnosis

If there is evidence of systemic disease, laboratory tests may be indicated. Orthogonal radiographs of at least 1 of the long bones that show discomfort should be performed to confirm the presence of panosteitis, recognizing that in the early stages of disease

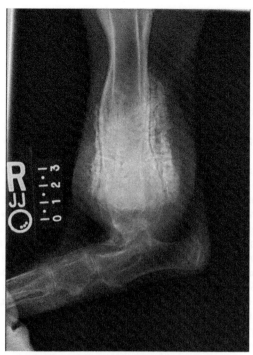

Fig. 7. The corresponding lateral projection of the dog in Fig. 4.

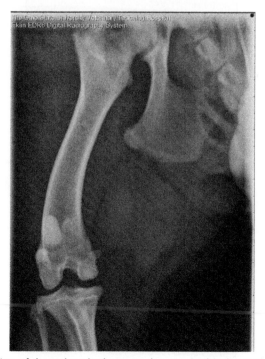

Fig. 8. Slight blurring of the trabecular bone can be seen in this dog with early evidence of panosteitis. This can easily be missed, and films read as normal.

changes may be minimal (as discussed elsewhere in this article). Additional imaging of the joints that are uncomfortable to rule in or rule out concurrent orthopedic disease should also be performed. This practice may include advanced imaging such as a computed tomography scan for the evaluation of disease, such as elbow dysplasia.

Radiographic signs of panosteitis varies with the stage of disease. Although panosteitis is often evident radiographically, early in the disease radiographs may be normal. Lesions can affect any portion of the diaphysis and can be solitary or affect multiple sites in a single bone or affect multiple long bones at the same time. Radiographic changes seen with panosteitis can be broken into 3 stages: early, middle, and late.[11,17,21]

Early on, the disease is often not noted, but if critically evaluated, radiographs will show blurring and accentuation of the trabeculae with radiolucency of the medullary canal (**Fig. 8**). These changes occur 10 to 14 days after the onset of clinical signs.[25] Quality radiographs with good technique must be made to see these early changes. As disease progresses, well-demarcated nodular opacities within the medullary cavity, of similar opacity to cortical bone, will be seen. Typically, this finding is centered around the nutrient foramen. These lesions may be small or be quite extensive, filling the entire diaphysis (**Figs. 9–11**). This feature is the hallmark of panosteitis, with lesions remaining evident for approximately 4 to 6 weeks.[11] Approximately 33% to 50% of cases will have changes to the periosteum, as well as consisting of a smooth continuous periosteal new bone growth. This growth begins as a subtle roughening that becomes denser over time, eventually becoming as dense as the cortex. As the disease resolves, the medullary cavity will return to a normal density, although a coarse trabecular pattern will remain. Approximately one-third of cases may continue

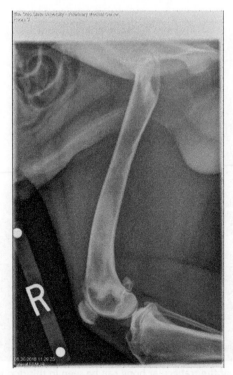

Fig. 9. A lateral projection of a femur showing patchy sclerosis of the femur.

to have thickening of the cortex at this time. Full radiographic resolution may take several months to occur.[17,26] The severity of radiographic changes does not correlate with clinical signs in all cases.[27] In addition to radiography, a computed tomography scan and a MRI as well as nuclear scintigraphy have been used to diagnose panosteitis (see **Fig. 11**).

The differential diagnoses for panosteitis include other developmental disease such as osteochondrosis or osteochondritis dissecans, elbow dysplasia, hip dysplasia, and cruciate disease. If there are multiple limbs affected, consideration should be given to rheumatoid arthritis and systemic lupus erythematosus.

Treatment

Pain relief can typically be accomplished with NSAIDs. No treatment has been found to decrease the duration of symptoms (Muir and associates[5]). Pain relief medication may be given as needed and may not be required for a significant duration of time in mild cases. The duration of the treatment varies with the course of the disease

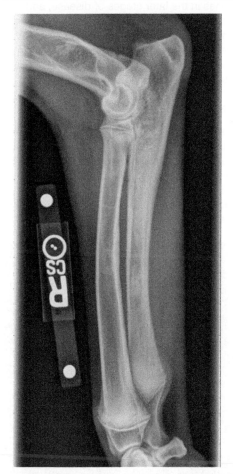

Fig. 10. This lateral projection of the antebrachium shows multifocal increased regions of mineral opacity within the medullary cavity of the ulna. There are similar but less pronounced regions within the mid radius and distal humerus. There is mild cortical irregularity of the distal metaphysis of the radius and ulna consistent with the cut back zone.

and may only be given for a few days, or in worse cases, a few weeks. Rest does not seem to affect comfort for the patient, with activity not worsening the signs of lameness; therefore, activity restriction is not required.[3] The use of corticosteroids for treatment has been reported in refractory cases,[3] but is rarely necessary and should not be a first choice treatment. If concurrent orthopedic disease is found, this disease must be treated separately, possibly after resolution of the symptoms from panosteitis to determine the degree of clinical impairment that is due to the concurrent disease. The prognosis is excellent, with the disease being self-limiting and causing no long-term impairment.

Summary

Panosteitis affects the bone marrow of the long bones of dogs causing the hematopoietic tissue to be temporarily replaced by fibrous tissue. Dogs will typically present with lameness of 1 or more limbs, or a shifting leg lameness over time. Pain on direct palpation of the long bones is found. Radiographic changes show increased medullary opacity of the long bones in the later stages of disease, and these changes are typically definitive for a diagnosis of panosteitis. However, in the early stages of disease radiographs may be normal with changes only being evident via a computed tomography scan. In more severe cases, the cortex and periosteum may be affected as well. Treatment with an NSAID for pain management is typically adequate treatment. Recurrence is not uncommon.

RETAINED CARTILAGINOUS CORE

Retained cartilaginous core is also known as retained hypertrophied endochondral cartilage or retained endochondral cartilage cores. It is primarily reported in the ulnar metaphysis and can lead to angular limb deformities of the forelimb, but has also been reported in the lateral femoral condyle.[28] The remainder of this discussion focuses on retained cores of the ulna only.

Retained cartilaginous cores are zones of viable hypertrophic chondrocytes, or growth plate cartilage that project proximally from the growth plate into the distal

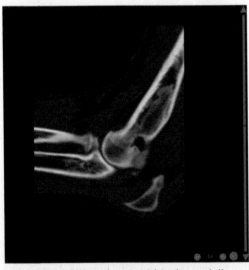

Fig. 11. This sagittal slice shows lobular sclerosis within the medullary canal of the distal humerus consistent with panosteitis.

metaphysis.[28] They are distinctively shaped like cones (**Fig. 12**). They occur when there is abnormal endochondral ossification of the distal ulnar physis, leaving cartilage where there should be conversion to normal bone. It is considered a manifestation of osteochondrosis by some.[29] An underlying cause for the development of retained cartilaginous cores is unknown. Great Danes seem to be over-represented; however, other large and giant breed dogs have been reported to develop the disease.

Histologically, the cores are made of hypertrophied hyaline cartilage cells. These cones themselves do not cause pain or clinical signs to the patient and may be an incidental finding on radiographs made of the forelimb for another reason. However, if the cone causes reduction of ulnar length during growth owing to the disruption of the distal ulnar physis, an angular limb deformity may be a sequela of the disease. With retardation of growth of the ulna, the styloid process does not extend to the ulnar carpal bone allowing the manus to abduct owing to the loss of lateral support. Ultimately, the radius will bow cranially exhibiting excessive procurvatum. In severe cases, there can be subluxation of the carpal and elbow joints.

Clinical Signs

Many dogs are asymptomatic. If, however, an angular limb deformity ensues, dogs will be presented for varying degrees of angular limb deformities and associated lameness.

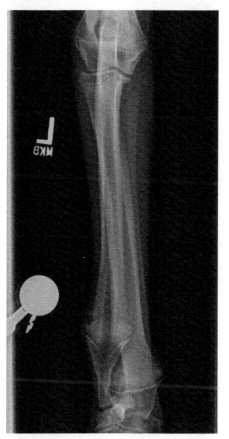

Fig. 12. Craniocaudal projection of the antebrachium with a triangular radiolucent region in the distal ulnar metaphysis, with a thin rim of sclerosis.

Diagnosis

Radiographically, the cores seem to be as radiolucent triangles, or "candlesticks," extending 3 to 6 cm proximally into the metaphysis of the ulna (see **Fig. 12**; **Fig. 13**). In some cases, this radiolucent lesion will be surrounded by a narrow zone of sclerosis.[30] There is no correlation between the size of the lesion and the severity of the angular limb deformity that may develop. The lesions have been reported to spontaneously disappear.[31] If there is disruption of the distal ulnar physis, radiographic changes will also show deformity, along with possible secondary osteoarthritic changes to the carpus and/or elbow joints (**Figs. 14** and **15**).

Treatment

If no angular limb deformity has developed, no treatment is required. However, if noted at a young age when the dog has significant growth potential left, ongoing monitoring

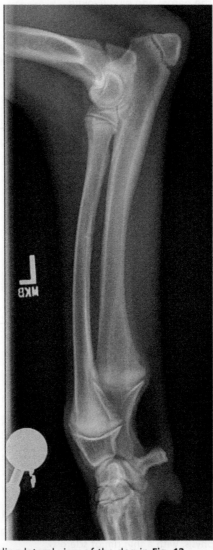

Fig. 13. The corresponding lateral view of the dog in **Fig. 12.**

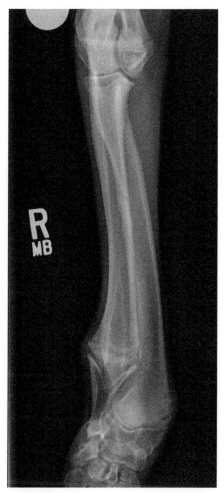

Fig. 14. This craniocaudal projection of the antebrachium with a triangular radiolucent region in the distal ulnar metaphysis, with a thin rim of sclerosis as in **Fig. 12**. However this, dog also developed an angular limb deformity secondary to the retained cartilaginous core causing the distal antebrachium to curve caudally and the distal radius to angle laterally with a valgus deformity.

is recommended to ensure any changes in limb angulation are noted in early stages, so surgical intervention can be performed. If a significant angular limb deformity has already occurred, it will need to be addressed in the same way one would address other angular limb deformities that have developed for other reasons (ie, premature closure of the distal ulnar physis owing to trauma) with an appropriate corrective osteotomy. Some investigators have advocated for decreasing nutritional intake in young puppies if retained cartilaginous cores are noted in an attempt to prevent angular deformities from occurring.[17] Prognosis is good if no severe angular limb deformity with elbow or carpal subluxation develops.

Summary

Retained cartilaginous cores develop owing to a failure of endochondral ossification. They are diagnosed radiographically as a radiolucent triangle extending into the

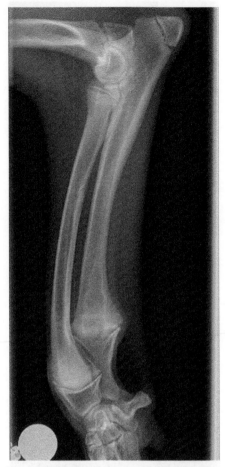

Fig. 15. The corresponding lateral view of the dog in **Fig. 14**.

metaphysis from the distal ulnar physis. They do not cause clinical signs, unless the distal ulnar physis growth is disrupted, in which case an angular limb deformity may develop that could require a corrective osteotomy to treat subsequent carpal or elbow joint issues.

CLINICS CARE POINTS

- HOD is a disease of young, growing dogs.
  - Radiographs are diagnostic for HOD with a double physis being seen.
  - Most dogs respond to supportive care with pain management at home, but can require hospitalization in severe cases.
  - HOD can lead to the formation of antebrachial and crural deformities in some cases.
  - Weimaraners may best be treated with corticosteroids versus NSAIDs.
- Panosteitis is a developmental inflammatory disease of the adipose component of the bone marrow of long bones.
  - Panosteitis is typically self-limiting.

- German Shepherd dogs are overrepresented.
- Clinical presentation of shifting leg lameness is common.
- Treatment consists of pain management with an NSAID.

- Retained cartilaginous cores develop owing to a failure of endochondral ossification.
  - Dogs may be asymptomatic.
  - If secondary angular limb deformities occur, corrective osteotomy may be indicated.

DISCLOSURE

The author has no conflicts of interest to disclose in regard to this article.

REFERENCES

1. Grondalen J. Metaphyseal osteopathy (hypertrophic osteodystrophy) in growing dogs: a clinical study. J Small Anim Pract 1976;17(11):721–35.
2. Munjar TA, Austin CC, Breur GJ. Comparison of risk factors for hypertrophic osteodystrophy, craniomandibular osteopathy, and canine distemper virus infection. Vet Comp Orthop Traumatol 1998;11:37–43.
3. Lenehan TM, Fetter AW. Hypertrophic osteodystrophy. In: Newton CD, Nunamaker DM, editors. Textbook of small animal orthopaedics. Philadelphia: JB Lippincott; 1985. p. 597–601.
4. Alexander JW. Hypertrophic osteodystrophy. Canine Pract 1978;5:48–52.
5. Muir P, Dubielzig RR, Johnson KA, et al. Hypertrophic osteodystrophy and calvarial hyperostosis. Compend Contin Educ Pract Vet 1996;18:143–51.
6. LaFond E, Breur GJ, Austin CC. Breed susceptibility for developmental orthopedic diseases in dogs. J Am Vet Med Assoc 2002;38:467–77.
7. Montgomery R. Hypertrophic osteodystrophy. In: Bojrab MJ, editor. Disease mechanisms in small animal surgery. 3rd edition. Jackson (Wyoming): Teton New Media; 2010. p. 564–70.
8. Towle Millard HA, Breur GJ. Miscellaneous orthopedic conditions. In: Johnston SA, Tobias KM, editors. Veterinary surgery: small animal. 2nd edition. St. Louis (MO): Elsevier; 2018. p. 1299–315.
9. Alexander JW. Selected skeletal dysplasia: craniomandibular osteopathy, multiple cartilaginous exostosis, and hypertrophic osteodystrophy. Vet Clin North Am Small Anim Pract 1983;13(1):55–70.
10. Abeles V, Harrus S, Angles JM, et al. Hypertrophic osteodystrophy in six Weimaraner puppies associated with systemic signs. Vet Rec 1999;145(5):130–4.
11. Bohning R, Suter P, Hohn RB, et al. Clinical and radiographic survey of canine panosteitis. J Am Vet Med Assoc 1970;156:870–84.
12. Mee AP, Webber DM, May C, et al. Detection of canine distemper virus in bone cells in the metaphysis of distemper infected dogs. J Bone Miner Res 1992;7(7):829–34.
13. Mee AP, Gordon MT, May C, et al. Canine distemper virus transcripts detected in the bone cells of dogs with metaphyseal osteopathy. Bone 1993;14(1):59–67.
14. Schulz KS, Payne JT, Aronson E. Escherichia coli bacteremia associated with hypertrophic osteodystrophy in a dog. J Am Vet Med Assoc 1991;199(9):1170–3.
15. Watson ADJ, Blair RC, Farrow BRH, et al. Hypertrophic osteodystrophy in the dog. Aust Vet J 1973;49(9):433–9.
16. Safra N, Hitchens PL, Maverakis E, et al. Serum levels of innate immunity cytokines are elevated in dogs with metaphyseal osteopathy (hypertrophic osteodystrophy) during active disease and remission. Vet Immunol Immunopathol 2016;179:32–5.

17. DeCamp CE, Johnston SA, Dejardin LM, et al. Disease conditions in small animals. In: Brinker, Piermattei, and Flo's handbook of small animal orthopedics and fracture repair. 5th edition. St Louis (MO): Elsevier; 2016. p. 821–37.
18. Safra N, Johnson EG, Lit L, et al. Clinical manifestations, response to treatment, and clinical outcome for Weimaraners with hypertrophic osteodystrophy: 53 cases (2009-2011). J Am Vet Med Assoc 2013;242:1260–6.
19. Montgomery R. Panosteitis. In: Bojrab MJ, editor. Disease mechanisms in small animal surgery. 3rd edition. Jackson (Wyoming): Teton New Media; 2010. p. 570–6.
20. McLaughlin RM. Hind limb lameness in the young patient. Vet Clin North Am Small Anim Pract 2001;31(10):101–23.
21. Stead AC, Stead MC, Galloway FH. Panosteitis in dogs. J Small Anim Pract 1983; 24:623–35.
22. Turnier JC, Silverman S. A case study of canine panosteitis: comparison of radiographic and radioisotopic studies. Am J Vet Res 1978;39(9):1550–2.
23. Barrett RB, Schall WD, Lewis RE. Clinical and radiographic features of canine eosinophilic panosteitis. J Am Anim Hosp Assoc 1968;4:94–104.
24. Van Sickle DC. Canine panosteitis, a skeletal disease of unknown etiology. Proceedings of the 4th Kal Can Symposium, Ohio University Columbus (Ohio): October 11-12, 1980. p. 67–71.
25. Lewis DD, McCarthy RJ, Pechman RD. Diagnosis of common developmental orthopedic conditions in canine pediatric patients. Compend Cont Educ Pract Vet 1992;14:287–301.
26. Pollard RE, Phillips KL. Orthopedic disease of young and growing dogs and cats. In: Thrall D, editor. Textbook of veterinary diagnostic radiology. 7th edition. St Louis (MO): Elsevier; 2018. p. 348–65.
27. Lee R. Legg-Perthes disease in the dog: the histological and associated radiological changes. Vet Radiol Ultrasound 1974;15:24–7.
28. Johnson KA. Retardation of endochondral ossification at the distal ulnar growth plate in dogs. Aust Vet J 1981;57(10):474–8.
29. Montgomery R. Miscellaneous orthopedic diseases. In: Bojrab MJ, editor. Disease mechanisms in small animal surgery. 3rd edition. Jackson (Wyoming): Teton New Media; 2010. p. 590–601.
30. Johnson AL. Growth deformities. In: Olmstead ML, editor. Small animal orthopedics. Columbus (OH): OH Mosby; 1995. p. 293–309.
31. Stogdale L. Foreleg lameness in rapidly growing dogs. J S Afr Vet Assoc 1979; 50:193–200.

Advanced Imaging of the Forelimb: Use of Musculoskeletal Ultrasound and MRI of the Shoulder and Brachial Plexus

Ryan King, DVM

KEYWORDS

• MRI • Ultrasound • Supraspinatus • Infraspinatus • Biceps • Brachial plexus

KEY POINTS

- Obtaining high-quality images requires knowledge of the capabilities and limitations of the image modality, including recognition of, and strategies to overcome, common image artifacts.
- Patient preparation, positioning, and selection of appropriate equipment (ultrasound transducers, MRI coils) is necessary to obtain diagnostic images.
- Image interpretation depends on knowledge of regional anatomy of tendons, ligaments, muscles, and osseous structures, as well as recognition of normal structural morphology on each modality. In addition, for MRI, a working knowledge of signal characteristics of each of the common sequences, as well as common pathology is necessary.
- MRI gives a more "global" view of the region of the brachial plexus and shoulder and is less operator dependent than ultrasound; however, it requires general anesthesia and may take up to 1 hour to obtain all of the necessary sequences and images.
- Ultrasound allows for minimally interventional, rapid evaluation of tendon morphology and is readily available for follow-up examinations to track lesion resolution/progression. However, its use in imaging the brachial plexus is limited by complex anatomy and lesion diversity.

INTRODUCTION/HISTORY/DEFINITIONS/BACKGROUND

Although developmental and acquired skeletal diseases occur at all levels of the forelimb, the proximal forelimb has a higher predisposition to disease of ligamentous, muscular, and nervous tissues, limiting the utility of radiography and computed tomography (CT) due to poor soft tissue resolution.[1–3] Ultrasound and MRI are

Cummings School of Veterinary Medicine, Tufts University, 200 Westboro Road, North Grafton, MA 01536, USA
E-mail address: ryan.king@tufts.edu

Vet Clin Small Anim 51 (2021) 383–399
https://doi.org/10.1016/j.cvsm.2020.11.005
0195-5616/21/© 2020 Elsevier Inc. All rights reserved.

particularly sensitive to changes in structure, morphology, and pathology of these structures.[4] Both have the additional benefit of being nonionizing.

Structures commonly targeted for shoulder ultrasound and MRI evaluation include muscle, tendon and joint structures (ligaments, capsule), regional nerves, and fascia. In addition, MRI evaluation may include the cervical spinal cord and nerve roots, imperative in a complete examination of the brachial plexus.

SHOULDER TENDON PATHOLOGY

The normal tendon structure has been well described in human and veterinary literature.[4] Normal tendons have a high percentage of type I collagen in a proteoglycan-water matrix.[4] Collagen fibrils are arranged into highly organized collagen fibers, then fascicles, which are organized along the length (axis) of tendon. Tendon fiber organization depends on the individual tendon, how it forms along the muscle, and the number of muscles supplying the tendon, as well as location within the tendon (proximal vs distal, musculotendinous junction, insertion).

Pathology commonly takes one of the 2 forms: enthesitis (inflammation at insertion on bone) or tendinopathy (mechanical, degenerative, or overuse). Enthesitis results in disruption of fiber organization and increased calcium deposition/mineralization within the tendon insertion.[5]

Tendinopathy results in degeneration and disorganization of collagen fibers and an increase in water (and ground substance/proteoglycan) content.[6,7] Increased calcium content may also occur.[8] Following fibril tearing, vascular ingrowth can occur.

These changes disrupt the normal homogenous, well-defined architecture on both ultrasound (hypoechoic, well-defined fiber pattern) and MRI (hypointense, homogenous). The degree of disruption may correlate with the degree of disease.[9,10]

MUSCULOSKELETAL ULTRASOUND
Anatomy of Interest and Associated Pathology

Shoulder:
- Biceps brachii
- Supraspinatus tendon
- Infraspinatus tendon
- Stabilizing structures and joint capsule
- Repetitive stress injury, acute injury of the tendinous structures (see The Shoulder Joint and Common Abnormalities by Stokes and Dycus)

Brachial plexus:
- C5–7 nerve roots (very limited evaluation)
- Nerve path to axilla (limited evaluation)
- Axillary region
- Nerve sheath tumors, lymphoma, neuritis (see Neurologic Causes of Thoracic Limb Lameness by Kerwin and Taylor)

Ultrasound is particularly useful in defining the tendinous structures of the shoulder, a common source of lameness in young to middle-aged, active, medium to large breed dogs. Pathology of these structures, including core lesions (disruption of tendon fibers), tears, significant swelling, and chronic changes including fibrosis and mineralization, are commonly noted. Ultrasound is of limited utility in evaluating the osseous structures, except in cases of severe disease. Similarly, ultrasound is of limited utility in assessment of disease of the proximal aspects of the brachial plexus. More commonly, ultrasound is used as a screening technique for nodules/masses in the more distal axillary brachial plexus and to guide lesion sampling at any level.

Technique

Appropriate patient preparation, including adequate sedation, is key to acquiring appropriate ultrasound images of the structures of the shoulder and axilla. Dexmedetomidine with butorphanol is commonly used in young, otherwise healthy patients. In older patients, or patients with concomitant disease, sedation and anesthesia should always be tailored to minimize patient risk, while limiting patient motion.

Preparation of the patient will depend on the area of interest, although clipping of the cranial aspect of the shoulder joint is typically sufficient. Commonly both shoulders are imaged, either to define pathology (eg, in shifting leg lameness) or to provide a comparison to normal contralateral structures.

A high-frequency transducer, typically linear, from 8 to 15 MHz is key to obtaining quality images of the small structures of the shoulder. A curvilinear 5 to 8 MHz transducer is appropriate for localizing axillary lesions, although a high-frequency transducer is of utility in further defining lesions once identified.

Imaging is typically performed in a transverse and sagittal plane to the structure of interest.

As with all tendinous structures, care must be taken to image the structure of interest as close to perpendicular as possible; this can be particularly challenging with a large footprint, high-frequency transducer. On transverse images, simply rocking the transducer from perpendicular to off angle will markedly affect the echogenicity of the tendon. On sagittal images, care must be taken to only interpret anatomy in the region of the image where the ultrasound beam is perpendicular to the structure. Anisotropy will create false/artifactual "hypoattenuating lesions" in the nonperpendicular, adjacent tendinous tissue (**Fig. 1**).

Patients are typically imaged in lateral recumbency, with the affected leg up. Supination of the limb will greatly increase tendon visualization (**Fig. 2**).

Although personal preference plays a role in the order of obtaining images, a typical complete shoulder ultrasound examination will include the following[11–13]:

Biceps tendon and muscle: the biceps brachii origin is well visualized from its origin at the cranial extent of the supraglenoid tubercle, to musculotendinous

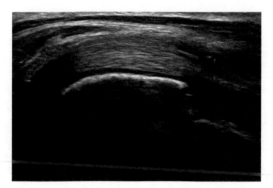

Fig. 1. Anisotropy. Biceps tendon in long axis (sagittal). Proximal is to the left. Note the decreased signal in the biceps tendon, as the tendon becomes increasingly tangential to the US beam (*red arrows*). Care must be taken not to interpret these hypoechoic regions as pathology.

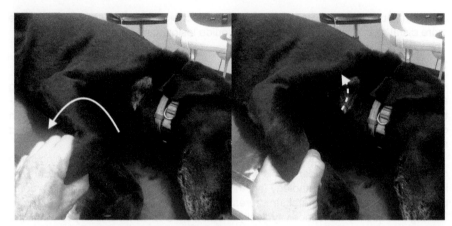

Fig. 2. Patient positioning for evaluation of the biceps, supraspinatus tendon, and infraspinatus tendon. Patient is placed in lateral recumbency with shoulder in a neural position, elbow at 90° (image above *left*). Image optimization of the BCT and supraspinatus tendon are achieved by supinating the limb (internal rotation of the manus at the level of the carpus) (image above, *right*). This will externally rotate the biceps groove, allowing for 90° probe orientation.

junction, running through the distal joint capsule extension (often referred to as the biceps bursa). Curvature of the tendon, as it traverses the intertubercular groove, requires constant manipulation of the transducer to maintain a perpendicular imaging angle.

Pathologic changes include tendon swelling, disruption of fiber pattern (core lesion), and mineralization of the tendon. Tendon mineralization may occur anywhere along the length of the tendon. Mineralization occurring at the origin on the supraglenoid tubercle may be a combination of fiber mineralization and enthesophytosis. Occasionally complete tearing of the tendon is noted secondary to trauma. Tendon size parameters are difficult to establish for all breed/sizes, and when possible the contralateral limb should be imaged for comparison (**Fig. 3**).

Supraspinatus tendon and muscle[13,14]: the supraspinatus tendon has the least well-organized fiber pattern of the structures of the shoulder. The insertion is broad,

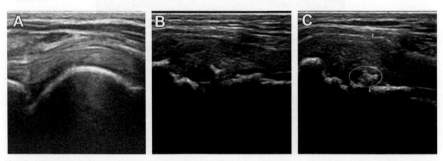

Fig. 3. Biceps tendon in long axis (sagittal plane). Proximal is to the left. Normal (*A*), minute mineral foci and thickening (*B*) and advanced disease (marked thickening, large mineral foci) (*C*). BCT is between blue arrows in the right image. Mineral foci are denoted by red arrows.

extending along the medial aspect of the greater tubercle. The musculotendinous junction is not well defined, as the tendon collects fibers from the deep aspect of the muscle along its distal extent. It is typically imaged in a sagittal plane by sliding the transducer laterally from the sagittal image of the mid-biceps tendon. The tendon and musculotendinous junction can be imaged in a transverse plane by locating the muscle cranial to the spine of the scapula and following the structure distally to its insertion.

The normal heterogeneity of the tendon makes interpretation of subtle fiber pattern changes difficult. Pathologic changes are typically mineralization of the tendon near the insertion and may vary from small pinpoint foci with minimal distal shadowing to large foci creating large regions of distal acoustic shadowing. Enthesophytes at the insertion on the greater tubercle are commonly noted in cases of advanced pathology (**Fig. 4**).

Infraspinatus tendon (IST) and muscle: this structure is easily imaged due to its uniform and highly structured distal tendon pattern. It inserts slightly distal to the supraspinatus tendon, often described as a "button-like" insertion in a small osseous divot (**Fig. 5**). The short tendon can be followed proximally into the muscle belly caudal to the scapular spine.

Pathologic changes are typically mineralization of the tendon near the insertion. Imaging pathology of IST contracture will depend on the stage of pathology. Hyperechoic disorganized regions within the muscle, secondary to hemorrhage and edema, are the hallmark of acute phase imaging. However, more commonly, these are imaged in the chronic stages, when there is muscle atrophy and muscle heterogeneity with hypoechoic fibrosis and mineralization of the tendon or muscle itself.[15,16]

Joint, joint capsule, and stabilizing structures: these structures are difficult to image via ultrasound in a complete fashion, as the medial aspect of the joint is particularly difficult to image.

The joint and joint capsule should be evaluated for excessive effusion and/or capsular thickening. The joint extension along the biceps tendon is a region that should be evaluated for effusion. Care must be taken not to overinterpret a small accumulation of joint fluid in the distal aspect of the capsule along the deep aspect of the biceps as pathology, but rather as a consequence of positioning, limb manipulation, and pressure on the joint from the ultrasound transducer (**Fig. 6**). The lateral and medial glenohumeral ligaments and the transverse humeral ligament/retinaculum are poorly visualized on ultrasound.

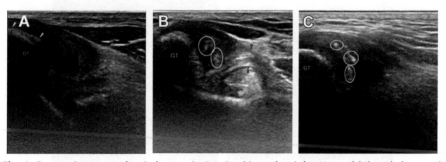

Fig. 4. Supraspinatus tendon in long axis. Proximal is to the right. Normal (*A*) and abnormal (*B, C*) tendon, with thickening, heterogeneity, and mineralization (*blue ovals*). Red arrows denote tendon before its expansion to attach on the greater tubercle of the humerus (GT, *blue arrows* in normal image).

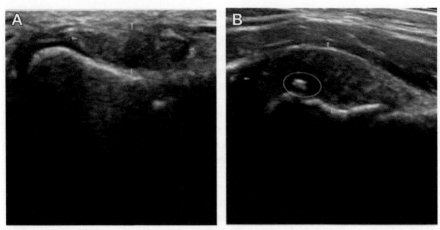

Fig. 5. Infraspinatus tendon in short axis (transverse plane). Normal (*A*) and abnormal (*B*) tendon (*blue arrows*) with enlargement and mineralization *(blue oval)*.

Brachial plexus[17]: imaging of the proximal brachial plexus is best left for MR evaluation, as the tissue is often poorly visualized on ultrasound due to its deep location and close association with vasculature. Ultrasound is more appropriate for regional scanning of the more distal brachial plexus, which is commonly imaged with the patient in dorsal recumbency, with the forelimb slightly abducted. Given the large region of anatomy, clipping/shaving of the region may only be performed on longer hair dogs. Often a cursory examination with alcohol is performed to define a region of interest, which is then clipped and prepped for more thorough ultrasound.

Because it is difficult to follow nerve structures in the region, a generalized "search" for nodules, masses, or regions of edema/cellulitis, using an overlapping series of passes in 2 planes is commonly used.

In general, ultrasound may be of low yield for small lesions due to complexity of anatomy and fascia in the region. Pathology will depend on the lesion type, although common findings associated with neoplasia of the brachial plexus include nerve thickening, nodules, or masses in the axillary or caudoventral neck region.

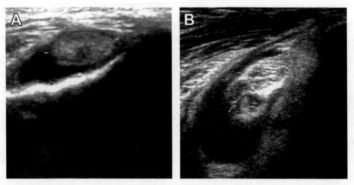

Fig. 6. Distal aspect of biceps tendon, slightly proximal to the musculotendinous junction, in transverse plane. Fluid accumulation (*red arrows*) in distal extension of joint capsule normal (*A*), pathologic (*B*) surrounding the medial aspect of the biceps tendon (*blue arrows*).

Ultrasound Benefits

Ultrasound examination of the shoulder has numerous benefits over other imaging modalities.

- Ultrasound is more readily available, fast, and noninvasive.
- Ultrasound has excellent tissue contrast, particularly for soft tissue structures, far superior to radiography and CT.
- Nonionizing radiation—benefit to pet and hospital staff.
- The cost is significantly less than that of MR. Although sedation is highly recommended, full anesthesia is rarely necessary, saving on cost and decreasing risk to the patient. Full anesthesia is of particular benefit in the follow-up setting, where a lesion may be tracked over weeks or months.
- A dynamic study can be performed in ultrasound, placing the leg through range of motion or in a position that best delineates a lesion, which is rarely possible in MR, in all but the most advanced research settings.
- May guide diagnostic sampling (aspiration, biopsy) and therapy (tendon injections, joint injections)

Ultrasound Challenges

- Requires advanced skill set with expertise in image acquisition
  - Imaging diagnosis depends on accurate depiction of lesions
- No "global" view of structures
- Minimal ability to adequately image osseous structures
- Minimal ability to image proximal brachial plexus
  - Distal brachial plexus limited evaluation
- Imaging artifacts may hamper interpretation
- Difficult to submit for teleradiology/second opinion

MRI

Anatomy of interest and associated pathology

Shoulder:
- Biceps brachii
- Supraspinatus tendon
- Infraspinatus tendon
- Stabilizing structures and joint capsule
- Repetitive stress injury, acute injury of the tendinous structures (see The Shoulder Joint and Common Abnormalities by Stokes and Dycus)

Brachial plexus:
- C5–7 nerve roots and regional/cervical spinal cord
- Nerve path to axilla
- Axillary region
- Nerve sheath tumors, lymphoma, neuritis (see Neurologic Causes of Thoracic Limb Lameness by Kerwin and Taylor)

Introduction: MR, with its remarkable soft tissue contrast resolution is the gold-standard imaging technique for soft tissue injury of the shoulder. Pathology of these structures, including core lesions (disruption of tendon fibers), tears, significant swelling, and chronic changes including fibrosis and mineralization are commonly noted.[9,10,18,19] In addition to those structures imaged on ultrasound, structures of the medial shoulder (ligaments) and transverse humeral ligament are better visualized.

Although CT may provide more anatomic detail of the osseous structures, MR is also the imaging technique of choice for evaluating acute bone injury, as well as bone marrow lesions.

MR is also the gold-standard imaging technique for evaluation of the brachial plexus including the nerve roots, their origin in the spinal cord, and plexi.[20] MR provides a "global view" of structures that allows for an evaluation of symmetry, aiding in lesion detection, as well as secondary changes (muscle atrophy, fibrosis etc.).

Equipment: image quality depends on the ability to obtain a high signal-to-noise ratio (SNR). SNR depends on many factors, with field strength (measured in Tesla [T]) tissue volume (size of structure) and coil selection being the primary determiners. Two types of MR scanners are available: high field (1–3 T) and low field (<0.3 T). As signal-to-noise ratio is proportional to field strength, high-field magnets have higher image quality.[21] New 3 T magnets provide resolution and osseous detail at the level of a CT, previously unachievable at 1.5 T and in low-field magnets. In addition, low-field magnets often have limited appropriate coil selection for canine shoulders.

Imaging sequences: to obtain the highest diagnostic yield, multiple scan sequences need to be performed. Each sequence requires 5 to 15 minutes to obtain images, and thus a balance must be struck between obtaining a thorough, complete examination and scan time. An entire examination may take between 45 minutes and 1.5 hours. in contrast to CT, where typically only 2 scans (of <30 seconds) need be obtained. Similarly, time-consuming MRI scan sequences (except for 3-dimensional (3D) sequences, discussed later) need to be performed in multiple imaging planes, in contrast to CT, where imaging can be reconstructed postacquisition. Sequence selection will depend on the capabilities of the scanning equipment, and personal preference, although it typically includes combinations of the following sequences:

- T1-weighted (T1w)—good to excellent anatomic detail, allows for comparison postcontrast administration
- T2w—low to moderate anatomic detail, with high lesion conspicuity (increased lesion detection)
- Proton density–weighted (PDw)—good anatomic detail with high lesion conspicuity
  ○ Note this sequence is "free" in that it is obtained during the T2w sequence, thus not increasing scan time
- Short tau inversion recovery (STIR)—fat suppression technique—excellent lesion conspicuity, particularly of bone, poor anatomic detail
- T1w C+ postcontrast imaging—contrast taken up by inflammatory and neoplastic lesion cause T1 shortening (increased signal), allowing for comparison to T1w images
- Fat saturation imaging—may be performed on any of the above sequences—suppresses the signal from fat in the bone marrow and fascia, greatly increasing lesion conspicuity. Time consuming
- 3D sequences—allow for postacquisition reconstruction in any plane with good to excellent anatomic detail

TECHNIQUE

Shoulder: the patient is typically positioned in lateral recumbency, with the forelimb in a neutral (standing) position. Imaging of the medial structures of the joint may be improved with slight extension (120°–150°).[19,22] The imaged limb may be placed dependently (on top of flex coil) or may be the nondependent limb with the coil draped over the patient. Occasionally, shoulder imaging is performed in ventral or dorsal recumbency, particularly if a bilateral study is being performed.

As with all musculoskeletal MRIs, coil selection is important. Typically, in combination with a spine coil, a surface or flexible coil is used to obtain the best image quality. A body coil may be used to image large fields of view to assess for muscular symmetry etc.

Arthrographic images, obtained following introduction of gadolinium (or other paramagnetic contrast medium) into the joint, may be of utility in defining adjacent tendon structures, although not commonly performed.[22–24]

Biceps tendon and muscle: the biceps is typically best visualized in a plane sagittal and transverse to the tendon. The highly organized collagen and tightly bound water cause the normal tendon to be hypointense on T1w and T2w imaging. The tendon becomes slightly more heterogenous at the level of the musculotendinous junction as muscle fibers originate. T2w images are generally of utility in imaging effusion surrounding the tendon at the distal intertubercular groove. Pathologic changes typically cause a loss of the hypointense signal, particularly on T2w and PDw images as fiber pattern becomes disrupted. Edema and hemorrhage manifest as increases in T2w, PDw, and STIR images. Enthesopathy at the tendon origin may be present. In extreme cases, tendon discontinuity with avulsion fragments may be visualized (**Fig. 7**).

Supraspinatus tendon and muscle: similar to the biceps tendon, the supraspinatus tendon is best visualized on sagittal and transverse T1w, T2w, and PD images. At its proximal extent the tendon becomes hypointense to muscle as it extends from the musculotendinous junction. The tendon then begins to fan out and become more broader as it inserts on the greater tubercle of the humerus. The normal tendon is described as having a trilaminar appearance on sagittal and transverse images, owing to the hyperintense central substance composition (of water-rich glycosaminoglycans interspersed among haphazardly arranged collagen bundles) surrounded by the more "tendon-like" makeup of the superficial and deep margins.[10]

Similar to ultrasound, the fibrocartilaginous makeup of the distal tendon creates signal heterogeneity and is normally T2w and PDw hyperintense. As most "normal" (highly organized) tendon is typically hypointense, care must be taken not to mistakenly misinterpret this hyperintensity in the distal tendon as a lesion.[10,18] Similarly, this intensity often may make detection of pathology in this location more difficult.

Pathologic features: as most tendons, the supraspinatus tendon becomes more heterogenous and hyperintense secondary to injury. However, the inherent comparative disorganization of tendon fibers, and the inherent normal intensity of the tendon, complicate interpretation. Recently, volume measurements have been proposed, with normalization to humeral head volume and width. Although the technique demonstrated a significant increased tendon volume in noncalcified supraspinatus tendinopathy, volume measurements can be difficult to obtain in practice.[7,10,25]

Impingement or displacement of the biceps tendon secondary to supraspinatus tendon enlargement has been suggested, although few publications exist. On MR, this manifests as medial displacement of the biceps tendon toward, or, in extreme cases, partially beyond the biceps groove onto, the lesser tubercle. Thickening of the transverse humeral ligament and joint effusion may be present[26] (**Fig. 8**A, B).

Infraspinatus tendon and muscle[9,22,27]: this tendon is typically evaluated in all 3 planes (transverse, dorsal, and sagittal) as it extends from the infraspinatus fossa, becoming hypointense at the musculotendinous junction and extending to its insertion on the distal greater tubercle. A hypointense band is often noted centrally and should not be mistaken for pathology.

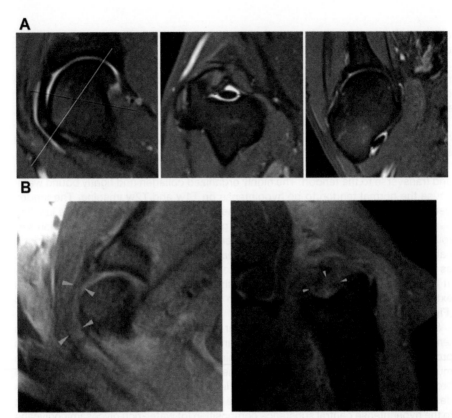

Fig. 7. (*A*) Normal PD fat-saturated images of the biceps tendon in sagittal (a) and transverse planes at 2 levels (b, c). Blue line indicates scan plane (transverse plane of forelimb) for distal biceps (*blue arrows*) just proximal to the musculotendinous junction. Red line indicates scan plane for proximal biceps (dorsal [oblique] plane of forelimb) tendon. Note both planes are transverse to the tendon. (*B*) Marked biceps tendinopathy in PDw sagittal plane (a) and transverse plane (b). Note the increased signal and heterogeneity of the tendon substance, with poor definition of the tendon compared with **Fig. 6**. Partial avulsion is suspected.

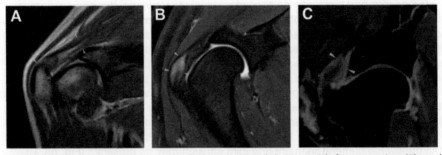

Fig. 8. Supraspinatus tendon in sagittal plane in PDw (*A*), PDw with fat saturation (*B*), and T1w 3D VIBE (*C*) sequences. Normal supraspinatus tendon (*A*), mild supraspinatus tendon enlargement and heterogeneity (*B*), moderate supraspinatus tendon enlargement, heterogeneity and mineralization (*C*). Blue arrows denote supraspinatus tendon. Red arrows denote mineralization. Note the heterogeneity in signal at the insertion in the normal tendon.

Pathologic features: in addition to tendinopathies common to all tendons, fibrotic muscle contracture has been described in the infraspinatus tendon. In the subacute phase, muscle swelling and heterogeneity are present, consistent with hemorrhage and edema. This manifests as increased T2w (and PD signal) within the muscle.[9,27] As the disease becomes chronic, the muscle returns to normal size, then becomes atrophied, often with large signal voids (hypointensities) on T1w and T2w imaging that may correspond to fibrous tissue,[27] or in even more chronic disease, mineralization (**Fig. 9**A, B).

Joint, Joint Capsule, and Stabilizing Structures

The transverse humeral ligament can be visualized crossing over the cranial aspect of the biceps between the greater (lateral) and lesser (medial) tubercles. The medial

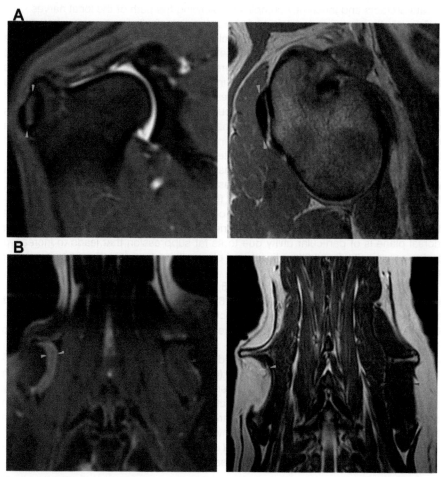

Fig. 9. (A) Infraspinatus tendon in transverse plane, PDw (A) sequence, T1w (B) transverse images. (B) Infraspinatus muscle contracture in the subacute (A) and chronic (B) phases. Note the atrophy and increased contrast enhancement of the right infraspinatus muscle (*blue arrows*) compared with the left (*red arrows*). Note the marked atrophy and loss of contrast enhancement in the chronic stage (B). Left limb is normal in both images. Note the concomitant ipsilateral supraspinatus muscle atrophy, without contrast enhancement, due to disuse.

glenohumeral ligament is typically difficult to distinguish from the adjacent joint capsule on nonarthrographic images but is best visualized on transverse T2w images.[18] The ligament is better visualized in the presence of joint effusion.

The lateral glenohumeral ligament and joint capsule can rarely be imaged as separate structures. Significant pathology must be present to identify lesions in these structures.[19] Joint capsule effusion or capsular thickening can be differentiated on MRI.[28] Glenohumeral ligament thickening has also been documented.[9,23]

Brachial Plexus

The brachial plexus is a difficult region to image because of several reasons: diversity of lesions (neoplastic to traumatic), overall anatomic region from spine to limb, complicated anatomy, and close association with arterial and venous structures, which both create artifacts and inherently complicate following the path of the local nerves.

As such, the approach to a brachial plexus lesion typically involves a systematic yet dynamic approach, beginning at the level of the nerve roots, extending down the length of the nerves and the cervical spine to the axilla, then following the nerves as distally as is possible into the proximal forelimb. Given the nature of brachial plexus lesions, and their large anatomic region, initial imaging is often designed to "cast a wide net" over the entire region of interest, while limiting scan time. Unlike some MR regions (eg, brain) that follow a fairly routine course of imaging, the brachial plexus often requires dynamic decision-making, as lesions of concern are identified on these early sequences. Additional sequences, in multiple planes, can then be performed through smaller regions of interest at the level of identified lesions.

Appropriate patient positioning, in sternal or dorsal recumbency with the forelimbs extended cranially, often provides the best opportunity for evaluation of symmetry. Depending on patient size, a body coil or flex coil is typically used.

Large field-of-view images are typically obtained in T1w, T2w, and STIR sequences to evaluate all of the length of the C5-T2 nerves. STIR, or fat-saturated, imaging in a dorsal plane is of particular utility due to its fat suppression that leads to increased lesion conspicuity. In addition, the dorsal plane allows for evaluation of symmetry of an inherently complicated region.

The brachial plexus nerve roots of the C6,7,8 and T1-2 can be well visualized on MR, exiting their respective foramina at C5-6, 6-7, C7-T1, and T1-2 and T2-3. *(Note that the cervical nerves are named with respect to the vertebral caudal to each nerve [1–8], whereas the thoracic nerves are named with respect to the vertebral cranial to each nerve.)

As mentioned, an STIR sequence in the dorsal plane aids in lesion detection. As potential lesions become identified, 3 plane (dorsal, transverse, and sagittal) images in T2w and T1w (+/− fat saturation) are often obtained. 3D sequences are particularly useful when endeavoring to follow the path of the nerve, as small modifications in angle can be made on the viewing software. Additional sequences may be added to suppress pure fluid (fluid-attenuated inversion recovery) or hemorrhage (T2*w) depending on the appearance of lesions of concern. Generally, T1w C+ imaging is acquired last and is often acquired with fat saturation.

PATHOLOGY

Neoplasia: the most common neoplastic lesions of the brachial plexus are peripheral nerve sheath tumors or lymphoma and may occur at the level of the root (spinal, foraminal), the plexus (postforaminal), or peripherally (distal to the plexus).[29,30] Lesions are typically isointense to muscle on T1w images, are T2w hyperintense or heterogenous, STIR hyperintense, and are moderately to markedly contrast enhancing. Ipsilateral regional muscle atrophy is present depending on the chronicity of the disease. Atrophied muscles are often heterogenous and hyperintense to the contralateral limb on T1w, T2w, and STIR images, with variable contrast enhancement. Lesions may be tubular thickening of the nerve, and follow the nerve over an extended distance, or reasonably well-circumscribed masses.

Inflammatory lesions of the brachial plexus are not common, although have been described in both dogs and cats. Bilateral nerve thickening with variable enhancement may occur.

Traumatic injuries of the brachial plexus are most often diagnosed before imaging evaluation based on clinical signs and history. These lesions can be particularly difficult to image due to regional tissue trauma, edema, and hemorrhage. Regions of inflammation may be STIR hyperintense with T2w hyperintensity of adjacent nerves secondary to edema or malacia. If ascending malacia is present due to an avulsion near the foramina, T2w hyperintensity may be noted extending into the vertebral canal (**Fig. 10**A, B).

Imaging pitfalls: the most common pitfalls are in image acquisition. Spin echo sequences (T1w, T2w, and STIR) are difficult to reconstruct in additional planes. Thus it is important to obtain ALL necessary images at the time of acquisition. 3D sequences have aided in the ability to postreconstruct images, although they may not have the inherent lesion conspicuity of other image sequences.

MR is quite sensitive to motion, and respiratory motion may be difficult to avoid, particularly in the deep brachial plexus region. Unlike CT, where only a single slice is affected, if motion occurs during acquisition in MRI, this often affects every image in the series, and the sequence must be repeated.

An imaging artifact unique to tendons is known as the "magic angle" artifact.[2,3,31] The hypointensity of tendons arises from rapid dephasing of water molecules. When the highly organized tendon collagen fibers are oriented at particular angles with respect to the main magnetic field (multiples of 55°), this dephasing slows, resulting in increased signal intensity from the structure. This increased signal (usually only noted on T1w, PD, and STIR images) is often misinterpreted as tendon pathology. Comparison with the T2w sequence, which is unaffected, can aid in differentiation of artifact from lesion[32] (**Fig. 11**).

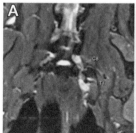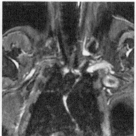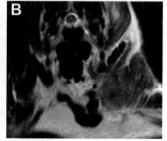

Fig. 10. (*A*) T1w C+ dorsal plane images of the axillary region. Brachial plexus nerve enlargement, suspect lymphoma, or peripheral nerve sheath tumor. Green arrows denote caudal cervical (C8, T1) nerves. (*B*). Transverse plane T1w C+ image at the cranial aspect of the axillary region. Brachial plexus avulsion. Avulsion and enlargement of the T1 nerve root (*red arrows*) as it enters a region of tissue edema and hemorrhage (*red oval*). Patient sustained trauma (hit by car). The nerve could not be traced into or beyond the region of cellulitis/hemorrhage.

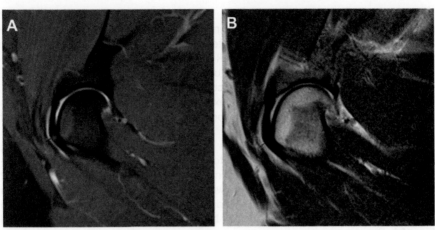

Fig. 11. (*A, B*) Sagittal images of the shoulder demonstrating magic angle artifact. Note the hyperintensity within the tendon on PDw image (*A*) that can be confirmed to be artifactual by evaluating the T2w sequence (*B*). *Red arrow* points to Pdw hyperintensity.

MRI Benefits

MR examination of the shoulder and brachial plexus has numerous benefits over other imaging modalities.

- Exquisite soft tissue contrast resolution
- Ability to view large area at one time—"global view" of structures of interest
- Can allow comparison with contralateral limb for a "built-in control"
- Nonionizing radiation—benefit to pet and hospital staff
- Ability to obtain images and view at a later time point or submit for interpretation

MRI Challenges

- Requires advanced interpretation skill set with expertise in image acquisition
  ○ Imaging diagnosis depends on accurate depiction of lesions
- Osseous structures may be more difficult to image than on CT
- Cost/availability
- Requires extended anesthesia
- Imaging artifacts may hamper interpretation

SUMMARY

A definitive/precise diagnosis of shoulder or brachial plexus injury often involves imaging beyond traditional radiographs or even CT. Ultrasound and MR can further evaluate lesions identified radiographically (eg, mineralization) or identify lesions not present on radiographic examination.

Given the common histologic pathology (tendon fiber/fibril disruption due to edema, hemorrhage, fibrosis, mineralization), tendinous lesions have a typical pattern on ultrasound and MRI with loss of the normal hypoechoic/hypointense appearance, regardless of the tendon involved.

Ultrasound, with its availability, low cost, and ease of use, is a valuable technique in further defining lesions of the tendons of the shoulder. This is not to undersell the knowledge of anatomy, normal appearance, and skill necessary to obtain diagnostic quality images.

The ability of MR to define pathology of soft tissues is of particularly utility in localizing lesions of the shoulder and brachial plexus, causing forelimb lameness.

A thorough evaluation of the biceps, supraspinatus, and infraspinatus tendons for regions of PD, STIR, and T2w hyperintensity and their corresponding musculature for signs of atrophy may lead to an accurate diagnosis.

Brachial plexus lesions involve a dynamic "wide-to-narrow" search pattern often starting with dorsal plane sequences to evaluate for tissue symmetry. Similar to ultrasound, a knowledge of anatomy, normal appearance, and knowledge of common artifacts is necessary to arrive at an accurate diagnosis.

CLINICS CARE POINTS

Ultrasound:
- Use the highest frequency probe available for shoulder tendons
- Plan to have the patient sedated—a pet with shoulder pain will resent pressure and manipulation
- Prep the region well—hair and debris hamper adequate image acquisition
- Be sure to only interpret the regions of tendon that are 80° to 100° to the probe footprint—tendon outside this angle may be artificially increased in echogenicity due to anisotropy
- Evaluate all major tendons for pathology—satisfaction of search on finding a lesion in one tendon does not rule out pathology in another
- Evaluate the contralateral limb, both for comparison and additional pathology

MR
- Develop a scan protocol for the shoulder—deciding which sequences to run after the fact is time consuming and increases anesthesia time
- Brachial plexus scans often require dynamic decision-making, and a predetermined/formulaic approach often results in increased scan time (scanning of non-lesion areas) or inadequate sequences through a lesion
- Recognize artifacts—motion, including motion of blood, will hamper image interpretation. "Magic angle" creates hyperintense regions in otherwise hypointense tendons.

DISCLOSURE

Nothing to disclose.

REFERENCES

1. Squire N, Canapp SO, Canapp D, et al. Assessment of magnetic resonance imaging, musculoskeletal ultrasound, and arthroscopy in the diagnosis of medial shoulder syndrome in canines. Vet Comp Orthopaed 2019;32:A13–24.

2. Sage JE, Gavin P. Musculoskeletal MRI. Vet Clin North Am Small Anim Pract 2016;46:421–51.

3. Gavin, P. R. Practical Small Animal MRI. 10–20 (2009) https://doi.org/10.1002/9780813810324.ch1c.

4. Weinreb JH, Chirag S, John A, et al. Tendon structure, disease, and imaging. Muscles Ligaments Tendons J 2014;4:66–73.

5. Iwona SS, Brygida K, Monika PS, et al. Enthesopathies and enthesitis. Part 1. Etiopathogenesis. J Ultrason 2015;15:72–84.

6. Khan KM, Cook JL, Bonar F, et al. Histopathology of common tendinopathies: update and implications for clinical management. Sports Med 1999;27:393–408.

7. Kannus P, Józsa L. Histopathological changes preceding spontaneous rupture of a tendon. A controlled study of 891 patients. J Bone Joint Surg Am 1991;73: 1507–25.

8. Lafuente MP, Fransson BA, Lincoln JD, et al. Surgical treatment of mineralized and nonmineralized supraspinatus tendinopathy in twenty-four dogs. Vet Surg 2009;38:380–7.

9. Murphy SE, Ballegeer EA, Forrest LJ, et al. Magnetic resonance imaging findings in dogs with confirmed shoulder pathology. Vet Surg 2008;37:631–8.

10. Pownder SL, Brian GC, Kei H, et al. Magnetic resonance imaging and histologic features of the supraspinatus tendon in nonlame dogs. Am J Vet Res 2018;79: 836–44.

11. Long CD, Nyland TG. Ultrasonographic evaluation of the canine shoulder. Vet Radiol Ultrasound 1999;40:372–9.

12. Barella G, Lodi M, Faverzani S. Ultrasonographic findings of shoulder tenomuscular structures in symptomatic and asymptomatic dogs. J Ultrasound 2018;21:145–52.

13. Lassaigne CC, Boyer C, Sautier L, et al. Ultrasound of the normal canine supraspinatus tendon: comparison with gross anatomy and histology. Vet Rec 2019; 186:e14.

14. Canapp SO, Canapp DA, Carr BJ, et al. Supraspinatus Tendinopathy in 327 dogs: a retrospective study. Vet Evid 2016;1:1–13.

15. Franch J, Bertran J, Remolins G, et al. Simultaneous bilateral contracture of the infraspinatus muscle. Vet Comp Orthop Traumatol 2009;22:249–52.

16. Siems JJ, Breur GJ, Blevins WE, Cornell KK. Use of two-dimensional real-time ultrasonography for diagnosing contracture and strain of the infraspinatus muscle in a dog. J Am Vet Med Assoc 1998;212:77–80.

17. Guilherme S, Benigni L. Ultrasonographic anatomy of the brachial plexus and major nerves of the canine thoracic limb: canine brachial plexus ultrasound. Vet Radiol Ultrasound 2008;49:577–83.

18. Schaefer SL, Forrest LJ. Magnetic resonance imaging of the canine shoulder: an anatomic study. Vet Surg 2006;35:721–8.

19. Zalcman, A. R. Cook, C. Mai, and W. Diagnostic MRI in Dogs and Cats. (2018). https://doi.org/10.1201/9781315121055. Chapter 4.

20. Kraft S, Ehrhart EJ, David G, et al. Magnetic resonance imaging characteristics of peripheral nerve sheath tumors of the canine brachial plexus in 18 dogs. Vet Radiol Ultrasound 2007;48:1–7.

21. Magee T, Shapiro M, Williams D. Comparison of high-field-strength versus low-field-strength MRI of the shoulder. Am J Roentgenol 2003;181:1211–5.

22. Agnello KA, Puchalski SM, Erik RW, et al. Effect of positioning, scan plane, and arthrography on visibility of periarticular canine shoulder soft tissue structures on magnetic resonance images. Vet Radiol Ultrasound 2008;49:529–39.

23. Schaefer SL, Baumel CA, Jamie RG, et al. Direct magnetic resonance arthrography of the canine shoulder. Vet Radiol Ultrasound 2010;51:391–6.

24. Rycke LMD, Gielen IM, Dingemanse W, et al. Computed tomographic and low-field magnetic resonance arthrography: a comparison of techniques for observing intra-articular structures of the normal canine shoulder. Computed tomographic and low-field magnetic resonance arthrography. Vet Surg 2015; 44:704–12.

25. Spall BF, Fransson BA, Martinez SA, et al. Tendon volume determination on magnetic resonance imaging of supraspinatus tendinopathy. Vet Surg 2016;45: 386–91.
26. Fransson BA, Gavin PR, Lahmers KK. Supraspinatus tendinosis associated with biceps brachii tendon displacement in a dog. J Am Vet Med Assoc 2005;227: 1429–33.
27. Orellana-james NG, Ginja MM, Regueiro M, et al. Sub-acute and chronic MRI findings in bilateral canine fibrotic contracture of the infraspinatus muscle. J Small Anim Pract 2013;54:428–31.
28. Carr BJ, Canapp SO, Canapp DA, et al. Adhesive capsulitis in eight dogs: diagnosis and management. Front Vet Sci 2016;3:55.
29. Brehm DM, Vite CH, Steinberg HS, et al. A retrospective evaluation of 51 cases of peripheral nerve sheath tumors in the dog. J Am Anim Hosp Assoc 1995;31: 349–59.
30. Zhalniarovich Y, Adamiak Z, Holak P, et al. Diagnosis of a brachial plexus tumour using magnetic resonance imaging assisted by fine-needle aspiration biopsy in a dog: a case report. Vet Med 2014;59:146–9.
31. Vahlensieck & Martin. MRI of the musculoskeletal system. (2000) https://doi.org/10.1055/b-0034-51218. Appendix 15-2.
32. Richardson ML, Amini B, Richards TL. Some new angles on the magic angle: what MSK radiologists know and don't know about this phenomenon. Skeletal Radiol 2018;47:1673–81.

Rehabilitation of the Canine Forelimb

Jennifer A. Brown, DVM[a],*, Julia Tomlinson, BVSc, PhD[b]

KEYWORDS

- Veterinary rehabilitation therapy • Photobiomodulation (laser therapy)
- Extracorporal shockwave therapy • Therapeutic ultrasound • Hydrotherapy
- Tissue healing • Therapeutic exercise

KEY POINTS

- The foundation of therapy is the utilization of structured and controlled tissue loading and manual therapy to help build strength and mobility in both affected and supporting structures.
- Therapeutic modalities are used with the goal of stimulating an appropriate healing response, and, in some cases, this involves the breakdown of abnormal tissue.
- Thorough knowledge of the inflammatory and repair response of each type of tissue will guide the rehabilitation plan.

INTRODUCTION

The goal of rehabilitation is to restore function and mobility and reduce pain associated with chronic disease such as osteoarthritis or following surgery or injury. In human medicine, physical therapy is standard of care for both acute and chronic injuries and an integral component of post-operative recovery; often implemented before the patient is discharged. While there is a dearth of evidence based veterinary medical studies in rehabilitation therapy and modalities for forelimb injuries in dogs, some extrapolation from human medicine can be made and applied to improve outcome and quality of life. What is important to consider when developing a rehabilitation and therapeutic plan is the biomechanics of the affected limb and timeline of tissue healing of the target tissue and/or joint.

THERAPEUTIC EXERCISE AND MANUAL THERAPY

The foundation of both in-clinic and at-home therapy is the utilization of structured and controlled exercise and manual therapy to help build strength and mobility in both

[a] Florida Veterinary Rehabilitation and Sports Medicine, 11016 North Dale Mabry Highway, #202, Tampa, FL 33618, USA; [b] Twin Cities Animal Rehabilitation & Sports Medicine Clinic, 12010 Riverwood Drive, Burnsville, MN 55337, USA
* Corresponding author.
E-mail address: dr.brown@floridavetrehab.com

affected and supporting structures. Components of this program include active and targeted exercise, range of motion (ROM), stretching, and joint mobilizations.

ROM can be passive, active, and active assisted and is utilized to maintain and restore normal joint kinematics and soft tissue flexibility. Passive ROM (PROM) is the act of applying an external force to the joint, taking it to its kinematic end range when the muscles are relaxed, and commonly is applied by a therapist or owner with the dog in a relaxed position. Stretching also is a component of PROM and, even when applied by the owner, this can help improve joint ROM. In a study of 10 Labrador retrievers with elbow osteoarthritis, PROM/stretching was performed daily for 3 weeks (10 repetitions of flexion and extension holding for 10 seconds at comfortable end range) and resulted in a statistically significant improvement in ROM.[1] ROM in this study was determined utilizing goniometry, which is a useful and reliable objective outcome measure.[2] Active and active assisted ROM in veterinary patients typically is facilitated by use of targeted therapeutic exercises focusing on the joints in question.

Therapeutic exercise aims to target both muscle activation and joint kinematics, although the specific effects of many targeted exercises used in veterinary rehabilitation currently are unknown. A few studies have given insight in both the forelimbs and hind limbs to help rehabilitation therapists design exercise programs appropriate for the injury, but more work needs to be done. In normal dogs, kinematic analysis of dogs walking down either stairs or a ramp evaluated peak extension and flexion as well as ROM were measured.[3] The investigators found no differences in the carpus, and, in the shoulder, increase in ROM was increased only on stair descent.[3] In the elbow, peak flexion and ROM were increased significantly with both stairs and ramp descent, but peak extension was maximal when trotting over a flat surface.[3] Comparing this to ascent up a similar grade of ramp or stairs, carpal, elbow, and shoulder flexion and extension were increased versus trotting over a flat surface.[4] Ramp ascent had more effect on shoulder ROM and stair ascent on carpus and elbow.[4] Another study in normal dogs looking at incline, decline walking, and stepping over obstacles showed that only stepping over obstacles significantly affected forelimbs' ROM.[5] Hurdles placed at carpal height resulted in increased elbow flexion and carpal flexion versus walking in the flat and increased carpal extension.[5] Weight also can be used to apply controlled loading to the forelimbs in the later stages of rehabilitation, because carrying a weight in the mouth increases load on the forelimbs.[6] Activation of specific muscle groups during therapeutic exercises utilizing surface electromyography has been evaluated in several studies.[7–9] Although similar work has not been done targeting forelimb musculature, future work in this area may help determine which therapeutic exercises would be of value in targeting specific muscle groups as it did in the hind limbs.

THERAPEUTIC MODALITIES AND THEIR EFFECTS ON TISSUE HEALING, FUNCTION, AND PAIN

Therapeutic modalities are used with the goal of stimulating an appropriate healing response, and, in some cases, this involves the breakdown of abnormal tissue. In addition to understanding how modalities work, timing of application relative to phase of healing and patient status should be considered.

Photobiomodulation (Low-Level Laser Therapy, Therapeutic Laser, and Cold Laser)

Ubiquitous in rehabilitation as well as in many general practices, photobiomodulation therapy probably is the modality applied most commonly for a plethora of problems.

Photobiomodulation therapy utilizes the properties of light delivered to tissues at a specific wavelength to affect cell function.[10–12] For pain modulation, mechanisms are through increasing endogenous opioid neurotransmitter production and increased adenosine triphosphate (ATP) production. Increased ATP production also plays a role in tissue healing via increases in mitochondrial metabolism.[13] Photobiomodulation therapy also aids in the dissociation of nitric oxide (NO) from cytochrome C oxidase, thereby improving cellular respiration.[14] Lasers also may stimulate DNA production and stem cell proliferation in various tissues.[15] Anti-inflammatory effects include increasing peripheral blood flow due to NO release as well as reducing prostaglandin E_2, cyclooxygenase (COX)-2, and inflammatory cytokines.[12]

Although photobiomodulation therapy use is widespread, little research has been performed in the veterinary field. In the laboratory setting and in clinical studies in human medicine, the use of photobiomodulation therapy has had mixed results in showing efficacy in musculoskeletal injuries.[16,17] Extrapolation from the multitude of studies in laboratory animals and humans for use in clinical veterinary medicine can be difficult because methodology varies widely in regard to dose, wavelength, and power of lasers used for treatment. In addition, penetration of photons may differ in the canine dermis compared with other species. In horses, skin thickness, coat color, and skin preparation were significantly associated with laser penetration to flexor tendons.[18,19] Factors, such as coat color and laser power and wavelength, appear to play a role in canines as well. In a recent study, dogs with darker skin showed significantly less penetration of laser light than those with lighter skin, and shaving increased the transmission in dogs with darker coats.[20] Wavelength and power also influenced laser transmission in the same study.[20] Appropriate dosage (measured in joules per square centimeter) for different tissues and pathology also may be a factor affecting clinical outcome. For example, in dogs with elbow osteoarthritis, the recommended dosage is 8.0 J/cm^2 to 10.0 J/cm^2; however, in a recent study, clinical improvement was not seen at this standard dose and doses up to 20.0 J/cm^2 were required.[21] It is not surprising that there likely are different dosage needs for different tissue types, pathology, and stage of healing as well as the goal of the treatment (pain modulation, anti-inflammatory, or tissue healing), but they have not been specifically defined in the literature. These factors all should be considered when applying photobiomodulation therapy. Simple crude outcome measures, such as palpation before and after photobiomodulation therapy to assess for a temporary analgesic effect, currently are indicated in practice.

Superficial Thermotherapy

Application of either heat or cold to injured tissues can help with pain, function, and inflammation control. Cryotherapy commonly is utilized postsurgery, after trauma, or following training. The goals of cryotherapy are to provide analgesia and decrease blood flow due to vasoconstriction. Decreasing blood flow to an area decreases edema formation and slow acute inflammation via decreasing metabolic rate and proinflammatory enzyme production. Application of cold packs has been shown to decrease intra-articular temperatures in a time-dependent manner up to 30 minutes of application.[22] In soft tissues, both superficial and deep muscles can be cooled effectively and blood flow decreased.[23,24] Superficial tissue layers are cooled more rapidly, but both retain the decreased temperature for up to 70 minutes after removal.[23,24] Compression cryotherapy has been shown to be beneficial in both humans and in dogs following knee surgery, with patients having decreased pain, improved ROM, and less edema in the acute phase.[25–27] In later stages, however, there is not an appreciable difference between compression cryotherapy and cryotherapy.[25]

The role of heat in physical rehabilitation is to reduce pain and improve tissue mobility, especially in conjunction with ROM and stretching. Extensibility of collagen containing tissue is increased significantly by the application of heat, allowing for elongation of the tissues.[28] In dogs with restrictions in ROM or loss of stretch, heat application in conjunction with manual therapy (PROM or stretching) may help therapist and owner achieve greater tissue mobility. The use of moist heat (either submersion or moist heat pack) over dry heat (heating pad) appears to achieve greater increases in heating deeper tissues in shorter periods of time.[29,30] Achieving the increase in temperature necessary to produce collagen extensibility can be difficult based on location, with areas that have significant fat layers substantially inhibiting heat transfer.[31] With an increase in 4°C as the temperature goal to increase collagen extensibility, this may be achieved only at depths less than 3 cm. In 1 study, after a 15-minute application of moist heat packs at 75°C, only a 0.75°C increase was observed at 3 cm, with a 3.83°C increase at 1 cm.[32] Another important component is the performance of PROM or stretching either during or immediately after the application of heat therapy. Multiple studies in people have shown that objective analysis of ROM and/or stretch was improved after heat application versus without, and a few studies showed that simultaneous heat application had more benefit.[33] Although superficial heat application is inferior to therapeutic ultrasound in heating deeper tissues, it can be useful especially to optimize an in-home therapeutic program to help restore normal ROM and stretch in affected tissues.

Therapeutic Ultrasound

Therapeutic ultrasound utilizes high-frequency sound waves applied to tissue for either thermal or nonthermal effects. One of the primary applications of therapeutic ultrasound is for heating of tissue. Heating tissue increases tissue elasticity, decreases spasm, and increases blood flow. Frequency (measured in hertz), intensity (measured in watts/square centimeters), duration, and tissue properties influence the amount and depth of tissue heating that can be achieved. In dogs, coat also can be an inhibiting factor. For thermal effects to be therapeutic, the tissue needs to be heated from 1°C to 4°C.[34] Frequency dictates depth of penetration, with 1-MHz heating at depths between 2 cm and 5 cm and 3.3-MHz heating between 0.5 cm and 3 cm. Intensity has the most influence on heat production in tissue; with increasing intensity, increased temperature change is noted in muscle tissue in dogs; 1.0-MHz and 3.3-MHz tissue heating within the proposed therapeutic heat range can be achieved between 1.0 W/cm^2 and 2.0 W/cm^2.[35,36] In order to utilize ultrasound for its therapeutic effects, clipping is required, no matter the coat length, and cannot be overcome by increasing the intensity. In 1 study, the hair coat was shown to absorb most of the heat with little to no heat produced in the underlying muscle tissue.[35]

Nonthermal effects focus on cavitation and acoustic streaming to improve collagen organization, decrease inflammatory cell migration, and increase tensile strength to tendon. The mechanisms of these actions and their outcomes in tissue healing have been studied widely in laboratory animals with mixed success, with some studies showing benefit in healing and strength of the tissue in experimental models and others showing no benefit.[37]

Extracorporeal Shock Wave Therapy

Extracorporeal shock wave therapy (ESWT) utilizes equipment designed to deliver high-intensity sound waves through tissue to relieve pain and stimulate tissue healing. In acute inflammation associated with wound healing, EWST has been shown to reduce apoptosis and reduce the expression of proinflammatory cytokines.[38,39]

When applied to tissue, EWST has mechanotransduction effects; stimulates growth factor production; and up-regulates tumor necrosis factor (TNF)-β, bone morphogenic protein, fibroblast growth factor (FGF)-2, and transforming growth factor (TGF)-β1.[40] Playing a role in treatment of insertionopathy, shock wave therapy increases type II collagen synthesis and neovascularization at the bone-tendon interface.[41] In animal models, ESWT slowed the progression of osteoarthritis via reduction in apoptosis and NO production and reduced expression of calcitonin gene–related peptide in dorsal root ganglion neurons, which are associated with hyperalgesia in osteoarthritis.[42,43] The mechanism behind the analgesic effects of shock wave therapy are not well understood but may be explained by calcitonin gene–related peptide expression or decreases in nerve conduction velocity from myelin sheath separation, as studied in horses.[42,44,45] These effects, however, may be only temporary.

There are 4 different types of shock wave that can be utilized: electrohydraulic, electromagnetic, piezoelectric, and radial. Radial is not considered true focused medical shock wave because it is a pneumatic delivery that does not penetrate the tissue but rather is dispersed across the tissue. Electrohydraulic is the most widely researched in human and veterinary medicine. Piezoelectric is becoming more popular in veterinary rehabilitation and unlike electrohydraulic does not require sedation for application. Unfortunately, there are no studies validating the efficacy of piezoelectric shock wave in veterinary medicine, but it has shown some efficacy in some musculoskeletal conditions in people.[46,47] In vivo evaluation of electromagnetic, electrohydraulic, piezoelectric, and radial shock wave on chondrocytes of normal and osteoarthritic cartilage did not identify any differences between the machines in the parameters studied.[48]

Clinically, 2 studies have retrospectively evaluated the use of electrohydraulic shock wave therapy on soft tissue pathology of the shoulder (supraspinatus, biceps, medial shoulder syndrome, and so forth). Successful outcomes were reported in 65% (n = 15) and 85% (n = 24) of dogs.[49,50] No published studies are available on the efficacy for other pathologies, such as arthritis in the forelimbs of dogs. In dogs with naturally occurring stifle arthritis, some improvement was noted, but there was not a significant difference compared with controls after 3 treatments.[51] In 2 studies using radial shock wave on dogs with hip arthritis, statistically significant differences were noted in peak vertical force and vertical impulse up to 3 months post-treatment, but changes were no longer significant by 6 months post-treatment. In the second study, improvements were noted using the same kinetic analysis but most parameters lacked significance.[52] In dogs treated with shock wave therapy postoperatively after tibial plateau leveling osteotomy (TPLO) surgery, investigators noted improvement in peak vertical force and vertical impulse, but again statistical significance was not achieved.[53] These studies indicate that there potentially is a place for shock wave therapy in rehabilitation therapy for tissue healing; however, its use in pain management for chronic conditions may be short-lived.

Targeted Pulsed Electromagnetic Field Therapy

Targeted pulsed electromagnetic field (tPEMFs) devices, which are Food and Drug Administration approved in human medicine for controlling postoperative pain and inflammation, use specific pulse widths, frequencies, and waveform bursts to affect tissue at a cellular level. One of the primary mechanisms is their effects on releasing intracellular Ca^{2+} and increasing calcium/calmodulin binding, which up-regulates NO release. This up-regulation of NO release produces anti-inflammatory effects as well as pain control.[54] It also causes up-regulation of growth factors VEGF, FGF, and TGF-β. In women who have had breast surgery, significant decreases in edema, fluid production postoperatively, and pain have been reported.[55,56] In rat models, tPEMF was shown to improve wound healing and tendon healing and produce more rapid neovascularization. Research in clinical veterinary medicine is sparse. Two recent studies evaluated a tPEMF therapy device in randomized placebo-controlled studies in dogs undergoing hemilaminectomies for intervertebral disc disease. In both studies, dogs had reduction in pain, evaluated either by measurement of mechanical sensory thresholds or reduction in pain medication usage in addition to improved wound healing compared with controls.[57,58] tPEMF devices have not been studied on other pathologies or other types of pain, but, based on human research showing benefits in treating patients with arthritis, their use may be able to be extrapolated to some degree for application in animals. Based on current research, tPEMF's role appears mainly in postoperative pain management, edema, and wound healing, but future research may validate it for additional applications.

Neuromuscular Electrostimulation

Along with transcutaneous electrical neuromuscular stimulation, microcurrent and neuromuscular electrostimulation (NMES) are forms of electrotherapy. Although the 2 forms are used primarily for analgesia, NMES is utilized primarily to stimulate muscular contractions. NMES stimulates muscle contractions by depolarization with subsequent activation of muscle tissue with recruitment of type I and type II muscle fibers. The therapeutic goal is to increase muscle strength and tone, stop or reduce atrophy, and improve ROM. NMES has been studied in dogs after TPLO surgery for cranial cruciate ligament deficiency, which often results in moderate atrophy of the affected limb. In dogs that received NMES, canine patients had less osteoarthritis, increased thigh muscle mass, improved lameness scores, and less cartilage damage compared with controls.[59] In humans, NMES used for increasing voluntary muscle strength in partially paralyzed muscle from spinal cord injury was shown to have some benefit.[60] It also is used therapeutically to facilitate standing in lower thoracic spinal cord injury, which resulted in increased blood flow and normalization of quadriceps circumference.[61]

Hydrotherapy

The utilization of water-based therapy, swimming, or underwater treadmill can be an important component of the rehabilitation of forelimb injury, but the choice of which method is dependent on the pathology. The properties of water make it an especially useful medium for rehabilitation therapy for a variety of injuries. Buoyancy of the body when in the water helps decrease load to limbs, which can be useful for dogs that are weak, with chronic orthopedic disease, or with injuries where decrease weight bearing is desired. It has been shown that standing vertical ground reaction force decreases by 62% when immersed into water at hip level.[62] At this water height, however, the distribution of the weight to the forelimbs does increase significantly, with the thoracic-to-pelvic ratio going from 64% on the forelimbs to 71%.[62] So, although buoyancy overall significantly decreases load in general, it increases it in particular for the forelimbs. This likely is not a significant issue due to the relative overall decrease in vertical ground reaction force but should be considered. Viscosity of water is another important characteristic of hydrotherapy. Viscosity creates resistance to movement of the body through the water, which in turn increases workload of the muscles via drag. This increase in workload also is water height dependent. There is an initial increase in muscle activity, as measured through surface electromyogram, of the gluteus medius and longissimus dorsi muscles, with water heights at the level of the tarsus, but, as water height is increased to the greater trochanter, this muscle activity decreases.[63] This change likely is due to increased buoyancy and its effects on stride parameters.[64]

Underwater treadmill has become a commonly used tool in rehabilitation for recovery from musculoskeletal injury, neurologic diseases, and obesity. Walking in water in an underwater treadmill has been shown to affect kinematics of stride and ROM around joints, which all can be manipulated to achieve a therapeutic goal. With increasing water heights, stride frequencies are decreased, and stride length, stance time, and swing time are increased.[64] ROM in the forelimbs also is impacted in a similar manner, with increased flexion achieved with a water height at or above the joint in question.[65] An advantage of underwater treadmill therapy over swimming is that a dog achieves near full walking extension due to ground contact that is not realized with swimming. In canines where extension is a concern, underwater treadmill therapy is preferred.

When dogs swim, they utilize a modified diagonal sequence gait, which is a modification of the gait used from walking over ground, termed *quadrupedal paddling*.[66] At initiation of the power phase of swimming, the shoulders and elbow are flexed and the carpus extended and then the limb extended rapidly through the shoulder and elbow and then swept vertically.[66] During the 2 kinematic phases of the gait, power and recovery, the forelimbs have a longer stroke phase and shorter recovery phase compared with the hind limbs.[66] Rehabilitation therapists need to use caution regarding use of swimming for soft tissue injuries of the forelimb because the repetitive nature of the swim stroke and rapid stretch of soft tissues through the power phase may have negative impacts on healing and pain. For pathologies that affect ROM, such as arthritis, the use of swimming may have more benefit to help restore ROM, but this has not been studied.

TIMELINE OF TISSUE HEALING AND TARGETS FOR REHABILITATION THERAPY

The acute inflammatory response lasts only a few days and is mediated by inflammatory cells from the local vascular supply as well as cells resident in local tissue, which produce cytokines. Prostaglandins change blood flow and sensitize nerves to pain as well as controlling cell growth, a consideration in the use of anti-inflammatory pharmaceuticals. NO relaxes vascular smooth muscle to increase blood flow to the area and it also is involved in oxidative damage and destruction of tissue to clear the path for deposition of healthy tissue. TNF-α and interleukin 1 are cytokines produced from macrophages that cause vasodilation and activate fibroblasts. The balance of tissue removal and of repair depends on how long these cytokines continue to be produced. During the acute inflammatory phase, rehabilitation therapy is focused on pain control and decreasing inflammation through implementation of therapeutic modalities, such as laser therapy and cryotherapy.

In the next phase of tissue healing, fibroblasts and other mesenchymal cells start to replicate to produce collagen, elastin, and ground substance (glycosaminoglycans) in the repair phase; endothelial (capillary lining) cells begin to replicate. Often a tissue in the repair phase is more vascular than necessary for the long term; this is a consideration in rehabilitation. Care is taken loading the tissue because blood vessels are friable and immature collagen easily is deformed. Strength of the tissue starts to increase as collagen is cross-linked and more ground substance is deposited.

The remodeling (maturation) phase is when controlled loading can help tissue strength and flexibility. Collagen fibers are reorientated along stress lines (gravity). Rehabilitation therapists use this to guide correct tissue repair. The maximum collagen amount is produced by 2 weeks to 3 weeks in many tissues; however, tensile strength continues to change and increase over a year. Most tissues do not heal to 100% of original strength, normal appearance, or with 100% elasticity. The aim is for a functional scar that withstands appropriate loads of everyday activities.

HEALING OF SPECIFIC TISSUES AND IMPACTS ON REHABILITATION PROTOCOLS

All tissues respond with inflammation when injured; some tissues have less response than others and that is reflective of their blood supply (eg, tendons and ligaments). These tissues can take longer to heal compared with those with a better blood supply. It is critically important that the rehabilitation therapist be familiar with healing time of the various tissue types because controlled loading as well as therapeutic modalities is used to aid healing (**Table 1**).

Bone

Bone is the only tissue that heals to 100% of original strength if conditions are correct. As bone heals, it is not shaped for normal stresses (callus), so osteoclasts remove bone from sides with less stress. Osteoblasts then are stimulated to make more bone where there is more stress (Wolff's law). Occasionally, healing of a fracture results in a deformity of the bone; this can affect the glide of soft tissues over the area, in which case modalities are used to stimulate bone remodeling with variable success; it is more important to free up soft tissue motion than to achieve remodeling.

With fractures, configuration and method of repair dictate rehabilitation therapy and therapists have to be cognizant of how much load to a fracture postrepair can be applied. One of the most significant morbidities associated with fractures of the forelimb is associated with the use of external coaptation. Immobilization or even lack of full weight bearing causes thinning of articular cartilage and subchondral bone with loss of matrix and thickening of connective tissues. Nerves and blood vessel walls lose elasticity and glide resulting in decreased tissue range of motion. There is thinning cortexes of long bones which can result in significant loss of bone density and osteoporosis. Muscles also atrophy and there is disorganization of fiber alignment in tendons and ligaments with weakened ligament attachment sites. Joint immobilization results in atrophy of cartilage, most marked in the highest weight bearing areas of the joint and often degenerative changes occur in conjunction with atrophy. The amount of synovial fluid in the joint decreases. Changes in cartilage depend on how the joint is immobilized; immobilization in extension leads to osteoarthritis whereas immobilization in flexion leads to disuse atrophy. Rigid fixation results in more cartilage and muscle atrophy. Age also affects how tissues respond to immobilization: young dogs tend to lose cartilage in the calcified zone (where production of new bone occurs in growth and so growth may be affected simply by immobilization) and mature dogs tend to lose cartilage in more superficial, uncalcified areas. Remobilization should be done cautiously, because it takes time for tissues to recover and they may not fully do so depending on the time immobilized and the tissue conditions prior to immobilization. For example, a dog placed in a rigid cast for 6 weeks needs 2 weeks of light weight bearing for cartilage to remodel close to normal strength. When remobilizing a patient's joint, avoid high stresses (more than a walk) and repeated mobilization (repetitive activity). Even daily PROM at this stage produces inflammatory mediators and this can be more than required for healing. When moving from a rigid cast to no support, often it is better to stage down support. Above all it is important to give tissues time to recover and to understand the longer the immobilization, the more likely changes will not be reversible.

The response of muscle to immobilization usually is atrophy, postural muscles are most at risk. These muscles are slow twitch and normally undergo sustained

Table 1
Tissue type and time frame for healing postinjury

Tissue Type	0 Days to 3 Days	4 Days to 14 Days	3 Weeks to 4 Weeks	Weeks	2 Months to 3 Months	3 Months to 6 Months	6 Months to 12 Months	Greater than 1 Year
Bone								
Muscle								
Exercise-induced muscle soreness								
Grade 1								
Grade 2								
Grade 3								
Tendon								
Acute								
Subacute								
Chronic								
Rupture/surgical repair								
Ligament								
Grade 1								
Grade 2								
Grade 3								
Intra-articular								Likely to not heal completely

Adapted from Kirkby Shaw K, Alvarez L, Foster SA, et al. Fundamental principles of rehabilitation and musculoskeletal tissue healing. Vet Surg. 2020;49(1):22-32; with permission.

contraction. Strength decreases rapidly within 1 week of immobilization and within 2 weeks of disuse. After 5 weeks' bed rest to simulate disuse atrophy, human patients lost 10% of their overall muscle mass.[67] The muscles crossing 1 joint and predominantly in slow twitch fibers were most at risk, for example, infraspinatus. Muscles crossing more than 1 joint but are predominantly slow twitch are the next in chronologic order to be adversely affected (eg, flexor carpi radialis). Muscles crossing multiple joints and mostly fast twitch are more resistant (eg, triceps long head). Knowledge of anatomy and muscle function is necessary for rehabilitation therapists, along with the fact that these are somewhat breed dependent.[68] Biochemical changes also occur in immobilized or poorly mobilized muscle. There is decreased glycogen storage, reduced oxidative enzymes available for energy, decreased calcium in the sarcoplasmic reticulum, and decreased protein synthesis.

Muscle remobilization takes time; medical doctors say that it takes twice the duration of immobilization for muscle to return to normal size and function. Higher levels of activity produce faster muscle building, but care needs to be taken about joint overload. Tendons and ligaments also lose strength after being immobilized or with disuse, and they need to remodel with remobilization as well. Ligament attachments to bone are areas that are particularly weakened. The rehabilitation therapist needs to factor this into the recovery plan. It should be 8 weeks' minimum of remobilization before jumping and high-speed turns are allowed.

Some rehabilitation modalities can be utilized to help promote fracture healing and prevent nonunions. Photobiomodulation (low-level laser therapy) has been shown in several studies to improve new bone formation and strength.[69] In a canine model for distraction osteogenesis, low-level laser therapy was shown to improve new bone formation and quality, collagen synthesis, and neovascularization.[70] Malunion and nonunion also are complications of fracture healing and can be a result of fracture configuration, infection, too much load, or motion during the healing process. Low-intensity pulsed ultrasound (LIPUS) has been utilized to speed fracture healing and healing of nonunion fractures, with mixed results in humans.[69,71] Use of LIPUS in dogs after TPLO did not show any enhanced healing radiographically.[72] Pulsed electromagnetic field therapy (PEMF) also may have some benefit in fracture healing. In the early stages, by decreasing edema as a primary role, PEMF increases osteogenesis, which may play a role in increasing fracture healing, and has been shown to improve healing in delayed and nonunions in humans through these mechanisms.[73–75] In a laboratory model of tibial fractures in dogs with 2-mm gap formation, PEMF improved parameters of fracture healing.[76] No studies of the effect of the common commercially available device used clinical veterinary medicine has been studied on fracture healing in dogs.

Muscle

Muscle strains occur in the face of a high intensity eccentric contraction that overloads the muscle causing tearing of the muscle fibers. In humans, pennate muscles that cross 2 joints and have a large percentage of type 2 muscle fibers are more prone to strain injury.[77,78] In the forelimb of dogs, these include the biceps and triceps muscles. Other pennate muscles crossing a single joint in the forelimb, such as the digital flexors and the flexor carpi ulnaris, also are susceptible to strain injury. Muscle injuries are termed, *strains*, and are graded 1 to 4, with grade 1 being disruption of a few fibers and grade 4 a complete rupture.[79] The muscle response to injury is spasm, to protect overload of fragile fibers. This is a resetting of muscle spindle cell tension, so the muscle has a shorter functional range. Muscle healing takes 4 weeks to 6 weeks to reach adequate repair. When a large portion of the muscle cells are damaged or when there is excessive motion between the cut ends of the muscle, fibroblasts make excess collagen and the area maintains some elasticity, but the tissue is not contractile. The overall effect is a change in muscle function with local weakening and a limit in functional length. Surrounding fibers of the same muscle can hypertrophy somewhat to compensate.

Rehabilitation aims to reduce the area of scar, ensure it is elastic, and increase the size of remaining muscle cells. Therapies depend on the stage of healing and grade of muscle strain. In the initial phase, the focus primarily is on pain reduction and reduction in the size of the hematoma for more severe strains. Hematomas can impede healing and application of cryotherapy or cold compression therapy can help decrease hematoma size in the acute phase (days 1–3), followed by heat therapy to speed absorption of the hematoma after day 3.[80] During the reparative phase, there is a delicate balance of applying load or stretch during the reparative phase because excessive load may lead to reinjury of the healing tissue or increased scar tissue formation. Load through therapeutic exercise is best documented with diagnostic ultrasound to assess reabsorption of the hematoma and changes in the organization of the muscle tissue and scar tissue formation. Therapeutic modalities can be utilized for treatment to help control pain and inflammation and proper healing. In 1 study, therapeutic ultrasound was found beneficial in muscle injury.[81] When appropriate scar tissue has formed, therapeutic exercises are focused on low-intensity eccentric contractions of the muscle, which enhances muscle and tendon stiffness.

Tendons and Ligaments

Tendon and ligament injuries are common presenting complaints in sports medicine and rehabilitation practice, with the shoulder the most common site in the forelimb. As covered elsewhere in this issue, soft tissue injuries to the shoulder often are complex and injuries to an isolated structure are rare. Because of the complexities of tendon and ligament healing, especially when intrasynovial, therapy is focused on decreasing inflammation, promotion of normal collagen formation, and strengthening supporting structures.

Tendon and ligaments are relatively avascular, which results in slow or poor healing. Most tendons are surrounded by paratenon (so can they glide over other structures) and blood supply branches from the adjacent muscle. The paratenon, bone, and muscle provide sources of neovascularization after injury. Some tendons or parts of tendons sit in a synovial fluid–filled sheath, and blood supply direct to the tendon is even lower.[82] Intra-articular ligaments are unlikely to heal, and the healing of sheathed tendons is similar to intra-articular ligaments and includes the tendon of origin of the biceps brachii.[83,84] Tendons and ligaments insert on bone by fibers blending with the periosteum, with some tendons having a zone of cartilage at the insertion.[82] Because cartilage also has a poor blood supply, healing at insertion sites of these tendons often is poor. There are few studies documenting healing progress of tendons in dogs. In 1 study of dogs that had their tendons cut and then resutured, healing took 6 weeks to 8 weeks to reach 60% tensile strength, and strength at 12 weeks was not much beyond this.[85]

Although healing of a tendon or ligament to maximal strength is approximately 12 weeks, remodeling occurs for up to 12 months and is in response to load. Acute laceration of the structure, or overload and avulsion of the bone at the insertion, with primary surgical repair generally heals more readily than a chronic repetitive overload injury. Chronic injury results in a tendinopathy or desmopathy with excess ground substance, disorganized collagen, and poor tensile strength, and therapists must intervene to reset the healing process. This is useful knowledge for rehabilitation therapists because it gives a therapeutic plan and time scale. Tendons and ligaments do not heal to their original strength, arising concerns about reinjury, but there is some redundancy in tissue strength, and this usually is enough even for running activity.

Because tendon and ligaments often also function to stabilize joints, immobilization techniques also often are utilized in the acute and reparative phases to allow therapists control of load placed on a healing tendon or ligament in addition to controlled exercise. Orthotics and braces can be completely rigid, rigid and hinged to allow load over time, or soft neoprene with and without thermoplastic splints applied over the top. For dogs affected with medial shoulder instability/medial shoulder syndrome, shoulder stabilization systems hobbles often are utilized to prevent abduction, but they also restrict cranial and caudal movement of the limb that results in restrictions in both extension and flexion of the shoulder and elbow that need to be addressed. The restrictive band can produce extra strain on limb flexors, in particular the biceps muscle and tendons. The advantage of orthotics and braces over casts and bandage/splints is that there is easier daily access to the limb for application of therapeutic modalities and importantly they allow for both therapist and owner to perform PROM and stretching.

Specific to optimizing tendon and ligament healing, therapeutic modalities can be utilized in conjunction with therapeutic exercise and manual therapies. Photobiomodulation therapy has been studied extensively in laboratory animals and human medicine for chronic tendinopathy. Results vary, with some studies showing improvement and others no effect in a variety of anatomic locations.[16] This is true with ESWT in people as well.[86] These review articles illustrate the necessity in both human and animal studies for some consistency in materials and methods in order to fully determine if a modality is effective and what equipment and dose will provide the desired therapeutic effect.

With increasing use of regenerative therapies, such as platelet-rich plasma (PRP) and mesenchymal stem cells (MSCs), to address both acute and chronic tendon and ligament injuries, the use of rehabilitation modalities has become a topic of concern. The use of therapies, such as therapeutic laser, ultrasound, ESWT, and PEMF postinjection, often has been discouraged because the effects on platelet activation and stem cell differentiation and migration were of concern. In vitro analysis of electrohydraulic ESWT on equine PRP showed an increase in growth factor expression, which could be a benefit after injection.[87] A recent review article evaluating the effect of low-level laser therapy on MSCs found that in 30 included studies there was a positive effect.[88] These effects included increased proliferation, viability, and differentiation of the MSCs at doses of 0.7 J/cm² to 4 J/cm² at wavelengths of 600 nm to 700 nm.[88] In equine tenocytes, low-level laser therapy in combination with growth factors promoted MSC differentiation toward tenocytes when combined with growth factors.[89] In vivo, laboratory animals with experimental tendon injuries have shown that the combination of low-level laser therapy and MSCs improved collagen organization.[90] The effect of laser therapy on PRP has not been extensively studied. LED laser application with PRP on sheep tenocytes did not have any negative effects at 4 J/cm².[91] Research on infrared lasers that are commonly used in veterinary medicine and their effects on both PRP and MSC applications needs to be done, but, based on current knowledge, they are unlikely to be detrimental at low doses and actually might optimize healing.

Cartilage

Cartilage is known for its metabolic inertness and its healing response varies with the extent of the injury. It has a relative absence of nerve and blood supply. Although adult animals remodel their cartilage matrix, they cannot replace cells embedded in the matrix when they die (via apoptosis or necrosis).

With a full-thickness cartilage defect, the subchondral bone is exposed and bleeding occurs. Blood is a ready source of mesenchymal regenerative cells as is the bone marrow, if uncovered. A clot forms followed by fibrocartilage and some bone formation; unfortunately, little to no hyaline cartilage is formed. This kind of defect (eg, after surgery to remove an osteochondrosis lesion in the humeral head) takes at least 2 months to heal; therefore, the rehabilitation therapist should control weight bearing for 2 months to avoid further subchondral bone damage. Hyaline cartilage normally varies in thickness and stiffness across the joint (weight distribution) but fibrocartilage lacks these properties and has a relatively poor response to tensile and compressive stresses and does not integrate with surrounding cartilage. These kinds of defects often are present after osteochondritis dissecans surgery and elbow dysplasia (cartilage débridement, subtotal coronoidectomy, and so forth). Partial-thickness areas of damage can be filled with matrix, but the repair response is minimal. Despite the presence of cartilage-derived and synovial membrane–derived MSCs, partial-thickness cartilage defects have no real repair capacity. Using exogenous stem cells may be a good solution to this problem, but generating mature cartilage of appropriate thickness and density from stem cells has not yet been possible. Knowledge of the effects of modalities on diseased or damaged cartilage is in its infancy. There are some promising results examining the effects of laser therapy on biomarkers of humans with knee osteoarthritis, and lasers can provide some pain relief along with improved function.[90–94] PEMF shows some promise in the healing of full-thickness cartilage defects in an experimental model.

Nerve

Mild nerve injuries, such as neurapraxia (failure of conduction due to crush) and axonotmesis, begin healing immediately; the inflammatory phase is less than for more severe injury. As long as a damaged axon has an endoneurial tube to direct growth down, functional recovery usually is complete. Nerves are extremely sensitive to oxygen and the glucose level of tissues. Therapists can work to help the body to provide optimal conditions for healing.[95]

More severe nerve injuries, such as brachial plexus avulsion, first undergo wallerian degeneration; the axon distal to the injury starts to die back and disintegrate 24 hours to 36 hours after injury. The remaining nerve cell lining is a guide for directing the sprouts coming from the end of the damaged axon after die-back. An axon sprout can grow into the empty nerve lining tube as fast as 1 mm per day if conditions are optimal. Endoneurium tubes in the end organ may narrow with time (>4 months) and impede axonal regeneration, although a human peripheral nerve retains the capacity to initiate a regenerative response at least 12 months after injury. Maturation time is needed after axon regeneration. This occurs at a slower rate than axon regrowth and continues for a protracted period because remyelination takes as long as 1 year. In more severe nerve injuries, where endoneurial tubes are disrupted, regenerating axons no longer are confined to their original sheaths and meander into surrounding tissue, thus failing to reinnervate their proper end organs. Neurologic recovery is compromised, generally to a degree proportional to the severity of the injury. Functional outcome also may be impaired by sensory deficits. After more severe injuries and nerve repair, sensory recovery is never complete; sensory cross reinnervation unfortunately is common.

Neurogenic atrophy of muscle is rapid (a mean 70% reduction of cross-sectional area by 2 months); the large fast twitch muscle fibers shrink first. The muscle cell losing its innervation undergoes a rapid loss in muscle cell size for up to 3 weeks postinjury; then, this stabilizes. If 15% or more of the nerve supply to the muscle motor units is intact, then reinnervation is possible and it is likely complete recovery will occur. If less than 15% of the nerve supply remains, there likely will be inadequate sprouting and incomplete recovery. Muscle cell metabolism decreases, and the end organ undergoes eventual fibrosis 6 months to 12 months after injury. It is the goal of the rehabilitation therapist to stimulate nerve recovery, but it also is vital to act rapidly to retain end organ function, keeping an ideal environment for reinnervation.

Electrical stimulation is the modality used most often to reduce muscle atrophy and fibrosis in conjunction with other therapies.[96] Photobiomodulation therapy can be used at the nerve root, the injury site, and the end organ and has been shown in several studies to enhance peripheral nerve regeneration.[97,98] PEMFs also have shown beneficial effects on peripheral nerve regeneration.[99,100]

Rehabilitation after nerve injury is a long process and decisions about possible future function should not be made in haste. Incomplete motor recovery is common after moderate to severe nerve injuries. Appropriate bracing and use of assistive devices can help an animal function and offset any disuse-related contractures that are common with nerve injury.

SUMMARY

Veterinary rehabilitation has the potential to optimize patient recovery after surgery or injury, provide pain management, restore function, and help maintain animals with chronic disease. The rehabilitation therapist takes into consideration healing times of affected tissues when developing therapeutic plans that promote proper healing and lead to successful outcomes.

DISCLOSURE

The authors have nothing to disclose.

REFERENCES

1. Crook T, McGowan C, Pead M. Effect of passive stretching on the range of motion of osteoarthritic joints in 10 labrador retrievers. Vet Rec 2007;160(16):545–7.
2. Jaegger G, Marcellin-Little DJ, Levine D. Reliability of goniometry in Labrador Retrievers. Am J Vet Res 2002;63(7):979–86.
3. Kopec NL, Williams JM, Tabor GF. Kinematic analysis of the thoracic limb of healthy dogs during descending stair and ramp exercises. Am J Vet Res 2018;79(1):33–41.
4. Carr JG, Millis DL, Weng H-Y. Exercises in canine physical rehabilitation: range of motion of the forelimb during stair and ramp ascent. J Small Anim Pract 2013; 54(8):409–13.
5. Holler PJ, Brazda V, Dal-Bianco B, et al. Kinematic motion analysis of the joints of the forelimbs and hind limbs of dogs during walking exercise regimens. Am J Vet Res 2010;71(7):734–40.
6. Bockstahler B, Tichy A, Aigner P. Compensatory load redistribution in Labrador retrievers when carrying different weights – a non-randomized prospective trial. BMC Vet Res 2016;12(1):92.
7. McLean H, Millis D, Levine D. Surface Electromyography of the Vastus Lateralis, Biceps Femoris, and Gluteus Medius in Dogs During Stance, Walking, Trotting, and Selected Therapeutic Exercises. Front Vet Sci 2019;6:211.

8. Bockstahler B, Kräutler C, Holler P, et al. Pelvic Limb Kinematics and Surface Electromyography of the Vastus Lateralis, Biceps Femoris, and Gluteus Medius Muscle in Dogs with Hip Osteoarthritis: Pelvic Limb Kinematics and Surface Electromyography in Dogs with Hip Osteoarthritis. Vet Surg 2012;41(1):54–62.

9. Breitfuss K, Franz M, Peham C, et al. Surface Electromyography of the Vastus Lateralis, Biceps Femoris, and Gluteus Medius Muscle in Sound Dogs During Walking and Specific Physiotherapeutic Exercises: Surface Electromyography in Sound Dogs During Walking and Specific Exercises. Vet Surg 2015;44(5): 588–95.

10. Chung H, Dai T, Sharma SK, et al. The nuts and bolts of low-level laser (light) therapy. Ann Biomed Eng 2012;40(2):516–33.

11. Mussttaf RA, Jenkins DFL, Jha AN. Assessing the impact of low level laser therapy (LLLT) on biological systems: a review. Int J Radiat Biol 2019;95(2):120–43.

12. Hamblin MR. Mechanisms and applications of the anti-inflammatory effects of photobiomodulation. AIMS Biophys 2017;4(3):337–61.

13. de Freitas LF, Hamblin MR. Proposed mechanisms of photobiomodulation or low-level light therapy. IEEE J Sel Top Quantum Electron 2016;22(3). https://doi.org/10.1109/JSTQE.2016.2561201.

14. Hamblin MR. Mechanisms and mitochondrial redox signaling in photobiomodulation. Photochem Photobiol 2018;94(2):199–212.

15. Yin K, Zhu R, Wang S, et al. Low-level laser effect on proliferation, migration, and antiapoptosis of mesenchymal stem cells. Stem Cells Dev 2017;26(10):762–75.

16. Tumilty S, Munn J, McDonough S, et al. Low level laser treatment of tendinopathy: a systematic review with meta-analysis. Photomed Laser Surg 2010; 28(1):3–16.

17. Clijsen R, Brunner A, Barbero M, et al. Effects of low-level laser therapy on pain in patients with musculoskeletal disorders: a systematic review and meta-analysis. Eur J Phys Rehabil Med 2017;53(4):603–10.

18. Duesterdieck-Zellmer KF, Larson MK, Plant TK, et al. Ex vivo penetration of low-level laser light through equine skin and flexor tendons. Am J Vet Res 2016; 77(9):991–9.

19. Ryan T, Smith R. An investigation into the depth of penetration of low level laser therapy through the equine tendon in vivo. Ir Vet J 2007;60(5):295.

20. Hochman-Elam LN, Heidel RE, Shmalberg JW. Effects of laser power, wavelength, coat length, and coat color on tissue penetration using photobiomodulation in healthy dogs. Can J Vet Res 2020;84(2):131–7.

21. Looney AL, Huntingford JL, Blaeser LL, et al. A randomized blind placebo-controlled trial investigating the effects of photobiomodulation therapy (PBMT) on canine elbow osteoarthritis. Can Vet J 2018;59(9):959–66.

22. Bocobo C, Fast A, Kingery W, et al. The effect of ice on intra-articular temperature in the knee of the dog. Am J Phys Med Rehabil 1991;70(4):181–5.

23. Vannetta M, Millis DL, Levine D, et al. The effects of cryotherapy on in-vivo skin and muscle temperature an intrauscular blood flow. J Orthop Sports Phys Ther 2006;36(1):A47.

24. Millard RP, Towle-Millard HA, Rankin DC, et al. Effect of cold compress application on tissue temperature in healthy dogs. Am J Vet Res 2013;74(3):443–7.

25. Song M, Sun X, Tian X, et al. Compressive cryotherapy versus cryotherapy alone in patients undergoing knee surgery: a meta-analysis. SpringerPlus 2016;5(1):1074.

26. Murgier J, Cassard X. Cryotherapy with dynamic intermittent compression for analgesia after anterior cruciate ligament reconstruction. Preliminary study. Orthop Traumatol Surg Res 2014;100(3):309–12.

27. Drygas KA, McClure SR, Goring RL, et al. Effect of cold compression therapy on postoperative pain, swelling, range of motion, and lameness after tibial plateau leveling osteotomy in dogs. J Am Vet Med Assoc 2011;238(10):1284–91.

28. Lehmann JF, Warren CG, Scham SM. Therapeutic heat and cold. Clin Orthop 1974;99:207–45.

29. Draper DO, Hopkins TJ. Increased intramuscular and intracapsular temperature via ThermaCare Knee Wrap application. Med Sci Monit 2008;14(6). PI7–11.

30. Petrofsky J, Berk L, Bains G, et al. Moist heat or dry heat for delayed onset muscle soreness. J Clin Med Res 2013. https://doi.org/10.4021/jocmr1521w.

31. Petrofsky JS, Laymon M. Heat transfer to deep tissue: the effect of body fat and heating modality. J Med Eng Technol 2009;33(5):337–48.

32. Draper DO, Harris ST, Schulthies S, et al. Hot-Pack and 1-MHz ultrasound treatments have an additive effect on muscle temperature increase. J Athl Train 1998;33(1):21–4.

33. Bleakley CM, Costello JT. Do thermal agents affect range of movement and mechanical properties in soft tissues? a systematic review. Arch Phys Med Rehabil 2013;94(1):149–63.

34. Draper DO, Castel JC, Castel D. Rate of temperature increase in human muscle during 1 MHz and 3 MHz continuous ultrasound. J Orthop Sports Phys Ther 1995;22(4):142–50.

35. Steiss JE, Adams CC. Effect of coat on rate of temperature increase in muscle during ultrasound treatment of dogs. Am J Vet Res 1999;60(1):76–80.

36. Levine D, Millis DL, Mynatt T. Effects of 3.3-MHz ultrasound on caudal thigh muscle temperature in dogs. Vet Surg 2001;30(2):170–4.

37. Tsai W-C, Tang S-T, Liang F-C. Effect of therapeutic ultrasound on tendons. Am J Phys Med Rehabil 2011;90(12):1068–73.

38. Davis TA, Stojadinovic A, Anam K, et al. Extracorporeal shock wave therapy suppresses the early proinflammatory immune response to a severe cutaneous burn injury. Int Wound J 2009;6(1):11–21.

39. Kuo Y-R, Wang C-T, Wang F-S, et al. Extracorporeal shock wave treatment modulates skin fibroblast recruitment and leukocyte infiltration for enhancing extended skin-flap survival. Wound Repair Regen 2009;17(1):80–7.

40. Chamberlain GA, Colborne GR. A review of the cellular and molecular effects of extracorporeal shockwave therapy. Vet Comp Orthop Traumatol 2016;29(2):99–107.

41. Wang C-J, Wang F-S, Yang KD, et al. Shock wave therapy induces neovascularization at the tendon–bone junction. A study in rabbits. J Orthop Res 2003;21(6):984–9.

42. Ochiai N, Ohtori S, Sasho T, et al. Extracorporeal shock wave therapy improves motor dysfunction and pain originating from knee osteoarthritis in rats. Osteoarthritis Cartilage 2007;15(9):1093–6.

43. Zhao Z, Ji H, Jing R, et al. Extracorporeal shock-wave therapy reduces progression of knee osteoarthritis in rabbits by reducing nitric oxide level and chondrocyte apoptosis. Arch Orthop Trauma Surg 2012;132(11):1547–53.

44. Bolt DM, Burba DJ, Hubert JD, et al. Determination of functional and morphologic changes in palmar digital nerves after nonfocused extracorporeal shock wave treatment in horses. Am J Vet Res 2004;65(12):1714–8.

45. Dahlberg JA, McClure SR, Evans RB, et al. Force platform evaluation of lameness severity following extracorporeal shock wave therapy in horses with unilateral forelimb lameness. J Am Vet Med Assoc 2006;229(1):100–3.
46. Razavipour M, Azar MS, Kariminasab MH, et al. The Short Term Effects of Shock-Wave Therapy for Tennis Elbow: a Clinical Trial Study. Acta Inform Med 2018;26(1):54–6.
47. Vaamonde-Lorenzo L, Cuenca-González C, Monleón-Llorente L, et al. Piezoelectric focal waves application in the treatment of plantar fascitis. Rev Espanola Cirugia Ortop Traumatol 2019;63(3):227–32.
48. Notarnicola A, Iannone F, Maccagnano G, et al. Chondrocytes treated with different shock wave devices. Muscles Ligaments Tendons J 2017;7(1):152–6.
49. Leeman JJ, Shaw KK, Mison MB, et al. Extracorporeal shockwave therapy and therapeutic exercise for supraspinatus and biceps tendinopathies in 29 dogs. Vet Rec 2016;179(15):385.
50. Becker W, Kowaleski MP, McCarthy RJ, et al. Extracorporeal shockwave therapy for shoulder lameness in dogs. J Am Anim Hosp Assoc 2015;51(1):15–9.
51. Dahlberg J, Fitch G, Evans RB, et al. The evaluation of extracorporeal shockwave therapy in naturally occurring osteoarthritis of the stifle joint in dogs. Vet Comp Orthop Traumatol 2005;18(03):147–52.
52. Mueller M, Bockstahler B, Skalicky M, et al. Effects of radial shockwave therapy on the limb function of dogs with hip osteoarthritis. Vet Rec 2007;160(22):762–5.
53. Barnes K, Faludi A, Takawira C, et al. Extracorporeal shock wave therapy improves short-term limb use after canine tibial plateau leveling osteotomy. Vet Surg 2019;48(8):1382–90.
54. Pilla AA. Nonthermal electromagnetic fields: From first messenger to therapeutic applications. Electromagn Biol Med 2013;32(2):123–36.
55. Rohde CH, Taylor EM, Alonso A, et al. Pulsed electromagnetic fields reduce postoperative interleukin-1β, pain, and inflammation: a double-blind, placebo-controlled study in TRAM flap breast reconstruction patients. Plast Reconstr Surg 2015;135(5):808e–17e.
56. Hedén P, Pilla AA. Effects of pulsed electromagnetic fields on postoperative pain: a double-blind randomized pilot study in breast augmentation patients. Aesthet Plast Surg 2008;32(4):660.
57. Alvarez LX, McCue J, Lam NK, et al. Effect of targeted pulsed electromagnetic field therapy on canine postoperative hemilaminectomy: a double-blind, randomized, placebo-controlled clinical trial. J Am Anim Hosp Assoc 2019;55(2):83–91.
58. Zidan N, Fenn J, Griffith E, et al. The effect of electromagnetic fields on postoperative pain and locomotor recovery in dogs with acute, severe thoracolumbar intervertebral disc extrusion: a randomized placebo-controlled, prospective clinical trial. J Neurotrauma 2018;35(15):1726–36.
59. Johnson JM, Johnson AL, Pijanowski GJ, et al. Rehabilitation of dogs with surgically treated cranial cruciate ligament-deficient stifles by use of electrical stimulation of muscles. Am J Vet Res 1997;58(12):1473–8.
60. de Freitas GR, Szpoganicz C, Ilha J. Does Neuromuscular Electrical Stimulation Therapy Increase Voluntary Muscle Strength After Spinal Cord Injury? A Systematic Review. Top Spinal Cord Inj Rehabil 2018;24(1):6–17.
61. Taylor PN, Ewins DJ, Fox B, et al. Limb blood flow, cardiac output and quadriceps muscle bulk following spinal cord injury and the effect of training for the Odstock functional electrical stimulation standing system. Paraplegia 1993;31(5):303–10.

62. Levine D, Marcellin-Little DJ, Millis DL, et al. Effects of partial immersion in water on vertical ground reaction forces and weight distribution in dogs. Am J Vet Res 2010;71(12):1413–6.

63. Parkinson S, Wills AP, Tabor G, et al. Effect of water depth on muscle activity of dogs when walking on a water treadmill. Comp Exerc Physiol 2018;14(2):79–89.

64. Barnicoat F, Wills AP. Effect of water depth on limb kinematics of the domestic dog (Canis lupus familiaris) during underwater treadmill exercise. Comp Exerc Physiol 2016;12(4):199–207.

65. Jackson A, Millis DL, Stevens M, et al. Joint kinematics of dogs walking on ground and aquatic treadmills. In: Proceedings of the Second International Symposium on Rehabilitation and Physical Therapy in Veterinary Medicine. University of Tennessee College of Veterinary Medicine, University of Tennessee at Chattanooga, Program in Physical Therapy, and University of Tennessee Department of Conferences, 2002; 2002.

66. Fish FE, DiNenno NK, Trail J. The "dog paddle": Stereotypic swimming gait pattern in different dog breeds. Anat Rec 2020. https://doi.org/10.1002/ar.24396.

67. Dirks ML, Wall BT, van de Valk B, et al. One week of bed rest leads to substantial muscle atrophy and induces whole-body insulin resistance in the absence of skeletal muscle lipid accumulation. Diabetes 2016;65(10):2862–75.

68. Guy PS, Snow DH. Skeletal muscle fibre composition in the dog and its relationship to athletic ability. Res Vet Sci 1981;31(2):244–8.

69. Bayat M, Virdi A, Jalalifirouzkouhi R, et al. Comparison of effects of LLLT and LIPUS on fracture healing in animal models and patients: A systematic review. Prog Biophys Mol Biol 2018;132:3–22.

70. Taha SK, El Fattah SA, Said E, et al. Effect of laser bio-stimulation on mandibular distraction osteogenesis: an experimental study. J Oral Maxillofac Surg 2018; 76(11):2411–21.

71. Rutten S, van den Bekerom MPJ, Sierevelt IN, et al. Enhancement of bone-healing by low-intensity pulsed ultrasound: a systematic review. JBJS Rev 2016;4(3):1.

72. Kieves NR, Canapp SO, Lotsikas PJ, et al. Effects of low-intensity pulsed ultrasound on radiographic healing of tibial plateau leveling osteotomies in dogs: a prospective, randomized, double-blinded study. Vet Surg 2018;47(5):614–22.

73. Daish C, Blanchard R, Fox K, et al. The Application of Pulsed Electromagnetic Fields (PEMFs) for Bone Fracture Repair: Past and Perspective Findings. Ann Biomed Eng 2018;46(4):525–42.

74. Streit A, Watson BC, Granata JD, et al. Effect on clinical outcome and growth factor synthesis with adjunctive use of pulsed electromagnetic fields for fifth metatarsal nonunion fracture: a double-blind randomized study. Foot Ankle Int 2016;37(9):919–23.

75. Shi H, Xiong J, Chen Y, et al. Early application of pulsed electromagnetic field in the treatment of postoperative delayed union of long-bone fractures: a prospective randomized controlled study. BMC Musculoskelet Disord 2013;14(1):35.

76. Inoue N, Ohnishi I, Chen D, et al. Effect of pulsed electromagnetic fields (PEMF) on late-phase osteotomy gap healing in a canine tibial model. J Orthop Res 2002;20(5):1106–14.

77. Maffulli N, Del Buono A, Oliva F, et al. Muscle Injuries: A Brief Guide to Classification and Management. Transl Med Unisa 2015;12:14–8.

78. Garrett WE. Muscle strain injuries: clinical and basic aspects. Med Sci Sports Exerc 1990;22(4):436–43.

79. Mueller-Wohlfahrt H-W, Haensel L, Mithoefer K, et al. Terminology and classification of muscle injuries in sport: The Munich consensus statement. Br J Sports Med 2013;47(6):342.

80. Smith TO, Hunt NJ, Wood SJ. The physiotherapy management of muscle haematomas. Phys Ther Sport 2006;7(4):201–9.

81. Tomlinson JE. The use of therapeutic ultrasound in the treatment of muscle injuries. In: Symposium of the American College of Veterinary Sports Medicine Adn Rehabilitatoin. Nashville (TN): 2015.

82. Benjamin M, Ralphs JR. Tendons and ligaments–an overview. Histol Histopathol 1997;12(4):1135–44.

83. Bray RC, Leonard CA, Salo PT. Correlation of healing capacity with vascular response in the anterior cruciate and medial collateral ligaments of the rabbit. J Orthop Res 2003;21(6):1118–23.

84. Garvican ER, Salavati M, Smith RKW, et al. Exposure of a tendon extracellular matrix to synovial fluid triggers endogenous and engrafted cell death: A mechanism for failed healing of intrathecal tendon injuries. Connect Tissue Res 2017; 58(5):438–46.

85. Gelberman RH, Manske PR, Akeson WH, et al. Flexor tendon repair. J Orthop Res 1986;4(1):119–28.

86. Zwerver J, Waugh C, van der Worp H, et al. Can shockwave therapy improve tendon metabolism?. In: Ackermann PW, Hart DA, editors. Metabolic influences on risk for tendon Disorders. Vol 920. Advances in experimental medicine and Biology. Springer International Publishing; 2016. p. 275–81. https://doi.org/10.1007/978-3-319-33943-6_26.

87. Seabaugh KA, Thoresen M, Giguère S. Extracorporeal Shockwave Therapy Increases Growth Factor Release from Equine Platelet-Rich Plasma In Vitro. Front Vet Sci 2017;4. https://doi.org/10.3389/fvets.2017.00205.

88. Fekrazad R, Asefi S, Allahdadi M, et al. Effect of Photobiomodulation on Mesenchymal Stem Cells. Photomed Laser Surg 2016;34(11):533–42.

89. Gomiero C, Bertolutti G, Martinello T, et al. Tenogenic induction of equine mesenchymal stem cells by means of growth factors and low-level laser technology. Vet Res Commun 2016;40(1):39–48.

90. Lucke LD, Bortolazzo FO, Theodoro V, et al. Low-level laser and adipose-derived stem cells altered remodelling genes expression and improved collagen reorganization during tendon repair. Cell Prolif 2019;52(3):e12580.

91. Alzyoud JAM, Al Najjar SA, Talat S, et al. Effect of light-emitting diodes, platelet-rich plasma, and their combination on the activity of sheep tenocytes. Lasers Med Sci 2019;34(4):759–66.

92. Makolinets KV, Makolinets VI, Morozenko DV, et al. Dynamics of biochemical markers of connective tissue metabolism in patients with knee osteoarthritis during conservative treatment with laser therapy. Wiadomosci Lek Wars Pol 1960 2019;72(5 cz 1):802–6.

93. Gworys K, Gasztych J, Puzder A, et al. Influence of various laser therapy methods on knee joint pain and function in patients with knee osteoarthritis. Ortop Traumatol Rehabil 2012;14(3):269–77.

94. Alayat MSM, Aly THA, Elsayed AEM, et al. Efficacy of pulsed Nd:YAG laser in the treatment of patients with knee osteoarthritis: a randomized controlled trial. Lasers Med Sci 2017;32(3):503–11.

95. Hashmi JT, Huang Y-Y, Osmani BZ, et al. Role of low-level laser therapy in neurorehabilitation. PM R 2010;2(12 Suppl 2):S292–305.

96. Nussbaum EL, Houghton P, Anthony J, et al. Neuromuscular electrical stimulation for treatment of muscle impairment: critical review and recommendations for clinical practice. Physiother Can 2017;69(5):1–76.

97. Rochkind S, Ouaknine GE. New trend in neuroscience: Low-power laser effect on peripheral and central nervous system (basic science, preclinical and clinical studies). Neurol Res 1992;14(1):2–11.

98. Rosso M, Buchaim D, Kawano N, et al. Photobiomodulation therapy (PBMT) in peripheral nerve regeneration: a systematic review. Bioengineering 2018; 5(2):44.

99. Raji AR, Bowden RE. Effects of high-peak pulsed electromagnetic field on the degeneration and regeneration of the common peroneal nerve in rats. J Bone Joint Surg Br 1983;65(4):478–92.

100. Sisken BF, Kanje M, Lundborg G, et al. Stimulation of rat sciatic nerve regeneration with pulsed electromagnetic fields. Brain Res 1989;485(2):309–16.

Humeral Intracondylar Fissure in Dogs

Andy P. Moores, BVSc, FRCVS

KEYWORDS

- Humeral condyle • Intracondylar fissure • Incomplete ossification • Elbow • Dog

KEY POINTS

- In most dogs this condition is thought to be a stress fracture of the humeral condyle, and so the descriptive term "humeral intracondylar fissure" is preferred to "incomplete ossification of the humeral condyle."
- Humeral intracondylar fissure has been reported in several breeds but is most commonly seen in spaniel breeds.
- Humeral intracondylar fissure predisposes dogs to condylar fractures that may occur with minimal or no trauma. It can also cause lameness without fracture.
- Computed tomography is more sensitive than radiography for diagnosis.
- Historic high surgical complication rates may be reduced by modifying technique and careful execution.

INTRODUCTION

Humeral intracondylar fissure (HIF), previously known as incomplete ossification of the humeral condyle (IOHC), is characterized by the presence of a midsagittal fissure in the humeral condyle, which may completely or partially separate the two halves of the humeral condyle. Such fissures weaken the humeral condyle and thus HIF predisposes affected dogs to complete condylar fractures. HIF may also cause clinical signs of lameness and elbow pain in its own right, without complete fracture. This article reviews the current understanding of this condition and treatment options.

HISTORY

In the 1980s, reviews of humeral condylar fractures in dogs indicated that spaniel breeds were at increased risk of these fractures compared with other breeds. In a study of 133 humeral condylar fractures from the United Kingdom, Denny[1] reported that 35% were in spaniel breeds with most being English Springer Spaniels (23% of all humeral condylar fractures). It was also recognized that these fractures often

Anderson Moores Veterinary Specialists, Bunstead Barns, Poles lane, Hursley, Winchester, SO21 2LL, United Kingdom
E-mail address: andy@andersonmoores.com

Vet Clin Small Anim 51 (2021) 421–437
https://doi.org/10.1016/j.cvsm.2020.12.006
0195-5616/21/© 2020 Elsevier Inc. All rights reserved.

occurred during normal activity. In a study of 20 dogs from the United States that fractured their humeral condyle during normal activity, Vannini and colleagues[2] reported that 11 (55%) of the dogs were Cocker Spaniels. It is worth noting that the breed referred to as the Cocker Spaniel in North America, is known as the American Cocker Spaniel in Europe to distinguish it from the European Cocker Spaniel, which is similar but has different breed standards. For the remainder of this review the two breeds are referred to as the American Cocker Spaniel and the Cocker Spaniel. Some of the American Cocker Spaniels identified by Vannini and colleagues[2] had been lame before fracture and some had radiographic evidence of remodeling of the lateral epicondylar crest.

The authors of both of these studies were unable to identify why these breeds were at increased risk of humeral condylar fracture but they proposed that it may be caused by a conformational issue or weakness in the distal humerus.[1,2] Denny[1] additionally proposed that it may be representative of English Springer Spaniels being active dogs that are frequently worked over rough ground.

The first description of HIF was made by Meutstege in 1989.[3] He described four dogs with chronic intermittent forelimb lameness. All four had a fracture line or fissure evident between the two halves of the humeral condyle, which was only visible on oblique craniocaudal radiographs. One of these dogs fractured the humeral condyle a short time after diagnosis and all four progressed well after lag screw fixation.

Marcellin-Little and colleagues[4] published the first detailed description of this condition, which they called IOHC. Because the term IOHC implies a developmental cause and more recent reports support this condition being the result of a stress fracture in some dogs,[5–7] the descriptive term HIF has been proposed and is used here.

ETIOPATHOGENESIS

Mineralization of the cartilaginous anlage of the humeral condyle is initiated at two separate centers of ossification at around 14 ± 8 days after birth. One goes on to form the capitulum and the lateral part of the humeral condyle and the other to form the trochlea and the medial part of the humeral condyle (**Fig. 1**). As mineralization progresses, the two centers of ossification are separated by a thin cartilaginous plate until they unite at 8 to 12 weeks of age.[8] The location of the fissure in dogs with HIF corresponds to the position of the cartilaginous plate that separates the two centers of ossification and thus in early reports of this condition it was proposed to be the result of the failure of the two centers of ossification to unite, hence the initial name of IOHC.[4]

The incomplete ossification theory has not adequately explained the clinical findings in many dogs with HIF. Biopsies from a small number of dogs identified fibrous tissue at the fissure, rather than the cartilaginous tissue that might be expected.[4] Also, clinical signs are often first recognized in adult dogs,[4,9–11] which would be unexpected if the weakness in the humeral condyle is present from a young age. Finally, failure of the two centers of ossification to unite does not fully explain complete HIFs, which extend to the supratrochlear foramen, because the cartilaginous plate does not extend that far proximal (see **Fig. 1**).

Over the past 10 years or so, with the increasing use of cross-sectional imaging, it has become apparent that, at least in some dogs, HIF is a form of stress fracture. Authors have reported not only the propagation of condylar fissures over time but also the development of intracondylar fissures in previously normal humeral condyles.[5–7,12] Additional support for the stress fracture theory comes from the adult onset of clinical signs in many dogs and the lack of association between fissure size and fracture risk, which would be consistent with the fissure size getting larger over time. If the fissure size

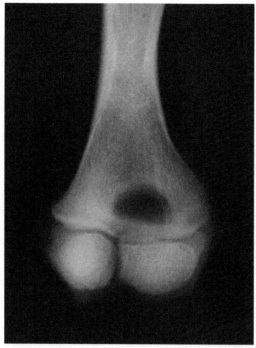

Fig. 1. Craniocaudal radiograph of the distal humerus from a 7-week-old Labrador.

was static then dogs with small partial fissures would be expected to be at lower risk of complete condylar fracture than dogs with complete fissures, but the evidence does not support this.[7,13] Assuming that HIF does represent a stress fracture, there is no evidence that these are insufficiency fractures, that is, associated with poor bone quality. Affected dogs are not predisposed to fractures elsewhere, which would be expected of a generalized bone disease. On the contrary, computed tomography (CT) imaging of HIF and surgical findings during open fracture repair of condylar fractures associated with HIF, confirm dense sclerotic bone adjacent to HIF lesions,[13–15] which is a characteristic of stress fractures in other locations.[16] A stress fracture in the presence of normal bone (ie, a fatigue fracture) implies repetitive mechanical overload. This might be expected in a breed, such as the English Springer Spaniel, which is known as an active breed and that is often worked as a gun dog. The American Cocker Spaniels reported with HIF, however, have been described as indoor dogs with a sedentary lifestyle.[13]

HIF does not universally present in adult dogs. HIF has been reported in dogs as young as 4 months of age.[7,11] It seems more likely that dogs of this age would have a developmental HIF (ie, incomplete ossification) rather than a stress fracture, so it is feasible that both theories are valid and HIF may result from two different mechanisms.

A microangiographic study of the humeral condyles of four American Cocker Spaniels without HIF reported that American Cocker Spaniels had reduced vascular density in the humeral condyle compared with mixed-breed dogs.[17] The significance of this finding in relation to HIF is unclear.

Irrespective of whether HIF develops as a failure of ossification or as a stress fracture, there may be a common underlying conformational issue that predisposes to both scenarios. In a CT survey of the elbows of English Springer Spaniels without a history of forelimb lameness, 50% of dogs had evidence of medial coronoid process pathology.[18] The same study reported an incidence of HIF of 14%. The high incidence of medial coronoid process pathology in a breed susceptible to HIF raises the intriguing possibility that the two conditions may share a common developmental or conformational abnormality. Radioulnar incongruity, for example, is a conformational abnormality that could plausibly predispose to HIF. There is conflicting evidence in relation to radioulnar incongruity and HIF, with one paper showing no evidence of incongruity in dogs with HIF[18] and another that reported significantly greater humeroulnar incongruity at the base and at the apex of the medial coronoid process in elbows with HIF, compared with unaffected elbows.[15]

A conformational abnormality of the elbow may have the effect of distorting weight-bearing forces acting on the elbow and predisposing the humeral condyle to either failure of the two centers of ossification to fuse or, in older dogs, a stress fracture. Arthroscopic findings suggest that it is not a pure axial force that stresses the humeral condyle. Eleven dogs with complete HIF were examined arthroscopically by the author, before placement of a transcondylar screw. The intracondylar fissure of each elbow was visualized arthroscopically while the elbow was put through a series of standardized manipulations. With the elbow at a weight-bearing angle, internal rotation of the lower limb caused the intracondylar fissure to visibly widen in 9 of 11 elbows. Pure axial force directed along the antebrachium and external rotation of the lower limb caused no visible change in the intracondylar fissure (A.P. Moores, unpublished data, 2020). The widening of the fissure seen during internal rotation is a consequence of the anconeal process putting a lateralized force on the lateral epicondyle and/or the medial coronoid process imparting a medially directed force on the trochlea (medial half of the humeral condyle). Sudden turning (which causes torque on the lower limb) may therefore play a greater role in stressing the humeral condyle than simple axial loading of the humeral condyle.

Pedigree analysis of eight affected American Cocker Spaniels has suggested that HIF may have a genetic basis with a recessive mode of inheritance in this breed.[4]

PRESENTATION

Breeds predisposed to HIF include the spaniel breeds (particularly the English Springer Spaniel in the United Kingdom and the American Cocker Spaniel in the United States, but other spaniel breeds may also be affected) and the German Wachtelhund,[11] which is also known as the German Spaniel. Other reported breeds include the German Shepherd Dog, Yorkshire Terrier, Tibetan Mastiff, Rottweiler, English Pointer, Siberian Husky, and Labrador Retriever.[9,14,19,20] Most studies report that male dogs are more commonly affected than female dogs.[4,7,11,21]

Dogs with HIF present in one of three ways. They may present with a weight-bearing forelimb lameness, they may present with a humeral condylar fracture associated with HIF, or they may present without lameness where HIF has been diagnosed as an incidental finding.

HIF should be considered in predisposed breeds that present with a forelimb lameness localizable to the elbow. The lameness is weight-bearing and may be mild and intermittent or be persistent and more severe. Elbow discomfort is most evident on full extension and there may also be discomfort on palpation over the lateral epicondylar crest. Often the lameness is poorly responsive to nonsteroidal anti-inflammatory drugs.

DIAGNOSIS

Diagnosis of HIF requires demonstration of a fissure in the midsagittal plane of the humeral condyle. Partial fissures extend part-way across the humeral condyle and originate from the articular surface.[15] Complete fissures extend across the entire humeral condyle. High-quality craniocaudal radiographs of the elbow may demonstrate the fissure (**Fig. 2**), which is radiolucent, although often the fissure is not evident unless the x-ray beam is directed exactly parallel to it. Several craniocaudal projections may therefore be required, each taken at slightly different angles of rotation. It has been suggested that a 15° craniomedial-caudolateral oblique projection is most likely to demonstrate the fissure and that rotation of the condyle greater than 5° away from this results in an inability to detect the fissure.[4] It is important that HIF is not mistakenly diagnosed based on seeing a Mach line, a visual anomaly created by the superimposition of one bone edge on another and that can appear as a radiolucent line through the condyle (**Fig. 3**). New bone, or a periosteal reaction, along the lateral margin of the lateral epicondylar crest may be seen in association with HIF (**Fig. 4**), which presumably represents a stress-adaptation of the lateral epicondylar crest caused by weakness in the condyle.

CT is the preferred diagnostic tool for HIF. Good quality transverse slices (typically 0.6–1.0 mm) readily demonstrate the hypoattenuating fissure (**Fig. 5**). In a CT study of 38 elbows with HIF all but two fissures were irregular (described as saw-tooth) rather than straight and all fissures were bordered by hyperattenuating bone (sclerosis). All of the partial fissures originated from the articular surface.[15] MRI also identifies HIF and is more sensitive than radiography.[12] If cross-sectional imaging is not available and radiography fails to identify HIF, many fissures are visible arthroscopically as an irregular

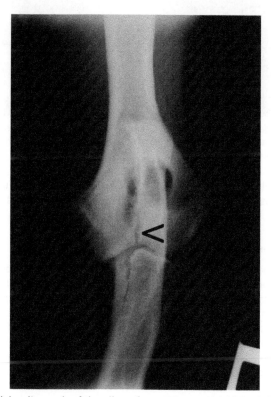

Fig. 2. Craniocaudal radiograph of the elbow from a 17-month-old English Springer Spaniel with humeral intracondylar fissure (*arrowhead*).

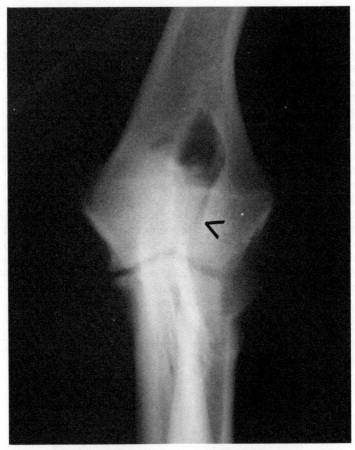

Fig. 3. Craniocaudal radiograph of the elbow. There is a Mach line present (*arrowhead*), because of superimposition of the axial edge of the lateral epicondyle and the lateral aspect of the anconeal process and olecranon.

midsagittal defect in the articular cartilage of the humeral condyle (**Fig. 6**),[11] although a CT-confirmed case without arthroscopic evidence has been reported.[22]

TREATMENT
The Dog with Lameness but No Fracture

These dogs are generally treated with a transcondylar screw to bridge the fissure and strengthen the condyle. The intention is to improve or eliminate the lameness and also to reduce the risk of future condylar fracture. A variety of implants have been described for this purpose. Initial reports described using standard AO-style cortical screws as either positional or lag screws (**Fig. 7**).[9,11] Although initial reports described reasonable outcomes, it was the experience of many surgeons that transcondylar screw placement is associated with a significant risk of complications. A multicenter UK study reported a 59.5% total complication rate after screw placement.[20] Seroma (32% incidence) and surgical site infection (30% incidence) were the two most common complications. The Labrador Retriever was at increased risk of a complication compared with other breeds and increasing body weight and the placement of the

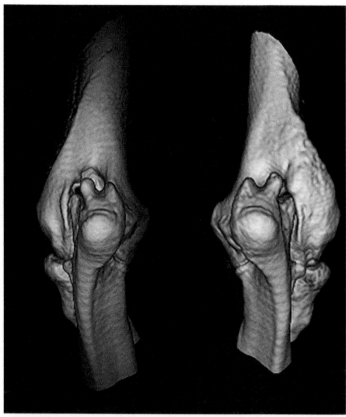

Fig. 4. Computed tomography three-dimensional reconstructions of the left and right elbows (caudal aspect) from a 3-year-old Working Cocker Spaniel with right-sided humeral intracondylar fissure. Note the remodeling of the lateral epicondylar crest of the affected elbow.

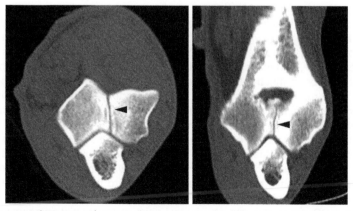

Fig. 5. Computed tomography scans (transverse on the *left*, reformatted frontal plane on the *right*) of the humeral condyle from a 5-year-old English Springer Spaniel with humeral intracondylar fissure (*arrowhead*).

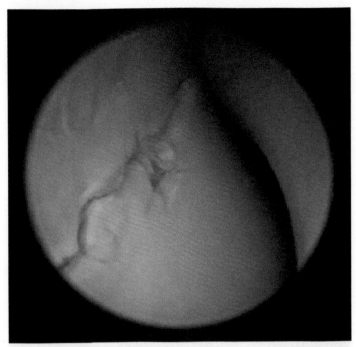

Fig. 6. Arthroscopic image of a humeral intracondylar fissure. Right elbow, medial portals, anconeal process on the right.

screw as a positional screw were risk factors for surgical site infection. Another study reported a surgical site infection rate of 42%.[21] At the time that the cases in these studies were managed, it was standard practice among UK surgeons to place transcondylar screws from lateral-to-medial and it is likely that this approach predisposes to wound complications and infection. In a study that compared both approaches, four of eight elbows treated via a lateral approach had a major complication, whereas zero of six treated via a medial approach did. This approached, but did not reach, statistical significance ($P = .085$).[10] Other studies have reported surgical site infection rates of 6% and 14% with a medial approach, which compare favorably with studies where a lateral approach was used.[23,24] The author's personal experience is that the lateral approach is associated with a significant risk of wound complications and surgical site infection, and that since adopting the medial approach these complications have not only been much less common but when they do occur, they have also resolved more readily. It is unclear why the lateral approach seems to predispose to such complications but poor soft tissue cover laterally and contact of the lateral aspect of the elbow with the ground when lying down are possibilities.

Transcondylar screws can be placed blind but this risks inadvertent intra-articular screw placement. It is preferable to use a self-aiming drill guide or intraoperative fluoroscopy to guide screw placement.[23,25] Safe entry/exit points for the medial and lateral epicondyles have been described.[26] Relative to the diameter of the humeral condyle (HCD) at its isthmus, its narrowest part, the medial point is 0.3 × HCD cranial and 0.2 × HCD distal to the most proximal point of the medial epicondyle and the lateral point is 0.3 × HCD cranial and 0.3 × HCD distal to the most proximal point of the lateral epicondyle. Patient-specific three-dimensional printed drill guides have

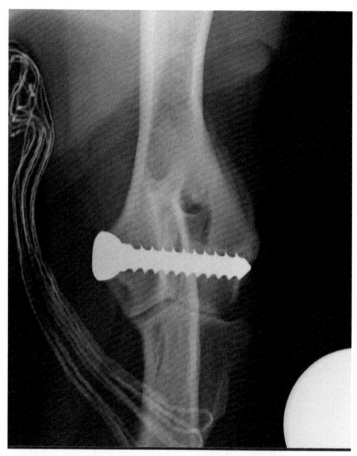

Fig. 7. Postoperative radiograph of a transcondylar 4.5-mm cortical lag screw. Note the re-modeling of the lateral epicondylar crest (this is the same dog as in **Fig. 4**).

also been described.[27] If a lagged implant is used, then the length of the glide hole is judged from preoperative imaging and drill stops are used to avoid inadvertent overdrilling.

Surgical treatment does not always result in bone healing across the fissure. The incidence of a persistent fissure after surgical management varies between reports. Collated data from several reports suggest that around 75% of fissures reduce in size or heal completely after conventional surgical management (**Table 1**).

Care should be taken in interpreting fissure healing data. The radiographic assessment of healing could be unreliable because of the difficulties of demonstrating fissures radiographically. CT assessment is preferable but could be hindered by implant-associated artifact. Finally, the act of compressing the fissure may alter its appearance, making comparisons with preoperative imaging problematic.

Failure (breakage) of transcondylar implants is well-recognized as a complication of HIF treatment with a reported incidence of 2.5% to 10%.[9,11,20,21,23] The reported incidence of implant failure is affected by the length of follow-up and whether imaging was performed or not (not all failed implants result in a recurrence of clinical signs[21]). The average time after surgery at which a failed implant is identified is 24 months (range,

Table 1
Reported data for persistence of a fissure after surgical treatment of HIF

	Imaging Technique	<3-mo Follow-Up			>3-mo Follow-Up		
		Fissure Unchanged	Fissure Smaller	No Fissure	Fissure Unchanged	Fissure Smaller	No Fissure
Meyer-Lindenberg et al,[11] 2002	Radiograph				2		5
Butterworth & Innes,[9] 2001	Radiograph	1	4			2	3
Moores et al,[10] 2014	CT		1		3	1	2
Chase et al,[21] 2019	Radiograph				6 (fissure present, but does not state if smaller or not)		3
Combined (Chase et al excluded)		1	5		5	3	10

Data from Refs.[9–11,21]

11–48 months).[9,11,28] Scanning electron microscopy of retrieved failed screws has revealed a multidirectional pattern of fatigue fracture that is presumed to result from persistent instability in the humeral condyle despite screw placement.[28]

One strategy to mitigate the risk of screw failure is to use the largest screw that can be safely placed across the humeral condyle. As a guide, a screw with a thread diameter of 30% to 50% of the diameter of the narrowest part of the humeral condyle is used.[14] Care should be taken not to overtighten AO cortical-style screws with domed screw heads; the author has seen a small number of medial epicondylar fissure fractures develop as screws are tightened, sometimes with an audible crack as the fissure occurs. These fractures initiate underneath the screw head, are nonarticular, and do not seem to require any specific treatment. (Jenkins G, Moores AP: Medial epicondylar fissure fracture as a complication during stabilization of HIF. Submitted for publication.)

Adult English Springer Spaniels typically require a 4.5-mm screw. Fully threaded 4.5-mm cortical screws can be used but these can break.[28] To provide additional strength at the midpoint of the humeral condyle the 4.5-mm shaft screw (Veterinary Instrumentation, Sheffield, UK) is used as a transcondylar implant.[10] This has a solid 4.5-mm diameter section that bridges the fissure (**Fig. 8**). The area moment of inertia (a geometric measure of a structure's resistance to bending) of the shaft of the 4.5-mm shaft screw is five times greater than that of a 4.5-mm cortical screw of the same material.[29,30] The author's experience is that fatigue failure of the 4.5-mm shaft screw is rare. The reduced surface area of the shaft screw compared with a fully-threaded cortical screw has, however, introduced an additional complication, namely screw back-out/loosening that is not associated with infection. Careful technique and screw length selection are important to maximize the engagement of the shaft screw threads in bone and thus reduce the risk of the screw backing out.[10]

Titanium has better fatigue resistance than stainless steel, although stainless steel is stronger. There may therefore be benefits to using titanium implants for treating HIF, although there are no studies comparing the two materials to confirm this.

Rather than simply using the largest implant possible, another strategy to avoid implant failure is to focus on encouraging bone healing across the fissure. Transcondylar bone tunnels used alone without an additional transcondylar screw did not result in bone healing in one report.[19] In another report bone tunnels were created alongside a transcondylar screw but bone healing at the tunnels was not assessed.[9] Autogenous corticocancellous dowels placed alongside a transcondylar screw resulted in bone healing at the site of the dowel in six dogs 11 to 16 weeks postoperatively.[31]

Implants specifically designed to manage HIF and to encourage bone healing have been described. One such implant has a 3-mm cannulated core designed to accept autogenous cancellous bone graft, with fenestrations in the implant to allow vascular access.[32] Another implant has a central 3-mm nonthreaded core that is placed within a 6-mm drill hole that crosses the fissure. The 1.5-mm void around the shaft of the implant is filled with demineralized bone matrix putty to encourage local bone healing.[33]

In managing HIF there will always be a trade-off between the amount of bone that can form across the fissure and implant size; strategies that aim to encourage large areas of the fissure to heal necessitate smaller implants. Strategies that rely on encouraging bone healing at the expense of implant strength are potentially flawed if the underlying cause of the fissure is a stress fracture and if the underlying stresses acting on the humeral condyle remain. A transcondylar implant may load-share sufficiently with any new bone that forms to avoid fatigue fracture of the new bone and the implant, but the ideal ratio of implant to new bone is not known. Currently, there are no

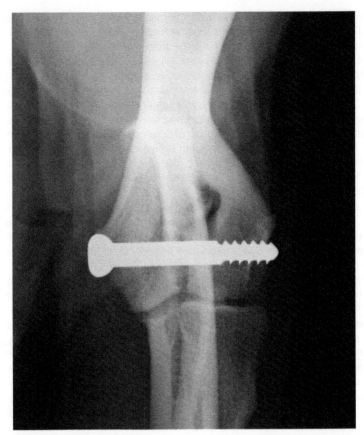

Fig. 8. Postoperative radiograph of a transcondylar 4.5-mm shaft screw, placed in a 2-year-old English Springer Spaniel.

long-term data to confirm the longevity of new bone that forms across the fissure with the novel screw types described previously.

Assessing studies that report outcomes after surgical management of HIF is problematic because of variable follow-up times and methodologies. Furthermore, breeds predisposed to HIF can also be affected by other conditions of the elbow, so long-term lameness may not be directly attributable to HIF in some dogs.[15,18,19] Nonetheless, outcome data with a minimum of 6-month follow-up, collated from several studies, indicate that around 70% of cases are expected to have good or excellent long-term function.[9–11,21,23]

The Dog with Fracture Associated with Humeral Intracondylar Fissure

Preexisting HIF should be suspected when dogs of at-risk breeds present with humeral condylar fractures after minor or no trauma. A history of weight-bearing lameness preceding fracture and/or HIF in the contralateral limb further support preexisting HIF. Confirmatory evidence includes hyperattenuating/sclerotic bone bordering the condylar part of the fracture or periosteal new bone/remodeling at the lateral epicondylar crest, evident on preoperative CT or at surgery.

Condylar fractures associated with HIF should be managed along the lines of all articular fractures; namely, accurate anatomic reduction and rigid fixation, typically using a transcondylar compression screw with additional epicondylar fixation. Surgeons should consider that the condylar part of the fracture may not heal[34] and a transcondylar implant that can withstand a prolonged period of stress should be chosen, similarly to nonfractured HIF.

Intracondylar (Y/T) fractures are typically double plated.[35] Lateral humeral condylar fractures associated with HIF are plated along the epicondylar crest rather than relying on an epicondylar Kirschner wire. Plating lateral humeral condylar fractures in this way should reduce the stress on the transcondylar implant and is associated with fewer complications than using a Kirschner wire, particularly in adult dogs.[34] Medial humeral condylar fractures are less common and are managed with epicondylar crest lag screws and/or plates.

The Dog with Nonsymptomatic Humeral Intracondylar Fissure

HIF may be diagnosed as an incidental finding, such as in the contralateral humeral condyle during the imaging assessment of a dog with a condylar fracture. In one survey 6 of 14 (43%) dogs presenting with a unilateral condylar fracture had a CT diagnosis of HIF in the contralateral humerus.[36]

In a study of 34 cases of nonsymptomatic HIF treated nonsurgically, six (18%) went on to fracture at a mean of 14 months after diagnosis (range, 5–24 months), and a further two cases had a transcondylar screw placed at 11 and 17 months to manage a progressive lameness presumed to relate to the HIF. The mean follow-up for cases not requiring surgery was 56 months (range, 29–79 months). Fissure size, body weight, age, and presence of a contralateral fracture were not associated with fracture.[7] These data suggest that a low number of nonsymptomatic HIFs will fracture following diagnosis and that if they do fracture then it is likely to be within 2 years of diagnosis, which is consistent with other data.[13]

The author's approach for nonsymptomatic HIF is to discuss the previously mentioned risks, and the risks of surgical management, with each owner. Some owners prefer early surgery to mitigate the risk of condylar fracture. Many prefer to avoid surgery. For those that decline surgery and have partial HIF there may be some value in a 4- to 6-month follow-up CT examination to assess if the fissure is progressing or not, with surgery being considered in those cases where it is. In a small number of cases followed by the author in this way the fissure has healed on follow-up CT examination.

It is not known if dogs with symptomatic HIF would have a similar risk of fracture to dogs with nonsymptomatic HIF. Most owners opt for surgical management to address their dog's lameness and so long-term data do not exist for conservatively managed symptomatic cases. It has been proposed that the pain associated with HIF relates to abnormal stresses on the lateral epicondylar crest,[9] and if this is the case then symptomatic dogs would be expected to be at a greater risk of fracture than nonsymptomatic dogs.

REVISION STRATEGIES

Removal of the screw tip of a transcondylar screw that has broken is problematic and is made a lot easier if a slightly longer screw than is needed is placed at the initial surgery, so that the tip of the screw can be gripped with pliers should the screw break. If the screw tip is buried and this is not an option then there are proprietary trephine systems available (eg, from DePuy Synthes) that can make the task of removal simple. Alternatively, bone is burred away from around the screw tip until a pair of pliers can be used to grip it.

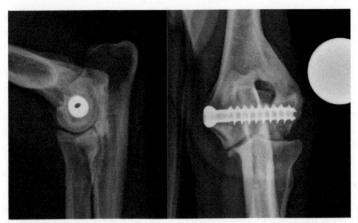

Fig. 9. Postoperative radiographs of a transcondylar 7.3-mm cannulated screw in a 4-year-old English Springer Spaniel, placed after staged removal of an infected shaft screw.

The simplest approach to a screw that has backed-out and has no bone loss around it and no infection present, is to retighten the screw. Sometimes the screw backs-out a second time in which case another solution should be considered, but often the screw remains secure the second-time around.

If a screw needs to be replaced, then as long as initial screw placement was central within the humeral condyle, a larger screw can usually be placed. For example, a fully-threaded 5.5-mm cortical screw (4.0-mm core) can be used to replace a 4.5-mm screw. This is particularly useful if there is minor bone loss around the original implant. If the bone loss is significant then even larger screws may be an option and the author has successfully replaced a 4.5-mm screw with a 7.3-mm cannulated screw (De Puy Synthes) in an English Springer Spaniel (**Fig. 9**). If there is no bone loss, then an alternate option is to replace the screw with a longer screw of the same size and secure the screw with a nut on the lateral aspect of the condyle (if medial screw placement).

It may be possible to resolve implant-associated infection with medical management only, but in some cases implant removal is required.[21] Some dogs can have a good outcome despite implant removal.[11] For those that remain lame or if the owner prefers to pursue further surgery to mitigate the risk of fracture, staged removal and replacement of the transcondylar implant is considered. The author has managed a septic and loose transcondylar screw in one dog with a lateral epicondylar crest plate alone (ie, with no transcondylar screw), with a resolution of lameness and no long-term complications.

CLINICS CARE POINTS

- Humeral intracondylar fissure (HIF) should be considered in spaniel breeds presenting with forelimb lameness and elbow pain.
- Computed tomography is more sensitive than radiography for diagnosis.
- Symptomatic cases (without complete condylar fracture) are treated with a transcondylar screw, which should be around 30% to 50% of the diameter of the isthmus of the humeral condyle.

- A medial approach is thought to reduce the complication rate and application of the screw as a lagged screw has been associated with a reduced risk of surgical site infection.
- Complete condylar fractures associated with HIF should be treated with standard AO principles of articular fracture repair.
- Lateral humeral condylar fractures should be repaired with a transcondylar compression screw and additional epicondylar crest plate, rather than a lateral Kirschner wire.
- Cases of nonsymptomatic HIF diagnosed as an incidental finding have an 18% risk of fracture, which typically occurs within 2 years of diagnosis.

DISCLOSURE

The author has no conflicts of interest to declare.

REFERENCES

1. Denny HR. Condylar fractures of the humerus in the dog; a review of 133 cases. J Small Anim Pract 1983;24:185–97.
2. Vannini R, Olmstead ML, Smeak DD. Humeral condylar fractures caused by minor trauma in 20 adult dogs. J Am Anim Hosp Assoc 1988;24:355–62.
3. Meutstege FJ. Incomplete condylar fracture in the canine humerus as a cause of obscure elbow lameness. In: 16th Annual Conference of the Veterinary Orthopaedic Society, Park City (Utah). 1989. p. 11.
4. Marcellin-Little DJ, DeYoung DJ, Ferris KK, et al. Incomplete ossification of the humeral condyle in spaniels. Vet Surg 1994;23:475–87.
5. Witte PG, Bush MA, Scott HW. Propagation of a partial incomplete ossification of the humeral condyle in an American Cocker Spaniel. J Small Anim Pract 2010;51: 591–3.
6. Farrell M, Trevail T, Marshall W, et al. Computed tomographic documentation of the natural progression of humeral intracondylar fissure in a Cocker Spaniel. Vet Surg 2011;40:966–71.
7. Moores AP, Moores AL. The natural history of humeral intracondylar fissure: an observational study of 30 dogs. J Small Anim Pract 2017;58:337–41.
8. Hare WC. The age at which the centers of ossification appear roentgenographically in the limb bones of the dog. Am J Vet Res 1961;22:825–35.
9. Butterworth SJ, Innes JF. Incomplete humeral condylar fractures in the dog. J Small Anim Pract 2001;42:394–8.
10. Moores AP, Tivers MS, Grierson J. Clinical assessment of a shaft screw for stabilization of the humeral condyle in dogs. Vet Comp Orthop Traumatol 2014;27: 179–85.
11. Meyer-Lindenberg A, Heinen V, Fehr M, et al. Incomplete ossification of the humeral condyle as the cause of lameness in dogs. Vet Comp Orthop Traumatol 2002;15:187–94.
12. Piola V, Posch B, Radke H, et al. Magnetic resonance imaging features of canine incomplete humeral condyle ossification. Vet Radiol Ultrasound 2012;53:560–5.
13. Marcellin-Little DJ. Incomplete ossification of the humeral condyle in dogs. In: Bonagura JD, editor. Kirk's current veterinary therapy XIII small animal practice. Philadelphia: W.B. Saunders Company; 2000. p. 1000–4.
14. Moores A. Humeral condylar fractures and incomplete ossification of the humeral condyle in dogs. In Pract 2006;28:391–7.

15. Carrera I, Hammond GJC, Sullivan M. Computed tomographic features of incomplete ossification of the canine humeral condyle. Vet Surg 2008;37:226–31.
16. Toal RL, Mitchell SK. Fracture healing and complications. In: Thrall DE, editor. Textbook of veterinary diagnostic radiology. Philadelphia: W.B. Saunders Company; 2002. p. 161–78.
17. Larsen LJ, Roush JK, McLaughlin RM, et al. Microangiography of the humeral condyle in Cocker Spaniel and non-Cocker Spaniel dogs. Vet Comp Orthop Traumatol 1999;12:134–7.
18. Moores AP, Agthe P, Schaafsma IA. Prevalence of incomplete ossification of the humeral condyle and other abnormalities of the elbow in English Springer Spaniels. Vet Comp Orthop Traumatol 2012;25:211–6.
19. Rovesti GL, Flückiger M, Margini A, et al. Fragmented coronoid process and incomplete ossification of the humeral condyle in a rottweiler. Vet Surg 1998;27:354–7.
20. Hattersley R, McKee M, O'Neill T, et al. Postoperative complications after surgical management of incomplete ossification of the humeral condyle in dogs. Vet Surg 2011;40:728–33.
21. Chase D, Sul R, Solano M, et al. Short- and long-term outcome after transcondylar screw placement to treat humeral intracondylar fissure in dogs. Vet Surg 2019;48:299–308.
22. Moores AP, Owen MR. Letter: Incomplete ossification of the humeral condyle as the cause of lameness in dogs - (Vet Comp Orthop Traumatol 2002; 15: 187-94). Vet Comp Orthop Traumatol 2002;15:VI.
23. McCarthy J, Woods S, Mosley JR. Long-term outcome following management of canine humeral intracondylar fissure using a medial approach and a cannulated drill system. Vet Rec 2019. https://doi.org/10.1136/vr.105403.
24. Clarke SP, Levy J, Ferguson JF. Peri-operative morbidity associated with mediolateral positional screw placement for humeral intra-condylar fissure. In: Proceedings of the British Veterinary Orthopaedic Association Spring Meeting. Birmingham (UK): 2012. p. 31–2.
25. Grand J-GR. Percutaneous screw fixation of incomplete ossification of the humeral condyle in three dogs (four elbows). J Am Anim Hosp Assoc 2017;53:45–51.
26. Barnes DM, Morris AP, Anderson AA. Defining a safe corridor for transcondylar screw insertion across the canine humeral condyle: a comparison of medial and lateral surgical approaches. Vet Surg 2014;43:1020–31.
27. Easter TG, Bilmont A, Pink J, et al. Accuracy of three-dimensional printed patient-specific drill guides for treatment of canine humeral intracondylar fissure. Vet Surg 2020;49:363–72.
28. Charles EA, Ness MG, Yeadon R. Failure mode of transcondylar screws used for treatment of incomplete ossification of the humeral condyle in 5 dogs. Vet Surg 2009;38:185–91.
29. Moores AP. Biomechanical basis of bone fracture and fracture repair. In: Gemmill TJ, Clements DN, editors. BSAVA manual of canine and feline fracture repair and management. 2nd edition. Gloucester: British Small Animal Veterinary Association; 2016. p. 20–31.
30. Muir P, Johnson KA, Markel MD. Area moment of inertia for comparison of implant cross-sectional geometry and bending stiffness. Vet Comp Orthop Traumatol 1995;8:146–52.
31. Fitzpatrick N, Smith TJ, O'Riordan J, et al. Treatment of incomplete ossification of the humeral condyle with autogenous bone grafting techniques. Vet Surg 2009;38:173–84.

32. Coggeshall JD, Lewis DD, Fitzpatrick N, et al. Biomechanical comparison of two implants for the stabilization of incomplete ossification of the humeral condyle lesions in dogs. Vet Surg 2014;43:58–65.
33. Walton B, Innes J. Initial clinical use of the Humeral Intracondylar Repair System (HIRS): complications and clinical and imaging outcomes. In: British Veterinary Orthopaedic Association, Spring Meeting. Birmingham (UK): 2018.
34. Perry KL, Bruce M, Woods S, et al. Effect of fixation method on postoperative complication rates after surgical stabilization of lateral humeral condylar fractures in dogs. Vet Surg 2015;44:246–55.
35. McKee WM, Macias C, Innes JF. Bilateral fixation of Y-T humeral condyle fractures via medial and lateral approaches in 29 dogs. J Small Anim Pract 2005;46:217–26.
36. Martin RB, Crews L, Saveraid T, et al. Prevalence of incomplete ossification of the humeral condyle in the limb opposite humeral condylar fracture: 14 dogs. Vet Comp Orthop Traumatol 2010;23:168–72.

Canine Elbow Dysplasia

Ununited Anconeal Process, Osteochondritis Dissecans, and Medial Coronoid Process Disease

Aldo Vezzoni, DVM, SCMPA[a],*, Kevin Benjamino, DVM[b]

KEYWORDS

- Elbow dysplasia • Medial coronoid process disease (MCPD)
- Ununited anconeal process (UAP) • Elbow OCD

KEY POINTS

- The genetic component that underlies the individual predisposition to develop elbow dysplasia is polygenic, involving multiple genes and without direct transmission.
- In association with medial coronoid process disease and persistent elbow incongruity, cartilage and subchondral bone changes involving the entire medial coronoid process and medial humeral condyle can be observed.
- Early diagnosis is possible in growing dogs; warning signs of dysplasia owing to medial coronoid process disease are represented by subtrochlear sclerosis of the ulna in the area of the affected medial coronoid process.
- In affected puppies and young dogs, the association of ulnar dynamic osteotomy to joint debridement is intended to improve the elbow congruity.
- Early treatment of ununited anconeal process has been widely shown to be effective in restoring the congruity, integrity, and biomechanics of the joint.

INTRODUCTION AND DEFINITION

Dysplasia of the elbow is a group of diseases involving the humeroradioulnar joint, including the injury or fragmentation of the medial coronoid process of the ulna (also referred to as fragmented medial coronoid process, osteochondritis dissecans (OCD) of the medial humeral condyle, the nonunion of the anconeal process of the ulna (ununited anconeal process [UAP]) and the joint incongruity, usually associated with medial coronoid process disease (MCPD), OCD, and UAP.[1–3] These orthopedic conditions can occur individually or in association with each other, further aggravating joint disease and affecting the long-term prognosis. Joint incongruity often accompanies the diseases listed, not only as a condition in itself, but also as a contributing factor to their development, in particular MCPD and UAP.[4–6]

[a] Clinica Veterinaria Vezzoni srl, via delle Vigne 190, Cremona 26100, Italy; [b] MedVet Medical and Cancer Centers for Pets, Columbus, 8155 Markhaven Drive, Columbus, OH 43235, USA
* Corresponding author.
E-mail address: aldo@vezzoni.it

Vet Clin Small Anim 51 (2021) 439–474
https://doi.org/10.1016/j.cvsm.2020.12.007

ETIOLOGY

The etiology of elbow dysplasia is considered to be multifactorial, with various causes, which determine its development to varying degrees. Incongruity, involving all 3 joint components, humeroradioulnar, asynchronous growth of radius and ulna and an endochondral ossification disorder, represent the most important pathogenetic factors in the determination of the different forms of elbow dysplasia.[2,3,7,8–10] The genetic component that underlies the individual predisposition to develop elbow dysplasia is polygenic, involving multiple genes and without direct transmission. Therefore, dysplasia is not expressed in all genetically predisposed subjects.[7,11–13] Environmental factors such as diet and type and amount of exercise which can worsen, but not cause dysplasia, are also involved in the expression of the severity of the disease. To date, the most recently published literature is not able to provide reliable data about the classification, etiology, or treatment of elbow dysplasia. One of the largest concerns is in regard to incongruity, because this is not necessarily a manifestation of elbow dysplasia, occurring also as a consequence of growth plates diseases, rather than being a main cause.[14–18]

In addition to the dysplastic forms, the elbow of the growing dog can be affected by other diseases, not included in the elbow dysplasia complex. Incomplete ossification of the humeral condyle, failed fusion of the medial condyle of the humerus, which is also described as ossification of the tendons and flexor muscles of the forearm.[2,3]

EPIDEMIOLOGY

Elbow dysplasia begins to occur in growing dogs, aged between 4 and 7 months of age, particularly in medium, large, and giant breeds. In adult dogs, the clinical signs are secondary to the osteoarthrosis that follows. Among the most affected breeds are the Labrador Retriever, Golden Retriever, German Shepherd Dog, Rottweiler, Bernese Mountain Dog, Great Dane, Dogue de Bordeaux, Chow-Chow, and Newfoundland.[9,19,20]

MEDIAL CORONOID PROCESS DISEASE AND OSTEOCHONDRITIS DISSECANS

By MCPD, we mean the formation of a separate osteocartilaginous fragment or a fissure or abrasion involving the cartilage and subchondral bone of the apex or incisor of the medial coronoid process[8] (**Fig. 1**). MCPD represents the most common form of elbow dysplasia; it can be observed as an isolated pathology or in association with OCD or less frequently with UAP.[21] The medial coronoid process of the ulna, completely cartilaginous at birth, reaches complete ossification around 20 weeks of age.[27] The disease becomes evident between the fourth and the seventh months, with differences regarding the species and the individuals. Both joints are commonly affected, many times with differing severity. Although the etiology is not fully known, most agree in considering joint incongruity in the early growing phase as a pathogenetic basis for the development of MCPD.[4–6]

In case of radioulnar incongruity with short radius and long ulna, the medial coronoid process is located slightly above the articular surface of the radius creating a step of 1 to 3 mm. In 2006, Lozier introduced a new pathogenetic theory, where it is possible to observe MCPD even if the ulna is shorter, because it develops later in growth.[23] According to the angular vector model, the radius (longer than the ulna) would cause an inclination of the humeral condylar axis to cause an increase in the load at the level of the medial humeral condyle and the medial coronoid process of the ulna. The radial head would dislocate proximally the lateral portion of the humeral condyle, forcing it

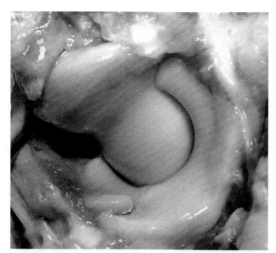

Fig. 1. Anatomic specimen of an elbow affected by MCPD, showing fragmentation of the apex of the medial coronoid process. Also shown are chondromalacia and erosion of the medial humeral condyle and of the trochlear notch of the ulna.

against the anconeous process, thus creating a fulcrum for rotation of the medial portion of the humeral condyle on the apex of the coronoid process. Regardless of the type of incongruity, the consequence is a maldistribution of the load forces, which are mainly directed toward the medial coronoid process of the ulna. In association with MCPD, cartilage and subchondral bone changes involving the entire medial coronoid process and medial humeral condyle can be observed, resulting in a "compartmental syndrome," [24]the maximum expression of an incongruent elbow joint (**Fig. 2**). The presence of MCPD is not always accompanied by an obvious joint incongruity at the time of diagnosis; the explanation could depend on an incongruity before fragmentation that resolved spontaneously during the residual growth of the dog.[24]

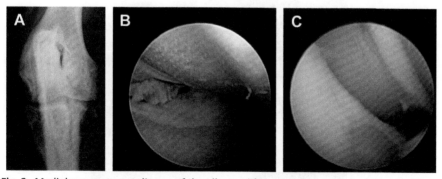

Fig. 2. Medial compartment disease of the elbow with severe erosion and subchondral bone exposure of the joint surfaces in the medial aspect of the joint. [A] Radiographic Cr-Cd view showing flattening of the medial condyle. [B] Arthroscopic view of the medial compartment with exposure of the subchondral bone. [C] Arthroscopic view of the neat separation between the lateral compartment with preserved cartilage and the medial compartment without cartilage.

Dissecting osteochondritis of the medial humeral condyle (OCD) is a manifestation of osteochondrosis (OC), or an enchondral ossification disorder, which results in a focal failure of the normal calcification process and vascular penetration into the epiphyseal cartilage.[25] This process results in cartilage thickening owing to a lack of evolution in bone tissue. Chondrocytes, given the lack of vascular supply, undergo necrosis and progressive weakening. At the articular level, this condition is manifested with initial cartilage fissure and formation of an osteochondral flap. The etiology is attributable to a set of genetic and environmental factors (rapid growth, nutrition, hormonal balance, physical activity, and microtrauma). The role of joint incongruity in the formation of elbow OCD is still unclear.[13] Often it overlaps with joint incongruity owing to a short radius, which causes an increase in weight loads at the medial humeral condyle level. The exposure of the subchondral bone in the synovial area and the degradation of the devitalized cartilage flaps trigger a series of reactive biochemical mechanisms that lead to synovial inflammation and arthritis. The breeds most likely to develop this disease are the Dogue de Bordeaux, Golden Retriever, Labrador Retriever, Bernese Mountain Dog, and Newfoundland.[19,20] Reported more often in males, OCD becomes evident between the fourth and the eighth months of life and affects both joints most frequently. When OCD is coexisting with MCPD and elbow incongruity, the prognosis is guarded (**Fig. 3**).

Diagnosis is made by palpation of the joint and radiographic examination. The prognosis varies from poor to good in relation to the severity of the lesion and the timeliness with which the treatment is initiated. In both MCPD and OCD, a medial collapse of the joint develops. Considering the offset of the ground reaction force with respect to the elbow, a straightforward conclusion follows that a medial larger offset will generate a larger moment in the frontal plane, which as an unavoidable consequence will cause compression of the medial compartment and tension on the lateral collateral ligament, leading to further medial friction.

Clinical Signs in Growing Dogs

The clinical presentation of dogs with MCPD and/or OCD is generally represented by lameness of varying degrees; the onset is progressive or acute. The first symptoms

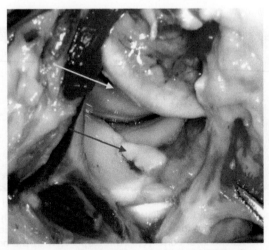

Fig. 3. Anatomic specimen of an elbow affected by both MCPD (*red arrow*) and OCD of the medial humeral condyle (*yellow arrow*).

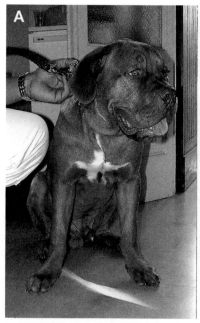
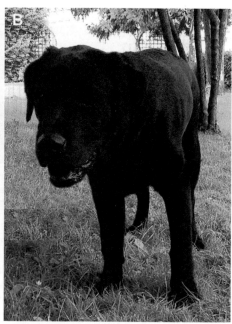

Fig. 4. (*A*) Dogue de Bordeaux, male, 8 months, affected by bilateral OCD of the humeral condyle, showing an alteration in posture in the standing position with external rotation of the distal limbs, as an analgesic behavior (pseudovalgus). (*B*) Labrador, male, 7 months, with left elbow MCPD, showing a shift of the center of gravity on the healthy right limb.

can appear during the first 4 to 6 months of life of the dog. An alteration in posture in the standing position can be observed, represented by analgesic behaviors, such as external rotation of the distal limb (**Fig. 4**A), which mimics limb alignment defects, or in case of unilateral involvement a shift of the center of gravity on the healthy limb is observed (**Fig. 4**B). When the pathology affects both joints, lameness becomes less evident, with exercise intolerance, until one of the elbows get worse and lameness occurs.[9] Bilateral conditions, which are frequent, have a more subtle symptomatology, characterized by the absence of a discreet lameness in the initial phase and by an uncertain gait with a tendency to sit; in these dogs, joint pain then becomes more evident with time, with the progression of joint inflammation and the appearance of lameness.

The clinical presentation and findings of the orthopedic examination in OCD cases can be superimposed on what is described in the paragraph relating to the MCPD. It is important to understand that the extent of synovitis depends on the degree of exposure of the subchondral bone. In the event that the osteochondral flap has not yet occurred, and this happens only in the initial stages of OC, clinical signs could be silent.[24]

Physical Examination in Growing Dogs

At the orthopedic examination, the affected dogs show a painful response to external rotation of the carpus of the affected limb. Swelling of the lateral joint capsule under the anconeal muscle can be observed, in relation to the amount of synovitis owing to exposed subchondral bone (**Fig. 5**A). In the most chronic forms, thickening of the medial compartment of the joint will be palpated (**Fig. 5**B). As the lesions become chronic, one will appreciate the rearrangement of the bony prominence typical of

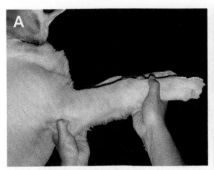
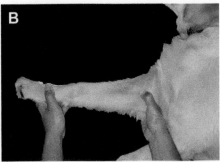

Fig. 5. (A) Swelling of the lateral joint capsule under the anconeal muscle can be observed in relation to the amount of synovitis owing to exposed subchondral bone. (B) In the most chronic forms, thickening of the medial compartment of the joint will be palpated.

the medial humeral epicondyle, which will be rounded and no longer pointed like in normal elbows. Variable reduction in joint excursion and crepitus during flexion and extension will be found related to the severity of the osteoarthritis that has developed. The physical findings of the orthopedic examination in OCD can be superimposed on what is described relating to the MCPD, elsewhere in this article. It is important to understand that the extent of synovitis depends the degree of exposure of the subchondral bone; therefore, of the osteochondral flap has not yet risen, and this happens only in the initial stages of OC, synovial ectasia could not be seen.[9]

Radiographic Findings in Growing Dogs

An early diagnosis is possible in growing dogs where the first warning signs of development of dysplasia owing to MCPD are represented by subtrochlear sclerosis (STS) of the ulna in the area of the affected medial coronoid process. STS is a bone reaction to joint inflammation and/or overloading. Owing to the frequency of bilateral disease, both elbows must always be examined, even in the case of apparent involvement of only 1 joint.

The following radiographic views are required:

- Mediolateral (ML) neutral view with the elbow at 120° (**Fig. 6**)
- ML neutral view with the elbow at 45° (**Fig. 7**)
- Craniocaudal (Cr-Cd) oblique view with pronation by 15° (**Fig. 8**)

It is necessary to carefully evaluate every detail regarding joint anatomy (**Fig. 9**) and congruity, subchondral sclerosis, and osteophytosis, taking into consideration that

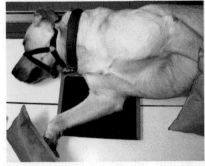
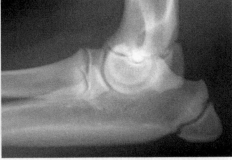

Fig. 6. ML neutral view with the elbow at 120°, keeping the carpus flexed to avoid supination.

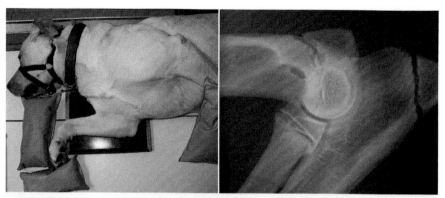

Fig. 7. ML flexed view with the elbow at 45°, keeping the carpus flexed to avoid supination.

slight signs during growth are most of the time a prelude to a dysplastic form that inevitably leads to more pronounced osteoarthritis signs.

ML view (**Fig. 10**)

- STS of the subtrochlear notch with loss of the trabecular pattern, obscured by a less defined increase in density.
- Loss of definition of the projection of the lateral coronoid process, obscured by the STS.
- Irregular silhouette of the projection of the medial coronoid process in the ML view
- Osteophytes formation starts over the profile of the anconeal process, the cranial border of the radial head, and on the profile of the lateral humeral condyle.
- Incongruity between the radius and ulna owing to a shorter radius can be seen in the neutral ML view. It is evidenced with a wider and uneven joint rim between the radial head and humeral condyle, and with a step between the radial head and the lateral coronoid process.

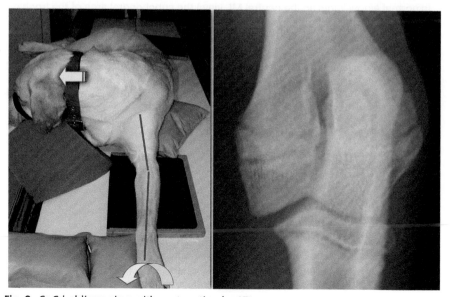

Fig. 8. Cr-Cd oblique view with protonation by 15°.

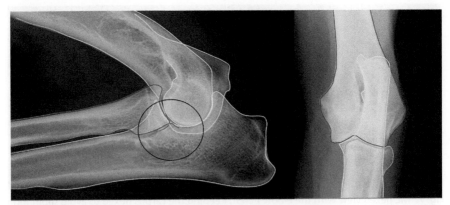

Fig. 9. Profiles of the bones in the elbow joint and their superimposition in the ML and Cr-Cd views. ML view: The *red line* delineates the radius; *yellow line* delineates the ulna, with medial coronoid process and anconeal process; *orange line* delineates the lateral coronoid process; and the *blue circle* indicates the subchondral trabecular pattern. The *pale green line* delineates the medial condyle and the *gray line* the medial humeral condyle. Cr-Cd view: The *red line* delineates the humerus, the *green line* the radius, and the *yellow line* the ulna.

- Less frequently, excessive narrowing of the radiohumeral joint associated to shorter ulna can be seen.

Cr-Cd oblique view (**Fig. 11**)

- Loss of density of the MCP projection and irregular profile
- Osteophyte formation with irregular profile over the profile of medial humeral condyle
- Incongruity between the radius and ulna owing to a shorter radius can be seen in the Cr-Cd view, with a step between the profile of the radial head and the profile of the ulnar articular surface

In normal elbow joints (in the neutral ML view) the subchondral area of the trochlear notch has a regular trabecular pattern without any bone sclerosis. In addition, the joint rim between the radius and the humeral condyle is thin and even (**Fig. 12**A). In the Cr-Cd view of normal elbows, the radial joint profile is continuous with that of the ulnar articular surface, without any step (**Fig. 12**B). The profile of the medial coronoid

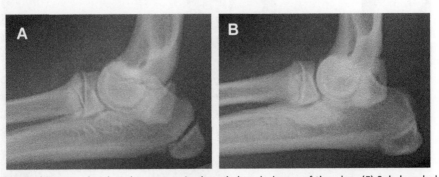

Fig. 10. (*A*) Normal trabecular pattern in the subchondral area of the ulna. (*B*) Subchondral sclerosis as a first sign of developing elbow dysplasia during growth.

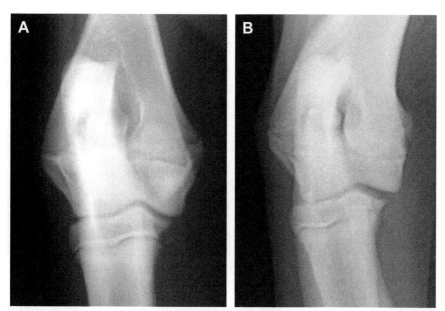

Fig. 11. (A) Normal profile of the medial humeral condyle and of the MCP of the ulna. (B) Loss of density of the MCP projection and irregular profile.

process and of the medial humeral condyle is well-defined and with a uniform radiographic density. Abnormalities, however minor, must be seriously considered because in most cases, these lesions will worsen as the dog grows.

Radiographic STS can be evaluated both visually and with objective measurement with digital assessment of bone mineral density using computer applications like the public domain application Image J (National Institute of Health, Bethesda, MD) (**Fig. 13**).[26–28] This process has been validated against dual energy x-ray absorptiometry studies in human studies,[29] comparing the bone density of 3 standard regions: the air, a metal bullet, and the subtrochlear region of the medial coronoid. Subtrochlear bone sclerosis is a consistent and direct sign of MCPD, owing to joint incongruity or malformation, as a consequence of joint inflammation and overloading of the MCP. In the elbow joint, it represents a very early and distinct sign of elbow dysplasia, regardless of whether incongruency is detected. Because elbow congruity can be altered by radiographic positioning, owing to physiologic joint laxity in growing dogs, subchondral bone sclerosis as a secondary sign of elbow incongruity is a more reliable sign that joint incongruity itself. As the lesion becomes chronic, the first osteophytes will become evident on the dorsal profile of the anconeal process of the ulna, on the head of the radius, on the medial coronoid process of the ulna in the ML view, and on the medial and lateral condyle in the Cr-Cd view (**Fig. 14**). In some cases, conventional radiology allows the observation of a fragment (**Fig. 15**). In questionable conditions, repetition of the radiographs after 2 to 3 weeks is usually diagnostic owing to the progression of the disease. A computed tomography scan, in contrast, provides a diagnosis of certainty in cases of doubtful radiographic diagnosis (**Fig. 16**).[30–32] A study is in progress correlating visual and digital evaluations of subtrochlear region in puppies and the final score of elbow dysplasia at adulthood. In **Fig. 17**, an example of a normal elbow joint at left of a 4-month-old Labrador (see **Fig. 17**A) is shown, compared with early signs of subtrochlear bone sclerosis in the center of a dog of

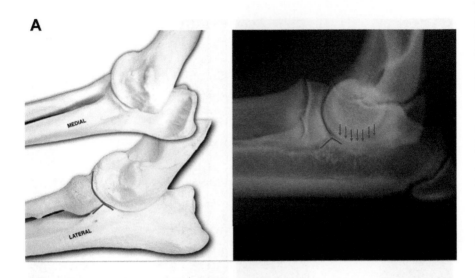

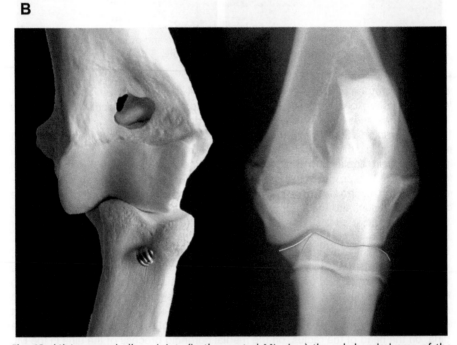

Fig. 12. (A) In normal elbow joints (in the neutral ML view) the subchondral area of the trochlear notch has a regular trabecular pattern without any bone sclerosis (*red arrows*). In addition, the joint rim between the radius and humeral condyle is thin and even, with congruity between the radial head and the lateral coronoid process (*red lines*). (B) In the Cr-Cd view of normal elbows, the radial joint profile is continuous with that of the ulnar articular surface, without any step.

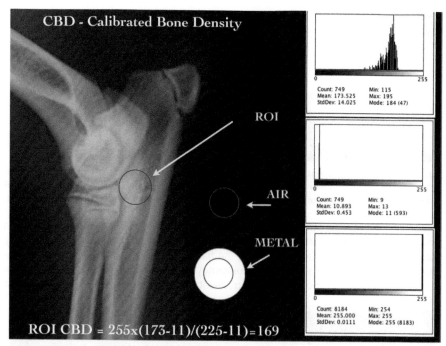

Fig. 13. Radiographic STS can be evaluated both visually and with objective measurement with digital assessment of calibrated bone mineral density using computer applications like the public domain application Image J. ROI, region of interest.

the same age and breed (see **Fig. 17**B), and a more advanced subtrochlear bone sclerosis at right of a 5-month-old Labrador (see **Fig. 17**C).

The radiographic study of OCD involves the execution of the same views described for the MCPD. Generally, the radiographic diagnosis of OCD of the medial humeral condyle does not present any difficulties.[33,34] We consider it extremely important to differentiate the initial forms of OC that do not require sudden treatment from forms

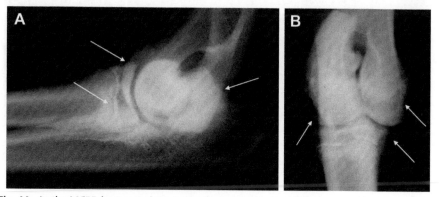

Fig. 14. As the MCPD becomes chronic, the first osteophytes will become evident on the dorsal profile of the anconeal process of the ulna, on the head of the radius, on the medial coronoid process of the ulna in the ML view, and on the medial and lateral condyle in the Cr-Cd view (*yellow arrows*). [*A*] ML view. [*B*] Cr-Cd view.

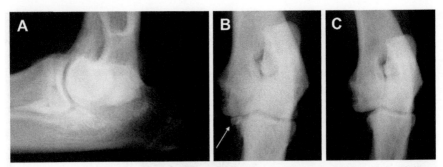

Fig. 15. In this case, conventional radiology allows the observation of a fragment of the coronoid process. [A] ML view with irregular shape of the MCP. [B] CrCd view showing the coronoid fragment. [C] CrCd view of the same elbow after removal of the coronoid fragment.

of OCD, in which a true osteocartilaginous flap has formed and is partly raised or still in place. In cases of OC, which can be seen in puppies 4 to 5 months of age, the only observable alteration is represented by the flattening of the profile of the medial humeral condyle, in the absence of radiolucency areas. In some cases, it is possible to highlight a real osteochondral flap associated with an underlying cuneiform

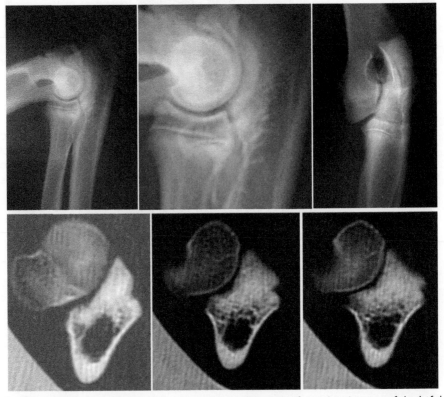

Fig. 16. A computed tomography scan provides a diagnosis of certainty in cases of doubtful radiographic diagnosis like in this Saint Bernard, female, 8 months, with doubtful STS in the radiograph, whereas the computed tomography scan shows the irregular shape and density of the MCP. (*Courtesy* Federica Rossi.)

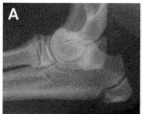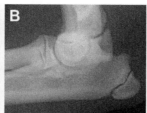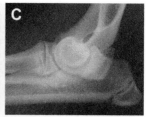

Fig. 17. (*A*) Normal elbow joint of a 4-month-old Labrador. (*B*) Early signs of subtrochlear bone sclerosis in a dog of the same age and breed. (*C*) More advanced subtrochlear bone sclerosis of a 5-month-old Labrador.

radiolucent area, whereas in other cases only the irregularity of the joint profile of the humeral condyle and slight radiolucency are observed (**Fig. 18**).

Treatment of Medial Coronoid Process Disease and Osteochondritis Dissecans in Growing Dogs

In view of a preventive medicine approach for all developmental skeletal diseases— other examples include hip dysplasia and patellar luxation—early diagnosis is critical for successful treatment.[27] Early diagnosis, when the dysplastic process is just starting, could intercept the disease process at its early stage, even before clinical signs have manifested. Thereafter early diagnosis of MCPD allows prompt surgical treatment, which is aimed at restoring joint congruity. MCPD is assumed to be underlying the observed sclerosis, such that the progression of the disease and osteoarthrosis may be prevented or reduced. Because MCPD starts developing at 3.5 to 5.0 months of age in the medium to large breeds, and approximately 1 month later in giant breeds, early diagnosis of elbow dysplasia is possible if a routine orthopedic examination is carried out in susceptible breeds at 4 months of age in medium to large breed dogs and at 5 months of age in giant breed dogs, and immediately when the first signs of forelimb lameness or abnormal gait occur in any breed of dog. The early orthopedic evaluation can be planned to be coordinated with vaccine protocols. The goal is to detect the disease as early as possible, without waiting for clinical signs. When no elbow dysplasia is detected, further evaluation 1 month later is advised because elbow disease can develop slightly later on. When elbow dysplasia is detected, the disease is confirmed, and proper countermeasures can be undertaken.[27]

Early treatment of developing mild elbow dysplasia medial coronoid process disease and osteochondritis dissecans at 4 to 5 months of age with distal dynamic ulnar ostectomy

In 4- to 5-month-old dogs, initial MCPD is suspected when subchondral bone sclerosis of the subtrochlear notch is observed on the ML radiographic view, with or without lameness.[35] OCD is diagnosed when flattening of the medial humeral condyle is seen in the Cr-Cd radiographic view. In affected dogs, a distal dynamic ulnar ostectomy only can be performed without joint treatment. It is believed that this practice releases the pressure on the medial and lateral coronoid processes (definitive peer-reviewed data to support this observation in vivo are lacking at this time). The distal dynamic ulnar ostectomy procedure is performed subperiosteally by removing 4 to 5 mm of ulna with a rongeur, bite by bite, approximately 2 to 3 cm proximal to the distal ulnar physis (**Fig. 19**A, B). The operated puppies are rechecked clinically and radiographically 3 to 4 weeks later. In cases with persistent clinical signs and worsening radiographic lesions with osteophyte formation or with development of

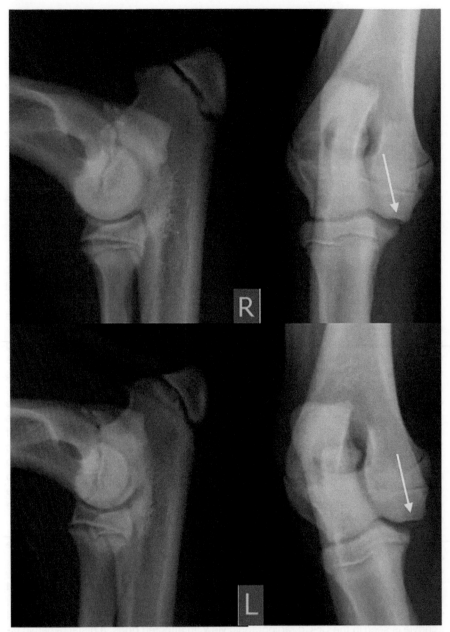

Fig. 18. Golden Retriever, female, 5 months, with a real osteochondral flap associated with an underlying cuneiform radiolucent area (*yellow arrows*).

an osteochondral flap, indicative of progression of the elbow dysplasia, conventional joint inspection and MCPD treatments are carried out with arthroscopy. In 4- to 5-month-old dogs with more severe clinical and radiographic signs suggesting advanced MCPD, we perform joint inspection and treatment with arthroscopy in

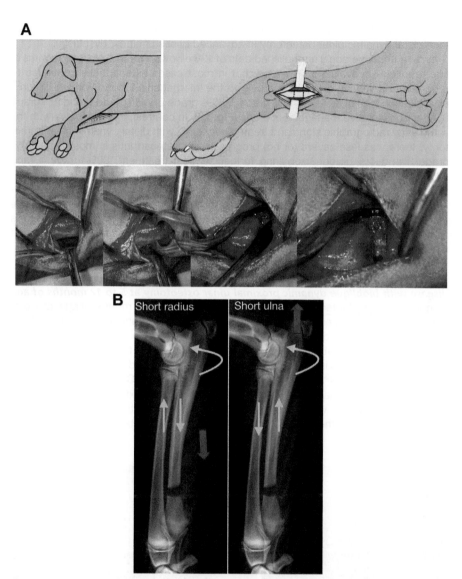

Fig. 19. (*A*) The distal dynamic ulnar ostectomy procedure is performed subperiosteally by removing 4 to 5 mm of ulna with a rongeur, bite by bite, approximately 2 to 3 cm proximal to the distal ulnar physis. (*B*) Spontaneous self-assessment of the joint congruity after distal dynamic ulnar ostectomy. In case of elbow incongruity owing to short radius, the weight bearing forces will lower the proximal ulna at the level of the radial head inside the joint. In case of short ulna, the pull of the triceps muscle will raise the ulna at the level of the radial head inside the joint. Torsional forces applied by muscles will improve joint congruity after distal dynamic ulnar ostectomy (*curved arrows*). [A] *Adapted from* Schultz KS, Hayashi K. Management of specific fractures. In: Fossum TW, editor. Small Animal Surgery. 2nd edition. Philadelphia (PA): Mosby; 2002:901-1022; with permission.

conjunction with proximal dynamic ulnar osteotomy (which we feel is more effective than distal dynamic ulnar ostectomy in advanced cases of elbow dysplasia).

In the authors personal unpublished data of 136 elbows with STS at 4 to 5 months of age, a follow-up evaluation revealed that in most cases osteoarthritis continued to progress to a varying degree according to the International Elbow Working Group[36] classification in 3° of severity (41% grade 3, 33% grade 2, 24% grade 1, and 2% grade 0) after conservative management alone (**Fig. 20**). In contrast, in 141 elbows with the same early radiographic signs and treated very early with distal dynamic ulnar ostectomy, there was less severe (or no) progression of osteoarthritis in most cases (4% grade 3 and 4% grade 2 requiring further surgical treatment, 80% grade 1, and 12% grade 0). Distal ulnar ostectomy is well-tolerated by patients and has no side effects when performed properly. This procedure entails a minimally invasive subperiosteal approach and the avoidance of injury to the radial periosteum and the interosseous vessels. Damage to the interosseous vessels may result in synostosis between the radius and ulna during the healing process. For this reason, no attempt is made to free the interosseous ligament.

Treatment of elbow dysplasia with moderate to severe medial coronoid process disease with bioblique dynamic proximal ulnar osteotomy at 5 to 12 months of age
In more severely affected puppies and in young dogs up to 12 months of age, presenting with different degrees of lameness, our approach is intended to improve elbow congruity and possibly decrease the unavoidable progression of osteoarthritis caused by the cartilage and subchondral bone lesions. Since 2012, the author has added a bioblique dynamic proximal ulnar osteotomy as suggested and later described by Fitzpatrick and colleagues[37] to the arthroscopic treatment of MCPD whenever cartilage damage is seen in the medial compartment. Oblique proximal osteotomy of the ulna, without fixation, will tend to lateralize the paw and thus unload the medial compartment. When the medial coronoid process fragmentation is the only lesion

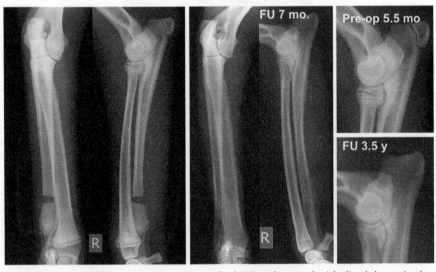

Fig. 20. Labrador, male, 5.5 months, with marked STS and treated with distal dynamic ulnar ostectomy. At 7 months, the STS is cleared and in the follow-up (FU) after 3.5 years the elbow has only minimal signs of osteoarthritis.

found in the joint, which is unusual, the treatment is limited to the arthroscopic removal of the fragments.[36]

In dogs up to skeletal maturity, between 5 and 12 months of age, without any medial compartment disease assessed at the arthroscopic inspection, being an unusual finding, fragmented coronoid process removal or regional debridement only is performed. In the more frequent condition where MCPD is associated with even mild medial compartment disease, bioblique dynamic proximal ulnar osteotomy can still improve joint congruity and the outcome. To decrease the morbidity and prolonged healing time associated with transverse proximal ulnar osteotomy, a maximal obliquity of the osteotomy (**Fig. 21**A, B) should be executed in the proximal midshaft of the bone, as described by Fitzpatrick and associates,[37] with a bioblique direction (caudoproximal to craniodistal and proximo-lateral to distomedial). This practice limits caudal and varus tilting of the proximal ulna under the triceps pull. With this bioblique dynamic proximal ulnar osteotomy performed at this range of age, we observed a quick healing of the osteotomy 1 to 2 months after surgery, with complete remodeling at 4 to 8 months. Although joint degenerative signs persisted at the follow-ups, a significant decrease of subtrochlear bone sclerosis and improved function were observed consistently. The varus deformity of the proximal ulna decreases the load on the ulnar joint surface.[37–39]

The author performed arthroscopic MCP debridement with bioblique dynamic proximal ulnar osteotomy on 117 dogs with MCPD with medial compartment disease between July 2012 and June 2015.[36] Eighty-three cases were reevaluated with a minimum of 6 months clinical and radiographic follow-up: 34 cases (41%) improved from grade 2 to grade 0 lameness, 27 cases (33%) improved from grade 1 to grade 0 lameness, 18 cases (22%) improved from grade 2 to grade 1 lameness, and 4 cases (5%) with grade 1 (2 dogs) and grade 2 (2 dogs) lameness did not improve. Thereafter, good outcome (no lameness) was obtained in 73% of the cases, improvement in 22%,

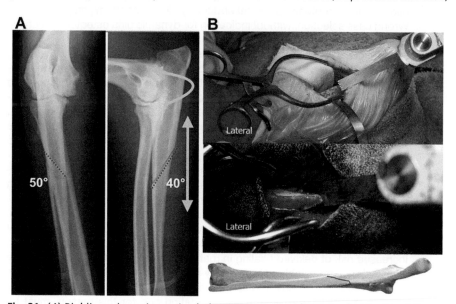

Fig. 21. (*A*) Bioblique dynamic proximal ulnar osteotomy with maximal obliquity of the osteotomy should be executed in the proximal midshaft of the bone, as described by Fitzpatrick and associates,[3] with a bioblique direction: at the left proximolateral to distomedial and at the right caudoproximal to craniodistal. (*B*) A long and narrow oscillating saw blade is required to perform the osteotomy with maximal obliquity in the 2 planes.

and a poor outcome in 5% of the cases. The poor outcome was seen in dogs with combined a fragmented coronoid process and OCD. Nevertheless, the long-term prognosis remains reserved and the owners should be instructed to perform regular rechecks, decrease high-impact physical activity, avoid any type of sporting or working activities, and maintain a slim body habitus.[36]

Complications after Dynamic Ulnar Osteotomies

- Complications in cases of distal ulnar ostectomy
  - Premature closure of distal ulnar physis can occur when the ostectomy is too close to the growth plate (<2 cm). In such a case, antebrachial deformity could occur with distal radial deviation in valgus and procurvatum, possibly requiring radial corrective osteotomy.
  - Synostosis can occur when the ostectomy involves the transcortex periosteum and the radial periosteum. This complication is more likely to occur when the ostectomy is performed with an oscillating saw blade instead of using a rongeur. Radioulnar synostosis impairs pronation and supination of the distal forelimb and can be a cause of lameness. When synostosis is limited to a small area and causes lameness, it can be removed surgically, but with the risk of secondary new synostosis.
  - Caudal tilting of the proximal segment could occur when the ostectomy is performed too proximal (>3 cm from the physis), favored by uncontrolled physical activity.
  - Nonunion or delayed union could occur when the ostectomy is performed in older dogs (>6 months of age).
  - A lack of efficacy in restoring joint congruity when the ostectomy is performed at 6 months of age or later, requiring further surgery (proximal dynamic bioblique ulnar osteotomy, proximal abducting ulnar osteotomy, etc).
  - Wrong case selection, without indication for dynamic ulna osteotomy because of misinterpretation of early signs of elbow dysplasia.[40]
- Complications in case of proximal ulnar ostectomy
  - The risk of causing excessive caudal and varus tilt and dislocation of the proximal ulnar segment can be secondary to the lack of owner compliance and consequently an excessive and uncontrolled physical activity or to surgical error, represented by a short oblique, or even worse, to a transverse ulnar cut. The use of a narrow and long blade, usually 9 cm long and 9 mm wide, is needed to obtain the required obliquity, which should be from 40° to 30° to the caudal ulnar surface. Severe tilt of the proximal segment could be associated with radial head luxation. This complication could result in a similar condition as a Monteggia fracture. The treatment of this type of complication depends on the amount of dislocation and on the timeline of diagnosis; reduction and fixation with an intramedullary pin, with or without tension band wiring, is required in the case of an early and severe dislocation. The cortical nature of the proximal ulnar segment predisposes this type of osteotomy to an increased risk of delayed healing in mature dogs. It is for this reason that the proximal dynamic bioblique osteotomy is not recommended after 12 months of age (skeletal maturity). Single session bilateral treatment dramatically increases the risk of proximal ulnar dislocation and for this reason, must be avoided. In case of bilateral condition, the 2 surgical interventions should be staged about 3 or 4 weeks apart, depending by the age of the dog.
  - Synostosis between radius and ulna could occur if the long interosseus ligament is involved, particularly in immature dogs.

o Inadvertent radial osteotomy could occur, either partial or complete. A proper surgical technique that protects the radius with a malleable retractor eliminates the risk of performing a radial cut and of radioulnar synostosis. A modest (15°) lateromedial direction of the osteotomy will help to avoid the radius distally. In cases of a partial radial incision, immediate radial plating could be required.

o Too rapid of healing of the osteotomy could prevent adequate improvement of joint congruity. It could occur in the case of an incomplete osteotomy or without cause, requiring a repeat of the osteotomy.

o Delayed union could occur in more mature dogs (>9 months of age), requiring 2 to 3 months to heal completely.

o Nonunion is unlikely to occur in dogs up to 12 months of age, but it could be a serious complication in adult dogs, requiring strong plate fixation and bone grafting, with a reserved prognosis.[40]

MEDIAL CORONOID PROCESS DISEASE AND OSTEOCHONDRITIS DISSECANS IN ADULT DOGS

Chronic osteoarthritis as a consequence of MCPD and OCD of the elbow is very frequent in dogs belonging to the breeds predisposed to develop elbow dysplasia. As with all degenerative joint diseases, the progression of osteoarthritis is correlated to the time and intensity of physical activity as well as increases in body weight. The main predisposing condition for the progression of osteoarthritis in elbow dysplasia is the persistence of joint incongruity with persistent uneven joint loading, leading to medial compartment disease. The collapse of the joint space in the medial compartment leads the dog to bring the limb into adduction, increasing the erosion of the medial compartment over time. Subchondral bone exposure owing to continuous contact and overloading of the joint surfaces causes heat with synovial necrosis and permanent stimulation of the biochemical factors of osteoarthritis.[24,41,42]

Clinical Signs in Adult Dogs

Forelimb lameness can be evidenced as an exacerbation of a chronic latent condition in relation to physical activity, stressful movements, or an increase in body weight. Bilateral conditions could be overlooked for several years owing to severe worsening of osteoarthritis in one of the elbows, leading to 1-sided lameness. In elderly dogs the condition could worsen to end-stage elbow dysplasia, with persistent lameness.

Physical Examination in Adult Dogs

On palpation, the elbow joint will seem to be thickened because of periarticular fibrosis and osteophytes. On manipulation, the amplitude of the range of motion will be decreased, especially in flexion. Crepitus could be present during flexion and extension, because of the osteophytes.

Radiographic Findings in Adult Dogs

The standard radiographic examination of the elbow joint involves 2 ML views, with the elbow in neutral position (about 110°) and flexed (about 45°), and a Cr-Cd view with about 15° of protonation the radiographic examination will show all the typical osteoarthritis changes induced by the underlying MCPD and/or OCD.[31]

In the ML views, the usual findings are (**Fig. 22**) as follows:

- Osteophytes on the ridge of the anconeal process
- Osteophytes on the cranial margin of the radial head
- Osteophytes on the ridge of the lateral condyle

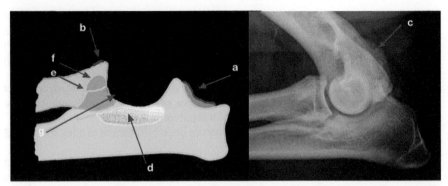

Fig. 22. In the ML views, the usual findings of MCPD are (a) osteophytes on the ridge of the anconeal process, (b) osteophytes on the cranial margin of the radial head, (c) osteophytes on the ridge of the lateral condyle, (d) STS, (e) abnormal silhouette of the medial coronoid process, (f) tip of the medial coronoid missing (blunting), and (g) uneven joint space between radius and ulna and between radius and humeral condyle.

- STS
- Abnormal silhouette of the medial coronoid process
- Tip of the medial coronoid missing (blunting)
- Uneven joint space between radius and ulna and between radius and humeral condyle

In the Cr-Cd view with 15° of protonation, the usual findings are (**Fig. 23**) as follows:

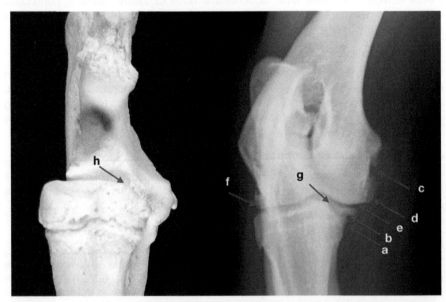

Fig. 23. In the Cr-Cd view with 15° of protonation, the usual findings of MCPD are (a) irregular profile of the medial coronoid process, (b) osteophytes on the medial surface of the medial coronoid, (c) irregular profile of the medial condyle, (d) loss of convexity (flattening) of the medial humeral condyle, (e) reduced joint space in the medial compartment, (f) increased joint space in the lateral compartment, (g) dislocated fragment of the medial coronoid process, and (h) incongruity between the radial head surface and the medial coronoid.

- Irregular profile of the medial coronoid process
- Osteophytes on the medial surface of the medial coronoid
- Irregular profile of the medial condyle
- Loss of convexity (flattening) of the medial humeral condyle
- Reduced joint space in the medial compartment
- Increased joint space in the lateral compartment
- Dislocated fragment of the medial coronoid process
- Incongruity between the radial head surface and the medial coronoid

The severity of the radiographic signs is variable according to the chronicity and severity of the disease. With MCPD, a real fragment is not always radiographically evident; more frequently, signs of secondary osteoarthritis are seen. Flattening of the medial humeral condyle can be due to chronic OCD or to erosion of the joint surface owing to medial compartment disease with medial collapse.[24,31,42]

Treatment of Medial Coronoid Process Disease and Osteochondritis Dissecans in Adult Dogs

The therapeutic approach differs based on the age of the dog, the degree of osteoarthritis present, the type of injury, and the choice of the surgeon.[43,44] The following is the approach used by the authors.[36]

- Conservative therapy is considered first in adult dogs with symptoms related to osteoarthritis evolution: weight reduction, limited activity and nonsteroidal anti-inflammatory drugs in cycles as needed. 15% reduction of body weight has been shown to be equivalent to nonsteroidal anti-inflammatory drug daily administration in a study published by Impellizzeri and colleagues.[45]
- Surgical treatment is performed when the conservative management is unsatisfactory. Joint inspection and local treatment can be performed by arthroscopy or traditional surgery. Arthroscopy allows one to view the joint in full, evaluate the extent of the cartilage damage associated with the MCPD and medial compartment disease, to distinguish different types of fragmentation, and to choose the best therapeutic approach. To date, the joint treatment involves the removal of the osteochondral fragment pertaining to the medial coronoid process or total/subtotal coronoidectomy. The MCPD, for the purposes of its treatment, should be considered not a pathologic form in its own right, but the symptom of a much more complex pathology, which unfortunately is still unclear to date. Persistent joint incongruity of the joint surfaces could be the end result. Whatever the treatment (removal of the fragment, coronoidectomy) and the method of execution (arthroscopy or arthrotomy), in most cases the osteoarthritis evolution secondary to the primary pathology will not be stopped, but only decreased at best.[44,46]
- In cases of OCD after the removal of the diseased cartilage, the sclerotic bone underlying the lesion can be activated by micropicking (few punctures with an awl, for a depth of 2 mm, spaced 2–3 mm apart) to favor the exit of mesenchymal cells and the formation of reparative fibrocartilage. It is not recommended to do this procedure when spurs of fibrocartilaginous tissue are already present.
- New surgical proposals for medial compartment disease are discussed in other sections of this issue. A number of different corrective osteotomies have been proposed and practiced to treat the condition. Most recommendations are based on observing incongruities within the joint, and are always meant to avoid the medial component of the ground reaction:
  - Elongation of the radius by an oblique proximal osteotomy (proposed by Slocum in 1998),[47] stabilized by a plate, will tend to lateralize the paw and thus

decrease the medial offset of the ground reaction and hence unload the medial compartment. This process will only occur if the interosseous ligament is sufficiently compliant—if not, the outcome may be the opposite.

○ Sliding humeral osteotomy, proposed by Mason and Schulz in 2008[48] and originally based on shifting the action of the triceps, incidentally, results in lateralization of the distal forelimb; Fitzpatrick and colleagues[49] have published a report suggesting a significant clinical improvement, but the risks of the procedure may be limiting its wider acceptance.

○ Proximal abducting osteotomy of the ulna proposed by Pfeil and Tepic in 2007.[50] Stabilized by a stepped plate, imposing a shift with abduction and incidental rotation of the ulna, which adds to lateralization of the distal limb and thus to unloading of the medial compartment (**Fig. 24**).

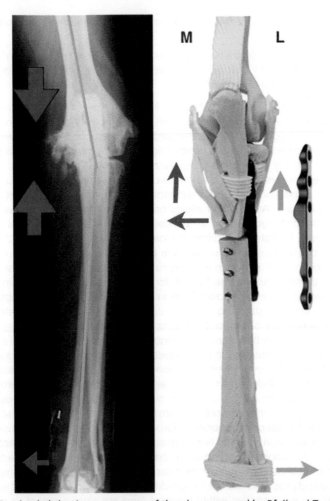

Fig. 24. Proximal abducting osteotomy of the ulna proposed by Pfeil and Tepic in 2007. Stabilized by a stepped plate, imposing a shift with abduction and incidental rotation of the ulna, adds to the lateralization of the distal limb and thus to unloading of the medial compartment.

- ○ Rotational osteotomy of the humerus (proposed by Tepic in 2011) aims at shifting the distal limb laterally—in vitro demonstration has yet to be confirmed by surgery in clinical cases.[51,52]
- ○ Midshaft radius abducting and elongating osteotomy (proposed by Tepic in 2011) fixed by medial plating is independent of the condition of the interosseous ligament and should, in all cases, led to lateralization of the distal limb and may be the method of choice in cases of the short radius.
- • Resurfacing techniques and joint arthroplasties will be presented in another section of this issue:, the most common being as follows:
  - ○ Canine unicompartmental elbow developed by Cook and Schulz in 2014[53,54]
  - ○ Total elbow arthroplasty (Randy Aker, 2007, Tate, BioMedtrix)[55]
  - ○ Partial elbow arthroplasty, involving the medial compartment only (Kirk Wendelburg, 2011, Kyon, still in clinical trials)[56,57]

End-stage medial compartment disease, occurring in older dogs, unresponsive to medical management as often seen in elderly age, can be treated with radiotherapy with a single application of 10 Gy with improved function for several months.[58] In another study lower dosage was used, 3 application every 48 hours of 2 Gy. Clinical improvement was observed in 92% of patients with median benefit duration of 356 days after the first treatment, and 418 days after the second treatment. No side effects were recorded.[59]

NONUNION OF THE ANCONEOUS PROCESS

UAP is a well-recognized disease affecting young growing dogs of several large and giant breeds. A high incidence has been reported in the German Shepherd Dog, and moderate to low incidence in Great Dane, Newfoundland, Black Russian Terrier (Tchorny Terrier), Saint Bernard, Basset hound, Greyhound, Italian Spinone, and Italian Cane Corso.[19,20,60] Unlike small breed dogs, which do not have a separate center of ossification,[61] a separate center for the anconeal process does exist in breeds such as the ones listed.[62,63] The anconeal process fails to unite with the proximal ulna during the first months of skeletal growth. In Greyhounds, this is ossified by 14 to 15 weeks but takes longer to ossify (16–20 weeks) in German Shepherd Dogs.[22,64] Failure to ossify after 20 weeks of age is termed "ununited." In a personal study performed in German Shepherd Dog puppies, the anconeal process was fused with the ulna at 15 weeks of age in females and at 16 to 17 weeks in males.[60] Nonunion of the anconeal process and persistent joint incongruity lead to joint instability, cartilage erosion and degenerative joint disease. An ununited anconeal process is the oldest known cause of elbow dysplasia and it was first described by Steirn, albeit under the term *patella cubiti*, in 1956.[65,66] The term UAP was first reported in 1959.[61] Several hypotheses regarding its pathogenesis have been proposed. The most accepted is asynchronous growth of the radius relative to the ulna in the early growing phase, which causes proximal displacement of the radial head and subsequent abnormal pressure on the anconeal process by the humeral trochlea when ulna is shorter than radius.[67] This process prevents bone union of its ossification center. Asynchronous growth may be related to genetic regulation and to rapid body growth. The antebrachial growth plates are different in the radius and ulna, with 2 distinct physes in the radius (proximal and distal) and 1 physis in the ulna, distally. Asynchronous growth of the radius and ulna can result in a shorter than normal ulna in the first phase of growth (up to 4–5 months of age) and a shorter than normal radius in the subsequent growth phase (5–6 months of age). Both may occur in the same dog, resulting in different diseases at different times of development (UAP and fragmented coronoid process).[21,64] Excision of the ununited process does not prevent the progression of degenerative joint disease because the permanent joint instability and incongruity are not corrected.[69,70] Screw fixation alone of the process without correction of the joint incongruity is not successful and usually leads to fixation failure. In accordance with the pathogenesis of UAP, a lengthening osteotomy of the proximal ulna has been shown to relieve the pressure on the anconeal process. This procedure allows the process to unite with the ulna, with or without screw fixation, depending on the stage of disease and different practitioners' preferences.[71,72] To achieve the same result without screw fixation, the anconeal process should still be firmly connected to the ulna by fibrocartilaginous tissue. The younger the dog, the greater the possibility that the process will fuse. With time and physical activity, the process will eventually become very loose or completely free in the joint, eliminating the possibility of fusion. The goals of treatment are fusion of the anconeal process and restoration of joint congruity before the establishment of osteoarthritis. Thus, an early diagnosis is essential for successful treatment of this condition and for preventing secondary degenerative joint disease associated with UAP.

Ununited anconeal process with persistent joint incongruity is a potentially devastating joint disease because of the risk of severe osteoarthritis over the time, which usually leads to chronic pain and functional impairment of the affected elbow. Early diagnosis and treatment of this condition is fundamental to obtain fusion of the anconeal process, restore joint congruity and prevent further osteoarthritis.[60] A complete understanding of the evolution of UAP aids in choosing the best treatment, which is aimed at fusion of the process and correction of joint incongruity.

Clinical Signs in Growing Dogs

The UAP manifests itself with a variable degree of lameness that occurs around 4 to 10 months of age of the dog. The symptoms could occur later in life, with acute onset without a previous history of lameness. In a standing dog, a constant shift of the center of gravity in unilateral cases and the abduction of the elbow is observed.[67,68]

Findings at Physical Examination in Growing Dogs

Lateralized joint effusion and distention is appreciated, and pain is observed at manipulation of the elbow, more with extension of the joint.[67,68]

Radiographic Findings in Growing Dogs and Staging the Disease

Early diagnosis of UAP is based on radiographic evidence of nonfusion of the anconeal process in the ML flexed view. This difference can be determined by comparing radiographs of the diseased and opposite elbows. In cases with bilateral disease, comparing the radiographs with those of healthy puppies of the same age and breed can be informative. Incongruity caused by a shorter than normal ulna can be better assessed in the extended (neutral) ML view. It is also possible to evaluate the mobility of the anconeal process, the degree of incongruity, and to stage the disease by comparing the extended and the flexed ML views. In the extended position, if the anconeal process is mobile, the humeral condyle pushes the process caudally and the gap widens, whereas in the flexed position, the pressure against the process is released, allowing it to return closer to the ulna. According to our personal experience, and in contrast with previous reports,[22,62–64] in most breeds, including German Shepherd Dogs, the anconeal process should be fused at 4 months of age, whereas in giant breeds, including Great Danes and Saint Bernards, union occurs between 4 and 6 months of age.[60]

UAP has different stages and clinical entities that can be differentiated by radiography and joint inspection (arthroscopy or miniarthrotomy) as suggested by Bardet in 1998.[73] In growing dogs, the disease can be differentiated into 5 entities according to radiographic aspects and intraoperative findings:[60]

1. The process is not fused but is still firmly attached; the joint can be congruent or incongruent with a longer than normal radius. Radiographically, the separation line of the anconeal process does not have a complete radiolucency zone and the anconeal process seems to be in its correct position. Intraoperatively, the anconeous process is strictly connected to the ulna by interposing fibrous tissue and does not seem to be mobile on palpation, with a minimal separation line (**Fig. 25**).
2. The process is not fused and moves slightly. It is hinged at its caudal part, creating a small cranial gap. The joint is usually incongruent with a shorter than normal ulna. Radiographically, the separation line has a complete radiolucency zone, but the process seems to be in place. Intraoperatively, it is possible to appreciate minimal mobility by means of palpation or by flexion and extension of the joint, and the anconeous process still seems to be in good condition and partially connected to the ulna (**Fig. 26**).
3. The process is not fused, but in place, with a radiolucent line of separation, with normal joint congruity and no signs of MCPD (**Fig. 27**).
4. The process is not fused and is completely loose; the joint is usually incongruent with a shorter than normal ulna. Radiographically the radiolucency area seems to be wider and is accompanied by bone resorption of the anconeal process and ulna, which shows irregularities. At this stage, the execution of 2 radiographs, in a midlateral neutral and midlateral hyperflexed position, allows to evaluate the mobility of the anconeal process. In surgery, a wide mobility of the anconeal process is appreciated (**Fig. 28**).
5. The process is not fused, the coronoid process is fragmented, and there is reversed joint incongruity (a longer than normal radius becomes a shorter than normal radius) (**Fig. 29**).

Treatment of Ununited Anconeal Process in Growing Dogs

Early treatment of UAP with dynamic ulnar osteotomy and screw fixation of the anconeal process has been widely shown to be effective in restoring the congruity, integrity and biomechanics of the joint. Personal experience confirms that, compared with

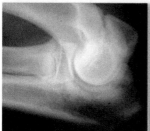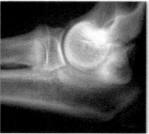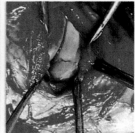

Fig. 25. UAP stage I. The process is not fused, but is still firmly attached. Radiographically, the separation line of the anconeal process does not have a complete radiolucency zone and the anconeal process seems to be in its correct position, not dislodged by the humerus in the extended elbow view. Intraoperatively, the anconeous process is connected to the ulna by interposing fibrous tissue and does not appear mobile on palpation, with a minimal separation line.

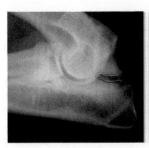
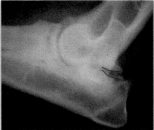
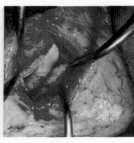

Fig. 26. UAP stage II. The process is not fused and moves slightly. It is hinged at its caudal part, creating a small cranial gap. The joint is usually incongruent, with a shorter than normal ulna. Radiographically, the separation line has a complete radiolucent zone, increased in the extended view under pressure by the humeral condyle, but the process seems to be in place. Intraoperatively, it is possible to appreciate minimal mobility by means of palpation or by flexion–extension of the joint, and the anconeal process still seems to be in good condition, partially connected to the ulna.

traditional treatment of UAP by removal of the process, better functional results are obtained with proximal ulnar osteotomy and screw fixation of the anconeal process to promote healing. The stability of the elbow joint is ensured by fusion of the anconeal process, which allows normal joint function and halts osteoarthritis progression. In contrast, in dogs that had undergone removal of the anconeal process osteoarthritis progressed, the range of motion was decreased and function was impaired. Reattachment of the UAP by means of a lag screw inserted from the ulna or from the process without dynamic ulnar ostectomy has been described.[75] However, this procedure does not eliminate the elbow incongruity that most likely caused the UAP in the first place, and, ultimately, fixation failure is highly likely. The prognosis of UAP treatment is influenced by the age of the dog at the time of surgery and by the condition of the anconeal process. The younger the dog, in term of months, the greater the likelihood that the UAP will heal, which emphasizes the importance of early diagnosis and treatment.[60] We found, as a general rule, that the prognosis in large breeds, such as German shepherd dogs and Rottweilers, was better when the surgery was done at 4 to 6 months of age. After 6 months of age, the prognosis deteriorates; in our own

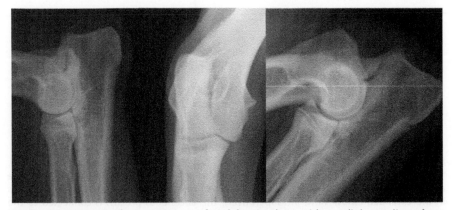

Fig. 27. UAP stage III. The process is not fused, but in place, with a radiolucent line of separation, with normal joint congruity and no signs of MCPD.

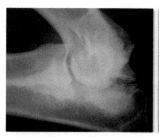
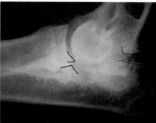
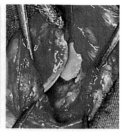

Fig. 28. UAP stage IV. The process is not fused and is completely loose; the joint is usually incongruent with a shorter than normal ulna. Radiographically the radiolucency area seems to be wider and is accompanied by bone resorption of the anconeal process and ulna, which shows irregularities. The execution of 2 radiographs, in a midlateral neutral and midlateral hyperflexed position, allows evaluation of mobility of the anconeal process. In surgery, mobility of the anconeal process is appreciated.

cases, we had only few successful outcomes in dogs in this older age group. In giant breeds, we found that an UAP can heal provided that surgery is carried out before 9 months of age.[60]

When dealing with lesions in both elbows, the patient will be more comfortable when 2 separate surgeries are carried out 2 to 3 weeks apart. However, by doing so, the dog will bear its weight after the first operation on the nonoperated leg, which increases the risk of loosening of the anconeal process. In selected cases of bilateral UAP at a very early age and with good owner compliance, both elbows can be operated at the same time. These dogs need more assistance during their daily routines and the owners should be made aware of this. However, it is critical to treat both elbows at an early age.

Concerning the osteotomy procedure, we have carried out osteotomies at different angles to determine which one was safest and most effective. Ideally, osteotomy should not change the final conformation of the ulna or its position relative to the radius in the joint. A cast or pin to stabilize the osteotomy should not be applied and weight bearing should be limited to promote physiologic realignment of the joint without unnatural or forced positioning. Because of the tension exerted by the triceps muscles on the olecranon and to avoid cranial tilting of the proximal ulna, an oblique osteotomy

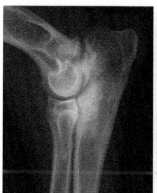
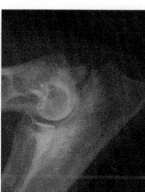
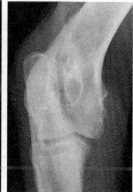

Fig. 29. UAP stage V. The process is not fused, the coronoid process is fragmented, and there is reversed joint incongruity (a longer than normal radius becomes a shorter than normal radius).

is preferred because the distal part of the proximal ulnar segment is stabilized by its contact with the distal ulnar segment. Moreover, an oblique osteotomy promotes bone healing because of the larger surface of bone interface. In contrast, a transverse osteotomy offers a smaller contact area, which prolongs the healing time, particularly in older puppies, and increases the risk of inclination of the proximal ulna. Driving a small smooth K wire from the tuber olecranon down the medullary canal across the osteotomy gap and into the medullary canal of the distal ulna has been suggested to reduce the cranial deviation of the proximal ulna and the instability of the osteotomy. In the author's experience, this is not necessary except in short legged dogs such as Basset hounds and in older dogs. In these cases, the pin must be removed after 3 to 4 weeks to prevent it from breaking owing to cycling fatigue. To decrease the risk of too rapid a bone healing, particularly in very young dogs, the removal of a thin segment of bone to create a wider gap and the insertion of an autologous fat graft into the defect have been described.[33] However, in our experience, these procedures are not necessary in most dogs and could lead to permanent nonunion. Dogs of giant breeds, such as the Saint Bernard, in which the growth period is much longer, should be closely monitored to determine whether additional procedures, such as repeated dynamic ulnar ostectomy or shortening of the radius, are required.

The osteotomy procedure can be accomplished using Gigli wire, an oscillating saw or an osteotome on a predrilled line.[61,75] Gigli wire is the safest and quickest, but only a transverse osteotomy can be easily achieved. With the oscillating saw, an oblique osteotomy can be made, but the risk of accidently notching the caudolateral cortex of the radius, which is very close to the ulna, must be considered.[70] With an osteotome, even when it is hammered on a predrilled line, the risk of causing a fissure in the cranial ulnar cortex is considerable.[73] In our experience, the use of an oscillating saw with a narrow long blade and isolating the entire circumference of the ulna with wet gauze sponges medially and with a malleable retractor laterally is the better choice.[74] The bioblique ulna osteotomy described by Fitzpatrick and colleagues[37] in 2013 for MCPD can be used for UAP too, at the level of the proximal third to the central third of the ulna.

The likelihood of finding concomitant lesions in the elbow of older puppies with elbow dysplasia is high, and a complete joint evaluation, possibly with computed tomography or arthroscopy/arthrotomy, is recommended.

Proximal dynamic ulnar ostectomy

A dynamic and lengthening ulnar osteotomy was shown to allow the anconeal process to unite spontaneously to the ulna in a varying percentage of cases.[60,71] The success rate was related to early treatment (4–7 months in large breed dogs and 6–9 months in giant breed dogs) and to the presence of a strong fibrocartilaginous connection between the process and the ulna. Varying angulations of the osteotomy line have been described. Transverse osteotomy is the simplest procedure and can be performed with Gigli wire. Because of the small osteotomy surface, the instability of transverse osteotomy is marked, resulting in greater morbidity for the patient. It can result in delayed bone union and in an excessive inclination of the proximal ulnar segment owing to the tension of the triceps brachii muscle and possible radial head subluxation.[70,73] Oblique osteotomy, in a proximal to distal direction, is the most indicated osteotomy and it must be performed with an oscillating saw with a narrow long saw blade. Because of the larger osteotomy surface, the instability of a very oblique osteotomy is decreased, resulting in less morbidity for the patient.[74] Bone union is faster and excessive inclination of the proximal ulnar segment is inhibited by bone contact of the cut surfaces. Some surgeons place a small intramedullary pin proximally to provide some stabilization.[76] However, fixation is not routinely undertaken to allow a sponta-neous anatomic realignment of the proximal ulna in the elbow joint, except in dogs that are more than 8 months of age and in Basset hounds. Although pin fixation of the osteotomy may speed recovery and decrease callus formation, it can also inhibit com-plete anatomic joint congruity and if not removed soon (after 3–4 weeks) it could break. A light padded bandage to protect soft tissues is applied for 10 days to make the pa-tient comfortable. Joint inspection, via arthroscopy or arthrotomy, is done before the dynamic ulnar ostectomy to ascertain the condition of the anconeal process.

Fixation of the anconeal process

Combining both dynamic ulnar ostectomy and lag screw fixation of the process has been shown to increase the probability of bony union of the anconeal process.[60,74–78] Fusion of the process can be achieved even when it is no longer firmly connected. Bone healing can be enhanced by curettage of the fibrous tissue in the gap and by filling it with a cancellous bone graft. Internal fixation of the anconeal process is achieved via a caudolateral approach, using an aiming device to drill the screw hole from the caudal ulnar cortex to the tip of the process (**Fig. 30**). One or 2 cortical 2.7-mm or 3.5-mm screws in lag fashion or one 4.0-mm partially threaded cancellous screw is inserted. With the latter, it is usually necessary to remove some of the prox-imal threads of the screw that would be engaged in the proximal ulna and thus, inhibit the lag effect. In a study by Meyer-Lindenberg,[42] a proximal dynamic ulnar ostectomy in association with screw fixation was carried out in all cases in which joint incongruity was evident radiographically and surgically. Otherwise, a middle or distal ulnar osteot-omy was chosen. In the authors' experience, a proximal ulnar osteotomy was always carried out when the anconeal process was fixed with a screw. When the treatment is successful, radiographic evidence of union of the anconeal process and ulna is seen within 5 to 8 weeks (**Fig. 31**). Several months are required for complete healing of the osteotomy and remodeling of the spontaneous hypertrophic callus. Dynamic ulnar osteotomy results in much better function because of the resulting improvement in joint congruity, even when anconeal bone union is not achieved. Fixation of a completely loose process is unlikely to be successful, and the failure of implants can be anticipated because of bone resorption of the process and remodeling of the trochlear notch, which causes an abnormal cycling load on the process by the

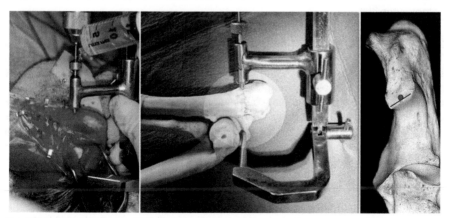

Fig. 30. Internal fixation of the anconeal process is achieved via a caudolateral approach, using an aiming device to drill the screw hole from the caudal ulnar cortex to the tip of the process.

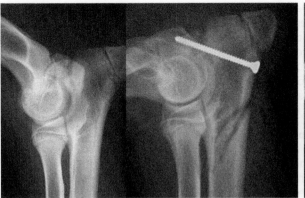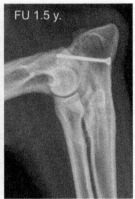

FU 1.5 y.

Fig. 31. When the treatment with proximal ulnar osteotomy and screw fixation of the anconeal process is successful, radiographic evidence of union of the anconeal process and ulna is seen within 5 to 8 weeks. FU, follow-up.

humeral condyle. In these cases, the loose anconeal process is removed together with the broken or loose implants. When a fragmented coronoid process is also present in growing dogs, the coronoid fragments are removed, the anconeal process is fixed, and proximal dynamic ulnar ostectomy is performed to improve joint congruity.

Clinical Signs in Adult Dogs

As for other forms of elbow dysplasia, front limb lameness can be evidenced as an exacerbation of a chronic latent condition in relation to physical activity, stressful movements, aging, or an increase in body weight. Bilateral conditions could be overlooked for several years owing to severe worsening of osteoarthritis in one of the elbows.[67,68]

Findings at Physical Examination in Adult Dogs

In adult dogs, it is possible to highlight hypomyotrophy of the affected limb, incomplete load and external rotation of the distal limb, reduction of the amplitude of the range of motion of the affected elbow, and pain and joint crepitus owing to osteophytes.[67,68]

Radiographic Findings in Adult Dogs

The radiographic examination of the elbow joint involves performing 2 ML views, with the elbow in extended position and flexed as much as possible, compatible with the decreased range of motion owing to osteoarthritis, and a Cr-Cd view with about 15° of protonation. The radiographic examination will show all the typical osteoarthritis changes induced by the underlying UAP and sometimes of concurrent MCPD. The severity of the osteoarthritis will be correlated to the age and to the persistency of short ulna incongruity (see **Fig. 33**). It is not unusual to find a UAP without severe osteoarthritis and without elbow incongruity (see **Fig. 27**).[60,67,68]

Treatment of Ununited Anconeal Process in Adult Dogs

In adult dogs, treatment of UAP becomes necessary when the anconeal process is loose or when it is suddenly dislodged from its fibrocartilaginous attachment by forced elbow extension. In such cases, removal of the free anconeal process is the only treatment.[60] In contrast, chronically degenerated joints with long-standing elbow

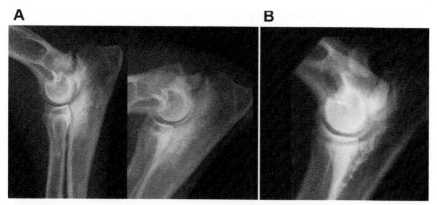

Fig. 32. Loose anconeal process, or sudden detachment and proximal dislodgment of the anconeal process owing to forced hyperextension in dogs with UAP without persistent joint incongruity, where the anconeal process is not fused but is firmly attached, causing acute lameness. Removal of the anconeal process is required.

incongruity and UAP do not benefit from any surgical treatment, apart from total elbow replacement (prosthesis) when conservative management is no longer feasible.

In adult dogs, the 4 most common conditions are:

1. UAP without persistent joint incongruity; the anconeal process is not fused but is firmly attached and there is no or only mild signs of osteoarthritis. This condition does not cause clinical problems and is incidentally diagnosed on routine radiographic examination. Usually, surgical treatment is not required (see **Fig. 27**).
2. Loose anconeal process, or sudden detachment and proximal dislodgment of the anconeal process owing to forced hyperextension in dogs with the condition described in point 1, causing acute lameness. Removal of the anconeal process is required (**Fig. 32**).
3. UAP with persistent joint incongruity with a shorter than normal ulna and severe osteoarthritis. Conservative management is recommended (**Fig. 33**).

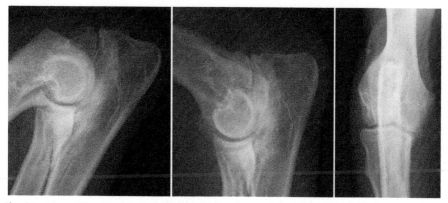

Fig. 33. UAP with persistent joint incongruity with a shorter than normal ulna and severe osteoarthritis. Conservative management is advised because the removal of the anconeal process will not improve elbow function.

4. UAP and severe degenerative joint disease with complete joint alteration such that joint incongruity can no longer be distinguished and with medial compartment alteration too. Conservative management is met with a poor prognosis.

PROGNOSIS FOR ELBOW DYSPLASIA

Elbow dysplasia has always had a variable prognosis depending on the severity of the disease. Nevertheless, the prognosis is always guarded because of the tendency of this disease to cause progressive osteoarthritis with time, exercise, and body weight increase. Early treatment of all forms of elbow dysplasia in the growing phase, before the development of osteoarthritis, looks to be the best way to mitigate the lifelong consequence of the disease.

CLINICS CARE POINTS

- The expression of elbow dysplasia is multifactorial, composed of both genetic aspects (polygenic involving multiple genes) and influenced by environmental factors such as diet, excessive exercise, and weight gain.
- A radiographic early sign of elbow dysplasia in the juvenile dog is STS of the ulna in the area of the medial coronoid process, this is in response to overloading of the medial compartment and inflammation.
- In many cases of juvenile dogs with MCPD, a dynamic ulnar osteotomy can improve elbow congruity and possibly decrease the progression of osteoarthritis.
- Early detection and treatment of elbow dysplasia (juvenile) is the key and in some cases can decrease the long-term degenerative changes seen with this debilitating disease.

DISCLOSURE

Dr A. Vezzoni is a paid instructor at PAUL Courses organized by Kyon. No other financial conflicts. Dr K. Benjamino has no commercial or financial conflicts.

REFERENCES

1. International elbow Working Group (I.E.W.G.). Protocol for Elbow Dysplasia screening. Adopted 1989 Davis, updated 1994, Philadelphia.
2. Nap RC. Pathophysiology and clinical aspects of canine elbow dysplasia. Vet Comp Orthop Traumatol 1996;9–58.
3. Hazewinkel HAW. Elbow dysplasia, definition and known etiologies. Proceedings of 22°IEWG Meeting, Munich 2007. p. 6–17.
4. Wind AP. Elbow incongruity and developmental elbow diseases in the dog. 1. J Am Anim Hosp Assoc 1986;22:711–24.
5. Wind AP, Packard ME. Elbow incongruity and developmental elbow diseases in the dog. 2. J Am Anim Hosp Assoc 1986;22:725–30.
6. Samoy Y, VanRyssen B, Gielen I, et al. Review of the literature: elbow incongruity in the dog. Vet Comp Orthop Traumatol 2006;19:1–8.
7. Corley EA, Carlson WD. Radiographic, genetic and pathologic aspects of elbow dysplasia. J Am Vet Med Assoc 1968;147:543–7.
8. Grondalen J, Grondalen T. Arthrosis in the elbow joint of young rapidly growing dogs: V.A. pathoanatomical investigation. Nord Vet Med 1981;33(1):1–16.

9. Kirberger RM, Fourie SL. Elbow dysplasia in the dog: pathophysiology, diagnosis and control. J S Afr Vet Assoc 1998;69:43–54.

10. Michelsen J. Canine elbow dysplasia: etiopathogenesis and current treatment recommendations. Vet J 2013;196:12–9.

11. Corley E, Sutherland T, Carlsson W. Genetic aspects of canine elbow dysplasia. J Am Vet Med Assoc 1968;153(b):543.

12. Breur GJ, Lambrechts NE, Todhunter RJ. The genetics of canine orthopedic traits. In: Ostrander EA, editor. The genetics of the dog. 2nd edition. Wallingford (United Kingdom): CABI; 2011. p. 136–60.

13. Padgett GA, Mostosky UV, Probst CW, et al. The inheritance of osteochondritis dissecans and fragmented coronoid process of the elbow joint in Labradors. J Am Anim Hosp Assoc 1995;31:327–30.

14. Murphy ST, Lewis DD, Shiroma JT, et al. Effect of radiographic positioning on interpretation of cubital joint congruity in dogs. Am J Vet Res 1998;59:1351–7.

15. Gemmill TJ. Clements DN Fragmented coronoid process in the dog: is there a role for incongruency? J Small Anim Pract 2007;48:361–8.

16. Blond L, Dupuis J, Beauregard G, et al. Sensitivity and specificity of radiographic detection of canine elbow incongruence in an in vitro model. Vet Radiol Ultrasound 2005;46:210–6.

17. Burton NJ, Warren-Smith CM, Roper DP, et al. CT assessment of the influence of dynamic loading on physiological incongruency of the canine elbow. J Small Anim Pract 2013;54(6):291–8.

18. Kramer A, Holsworth IG, Wisner ER, et al. Computed tomographic evaluation of canine radioulnar incongruence in vivo. Vet Surg 2006;35(1):24–9.

19. LaFont E, Breur GJ, Austin CC. Breed susceptibility for developmental orthopedic diseases in dogs. J Am Anim Hosp Assoc 2002;38:467–77.

20. Remy D, Neuhart L, Fau D, et al. Canine elbow dysplasia and primary lesions in German shepherd dogs in France. J Small Anim Pract 2004;45:244–8.

21. Meyer-Lindenberg A, Fehr M, Nolte I. Co-existence of ununited anconeal process and fragmented medial coronoid process of the ulna in the dog. J Small Anim Pract 2006;47:61–5.

22. Breit S, Kunzel W, Seiler S. Variation in the ossification process of the anconeal and medial coronoid processes of the canine ulna. Res Vet Sci 2004;77(1):9–16.

23. Lozier S. How I treat elbows in the older canine patient and new perspectives in elbow dysplasia. Proceedings 13° ESVOT Congress 2006, Munich. p. 93–6.

24. Coppieters E, Gielen I, Verhoeven G, et al. Erosion of the medial compartment of the canine elbow: occurrence, diagnosis and currently available treatment options. Vet Comp Orthop Traumatol 2015;28(1):9–18.

25. Lau SF, Wolschrijn CF, Hazewinkel HA, et al. The early development of medial coronoid disease in growing Labrador retrievers: radiographic, computed tomographic, necropsy and micro-computed tomographic findings. Vet J 2013;197(3):724–30.

26. Ohlerth S, Busato A, Gaillard C, et al. Early radiographic diagnosis of elbow disease and its predictability in a colony of Labradors. Proceedings 11th IEWG Meeting 2000, Amsterdam. p. 18–19.

27. Vezzoni A. Juvenile screening for elbow dysplasia. Proceedings 17° ESVOT Congress 2014, Venice. p. 317–23.

28. Burton NJ, Toscano MJ, Barr FJ, et al. Reliability of radiological assessment of ulnar trochlear notch sclerosis in dysplastic canine elbows. J Small Anim Pract 2008;49(11):572–6.

29. Small SR, Ritter MA, Merchum JG, et al. Changes in tibial bone density measured from standard radiographs in cemented and uncemented total knee replacements after ten years' follow-up. Bone Joint J 2013;95-B:911–6.

30. Gielen I, Villamonte-Chevalier A, Broeckx BJG, et al. Different imaging modalities in ED; what is their specific added value? Proceedings 31° IEWG Meeting 2017, Verona. p. 5–8.

31. Cook CR, Cook JL. Diagnostic imaging of canine elbow dysplasia: a review. Vet Surg 2009;38:144–53.

32. Rau FC, Wigger A, Tellhelm B, et al. Observer variability and sensitivity of radiographic diagnosis of canine medial coronoid disease. Tierarztl Prax Ausg K Kleintiere Heimtiere 2011;39(5):313–22.

33. Chanoit G. Comparison of five radiographic views for assessment of the medial aspect of the humeral condyle in dogs with osteochondritis dissecans. Am J Vet Res 2010;71:780–3.

34. Olsson SE. Pathophysiology, morphology and clinical signs of osteochondrosis in the dog. In: Bojrab MJ, editor. Disease mechanisms in small animal surgery. 2nd edition. Philadelphia: Lea & Febiger; 1993. p. 777.

35. Vezzoni A, Dynamic ulna osteotomy in treating canine elbow displasia. Proceedings of the 10 th ESVOT Congress 2000, Munich. p. 94–8.

36. Vezzoni A, Medial Coronoid Process Disease: my treatment algorithm and why. Proceedings ACVS Symposium 2015, Nashville. p. 205–9.

37. Fitzpatrick N, Caron A, Solano MA. Bi-Oblique ulnar osteotomy in dogs: reconstructed computer tomographic assessment of radioulnar congruence over 12 weeks. Vet Surg 2013;42:727–38.

38. Krotscheck U, Kalafut S, Meloni G, et al. Effect of ulnar ostectomy on intra-articular pressure mapping and contact mechanics of the congruent and incongruent canine elbow ex vivo. Vet Surg 2014;43(3):339–46.

39. McConkey MJ, Valenzano DM, Wei A, et al. Effect of the proximal abducting ulnar osteotomy on intra-articular pressure distribution and contact mechanics of congruent and incongruent canine elbows ex vivo. Vet Surg 2016;45(3):347–55.

40. Vezzoni A. Complications with dynamic ulna osteotomies in Elbow Dysplasia. Proceedings GEVO Congress 2019, Leon.

41. Van Ryssen B, van Bree H. Arthroscopic findings in 100 dogs with elbow lameness. Vet Rec 1997;140:360–2.

42. Fitzpatrick N, Smith TJ, Evans RB, et al. Radiographic and arthroscopic findings in the elbow joints of 263 dogs with medial coronoid disease. Vet Surg 2009a;38:213–23.

43. Fitzpatrick N, Yeadon R. Working algorithm for treatment decision making for developmental disease of the medial compartment of the elbow in dogs. Vet Surg 2009c;38(2):285–300.

44. Puccio M, Marino DJ, Stefanacci JD, et al. Clinical evaluation and long-term follow-up of dogs having coronoidectomy for elbow incongruity. J Am Anim Hosp Assoc 2003;39:473–8.

45. Impellizzeri JA, Tetrick MA, Muir P. Effect of weight reduction on clinical signs of lamenes in dogs with hip osteoarthritis. J Am Vet Med Assoc 2000;216:1089–91.

46. Vezzoni A. Radiographic aspects before and after surgery foe Elbow Dysplasia. Proceedings IEWG Verona 2017. p. 16–23.

47. Slocum B, Devine T. Proximal radial lengthening in elbow dysplasia with short radius. Proceedings AVORE Meeting 1998, Sunriver, OR.

48. Mason DR, Schulz KS, Fujita Y, et al. Measurement of humeroradial and humeroulnar transarticular joint forces in the canine elbow joint after humeral wedge and humeral slide osteotomies. Vet Surg 2008;37:63–70.

49. Fitzpatrick N, Yeadon R, Smith T, et al. Techniques of application and initial clinical experience with sliding humeral osteotomy for treatment of medial compartment disease of the canine elbow. Vet Surg 2009e;38(2):261–78.

50. Pfeil I, Tepic S. Proximal ulnar osteotomy for elbow dysplasia. Proceedings Kyon Symposium 2000, Zurich.

51. Tepic S. More on the osteotomies for the elbow. Kyon Symposium 2011, Boston.

52. Gutbrod A, Guerrero TG. Effect of external rotational humeral osteotomy on the contact mechanics of the canine elbow joint. Vet Surg 2012;41:845–52.

53. Franklin SP, Schulz KS, Karnes J, et al. Theory and development of a unicompartmental resurfacing system for treatment of medial compartment disease of the canine elbow. Vet Surg 2014;43:765–73.

54. Cook JL, Schultz KS, Karnes GJ, et al. Clinical outcomes associated with the initial use of the canine unicompartmental elbow (CUE) Arthroplasty System. Can Vet J 2015;56(9):971–7.

55. Acker R, van der Meulen GT. Resurfacing arthroplasty of the canine elbow. Proceedings 34th Annual Vet Orthop Soc Conference 2007, Sun Valley, ID. p. 55.

56. Wendelburg K, Tepic S. Kyon Elbow prosthesis project, Proceedings, Kyon Symposium, April 15–17, 2011. Boston.

57. Wendelburg KL. Kyon unicompartmental elbow replacement - Initial series. Proceedings 5th WVOC ESVOT/VOS Congress 2018, Barcelona. p. 514–6.

58. Kapatkin AS, Nordquist B, Garcia TC, et al. Effect of a single dose radiation therapy on weight-bearing lameness in digs with elbow osteoarthritis. Vet Comp Orthop Traumatol 2016;29:338–43.

59. Rossi F, Cancedda S, Leone VF, et al. Magavoltage radiotherapy for the treatment of degenerative joint disease in dogs: results of a preliminary experience in an Italian radiotherapy center. Front Vet Sci 2018;5:74.

60. Vezzoni A. How I treat ununited anconeal process. Proceedings 18th ESVOT Congress, London 2016. p. 282–6.

61. Cawley AJ, Archibald J. Ununited anconeal process of the dog. J Am Anim Assoc 1959;134:453.

62. Van Sickle DC. The relationship of ossification to canine elbow dysplasia. J Am Anim Hosp Assoc 1966;2:24–31.

63. Grondalen J, Rorvik AM. Arthrosis in the elbow joint of young rapidly growing-dogs 4. Ununited anconeal process – a follow up investigation of operated dogs. Nord Vet Med 1980;32:212–8.

64. Van Sickle DC. A comparative study of the post-natal elbow development of the Greyhound and the German Shepherd Dog. J Am Vet Med Assoc 1966;147:24–31.

65. Steirn RA. Ectopic sesamoid bones at the elbow (patella cubiti) of the dog. J Am Vet Med Assoc 1956;128:498.

66. Sumner Smith G. Variation in ages of growth plate fusion in the dog. Vet Comp Orthop Traumatol 2000;13:211.

67. Thacher C. Ununited anconeal process. In: Slatter D, editor. Textbook of small animal surgery. Philadelphia: WB Saunders; 1985.

68. Guthrie S. Some radiographic and clinical aspects of ununited anconeal process. Vet Rec 1989;124:661–2.

69. Roy RG, Wallace LJ, Johnston RA. A retrospective long term evaluation of un-united anconeal process excision of the canine elbow. Vet Comp Orthop Traumatol 1994;7:94.
70. Matis U. Treatment of Ununited anconeal process. Proceedings of 6° ESVOT Congress, Rome, 1992.
71. Sjostrom L, Kasstrom H, Kallberg M. Ununited anconeal process in the dog: pathogenesis and treatment by osteotomy of the ulna. Vet Comp Orthop Traumatol 1995;8:170.
72. Fox S, Burbidge HM, Bray JC, et al. Ununited anconeal process: lag-screw fixation. J Am Anim Hosp Assoc 1996;32:52.
73. Bardet J. Classification and treatment of ununited anconeal process in dogs. Proceedings 9th ESVOT Congress 1998, Munich.
74. Vezzoni A, Ferretti A, Abbiati G. Results of proximal ulna osteotomy as a treatment for ununited anconeal process (UAP). Proceedings of the IEWG Meeting 1998, Bologna.
75. Meyer-Lindenberg A, Fehr M, Nolte I. Short- and long-term results after surgical treatment of an ununited anconeal process in the dog. Vet Comp Orthop Traumatol 2001;14:101–10.
76. Pettit RA, Tattersall J, Gemill T, et al. Effect of surgical technique on radiographic fusion of the anconeus in the treatment of ununited anconeal process. J Small Anim Pract 2009;50:545–8.
77. Turner BM, Abercromby RH, Innes J, et al. Dynamic proximal ulnar osteotomy for the treatment of ununited anconeal process in 17 dogs. Vet Comp Orthop Traumatol 1998;11:76–9.
78. Krotscher U, Hulse DA, Bahr A, et al. Ununited anconeal process: lag-screw fixation with proximal ulnar osteotomy. Vet Comp Orthop Traumatol 2000;13:212–6.

Canine Elbow Dysplasia
Medial Compartment Disease and Osteoarthritis

Kenneth A. Bruecker, DVM, MS[a],*, Kevin Benjamino, DVM[b],
Aldo Vezzoni, Med Vet[c], Charles Walls, DVM[d],
Kirk L. Wendelburg, DVM[e], Christelle M. Follette, DVM[e],
Loïc M. Déjardin, DVM, MS[f], Reunan Guillou, Doc Vét[g]

KEYWORDS

- Elbow • Degenerative joint disease (DJD) • Osteoarthritis (OA)
- Medial compartment disease • Sliding humeral osteotomy (SHO)
- Proximal abducting ulnar osteotomy (PAUL) • Canine unicompartmental elbow (CUE)
- Partial elbow replacement (KYON BANC)

KEY POINTS

- Degenerative joint disease (DJD)/osteoarthritis (OA) of the elbow often is associated with elbow dysplasia or traumatic injury.
- DJD/OA of the elbow most commonly affects primarily the humeroulnar articulation or medial compartment. This has been termed, *medial compartment disease* or *medial compartment syndrome.*
- The degree of cartilage loss can be defined and categorized using a modified Outerbridge scoring system.
- When medical management is not effective in palliating signs of DJD/OA, surgical strategies include off-loading of the medial compartment by axis-shifting osteotomies, including proximal abducting ulnar osteotomy and sliding humeral osteotomy. Other strategies involve replacement of portions or all of the articular surface of the medial compartment with canine unicompartmental elbow or partial elbow replacement. With global elbow joint OA (medial and lateral compartment), a total elbow replacement may be required.

[a] Continuing Orthopedic Veterinary Education, Moorpark, CA 93021, USA; [b] MedVet Medical and Cancer Centers for Pets, Columbus, 8155 Markhaven Drive, Columbus, OH 43235, USA; [c] Clinica Veterinaria Vezzoni srl, via Massarotti 60/A, Cremona, Cremona 26100, Italy; [d] Veterinary Clinical Sciences, School Of Veterinary Medicine, Louisiana State University, Baton Rouge, LA 70803, USA; [e] VCA Animal Specialty Group, 4641 Colorado Boulevard, Los Angeles, CA 90039, USA; [f] Department of Small Animal Clinical Sciences, College of Veterinary Medicine, Michigan State University, 736 Wilson Road, East Lansing, MI 48824-1314, USA; [g] ACCESS Bone & Joint Center, 9599 Jefferson Boulevard, Culver City, CA 90232, USA
* Corresponding author.
E-mail address: kbruecker@me.com

Vet Clin Small Anim 51 (2021) 475–515
https://doi.org/10.1016/j.cvsm.2020.12.008
0195-5616/21/© 2020 Elsevier Inc. All rights reserved.
vetsmall.theclinics.com

INTRODUCTION

Erosion of the articular cartilage of the medial compartment of the elbow (the humeroulnar articulation) secondary to incongruency associated with elbow dysplasia (fragmented coronoid process/osteochondritis dissecans) or traumatic injury has been termed, *medial compartment disease (MCD)*.[1] The end result is degenerative joint disease (DJD) and osteoarthritis (OA) that primarily affects the medial compartment (humeroulnar articulation) while largely sparing the lateral compartment (humeroradial articulation) of the elbow joint.

The severity of cartilage loss has been described and quantified using a modified Outerbridge classification. This system assigns a grade of 0-IV based on severity of cartilage damage/loss.[2]

Modified Outerbridge scores (**Fig. 1**):

0—normal cartilage

I—chondromalacia

II—fibrillation and damage to the superficial matrix only

III—full-thickness fissure, thus loss of the cellular components

IV—full-thickness erosion of cartilage to the level of subchondral bone

Modified Outerbridge scores of grades I to II may be reversible. Due to the loss of cellular components, grades III to IV scores generally are thought to be irreversible and progressive (**Fig. 2**).

Nonsurgical strategies to palliate discomfort associated with OA include

- Weight control
- Activity restrictions (encourage low-impact activity and discourage high-impact activity)
- Joint supplements containing glucosamine, chondroitin, Polysulfate glycosaminoglycans (PSGAGs), and omega-3 essential fatty acid (EFA)
- Nonsteroidal anti-inflammatory drugs (NSAIDs)
- Nonopioid analgesics (eg, gabapentin and amantadine)
- Intra-articular injections (hyaluronate and corticosteroids)
- Regenerative medicine (intra-articular stem cells and platelet-rich plasma)
- External rehabilitation modalities, such as class 3 laser

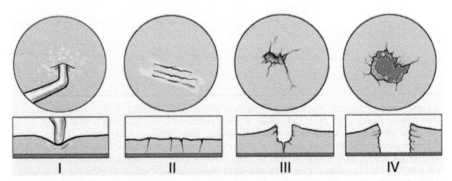

Fig. 1. Modified Outerbridge scores of articular cartilage damage. 0—normal cartilage, I—chondromalacia; II—fibrillation and damage to the superficial matrix only; III—full-thickness fissure, thus loss of the cellular components; and IV, —full-thickness erosion of cartilage to the level of subchondral bone. (*From* Lasanianos NG, Kanakaris NK. Chondral Lesions. In: Lasanianos NG, Kanakaris NK., Giannoudis PV, eds. Trauma and Orthopaedic Classifications: A Comprehensive Overview. London, UK: Springer-Verlag; 2015:501-504; with permission. (Org Fig 113.1).)

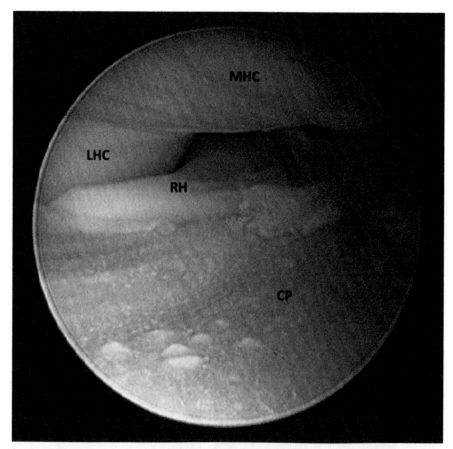

Fig. 2. MCD—arthroscopic image of left elbow with full-thickness cartilage loss of humer-oulnar joint surfaces consistent with grade 4 modified Outerbridge score. The lateral compartment is visually healthy. CP, coronoid process; LHC, lateral humeral condyle; MHC, medial humeral condyle; RH, radial head.

- External beam radiation and radiation delivery through intra-articular injection (Synovetin OA [Exubrion, Buford, Georgia, USA])

Surgical strategies to reduce pain through offloading of the medial compartment by load shifting osteotomies include Proximal Abducting Ulnar Osteotomy (PAUL) by KYON and Sliding Humeral Osteotomy (SHO) by New generations devices (DGD). Other strategies involve replacement of portions or all of the articular surface of the medial compartment. This article discusses the canine unicompartmental elbow (CUE) by Arthrex and the biomechanically anatomic, nonconstrained, and compartmental (BANC) partial elbow replacement (PER) system by KYON. With global elbow joint OA (medial and lateral compartment), a total elbow replacement (TER) may be required, with the TATE system by BioMedtrix being the focus.

SLIDING HUMERAL OSTEOTOMY
Rationale

The SHO was reported in 2009 in a pair of articles by Fitzpatrick and colleagues[3,4] as a technique used to decrease weight-bearing load within the medial compartment of the elbow joint. There were precursors to this more refined procedure in the early 2000s, evidenced by the humeral wedge and humeral slide osteotomies.[5,6] Further research was done looking at medium-term and long-term outcomes, gaining this procedure a spot in the armament against MCD.[7]

The goal of the SHO is to shift the weight-bearing axis of the forelimb (digits to shoulder) as it crosses the elbow joint (in particular, the humeroulnar contact) laterally. This decreases the weight-bearing load within the medial compartment of the elbow joint, because this is where the majority of pathology resides (**Fig. 3**). The exact cause of MCD largely is unknown; however, it is evidenced as advancing cartilage wear and

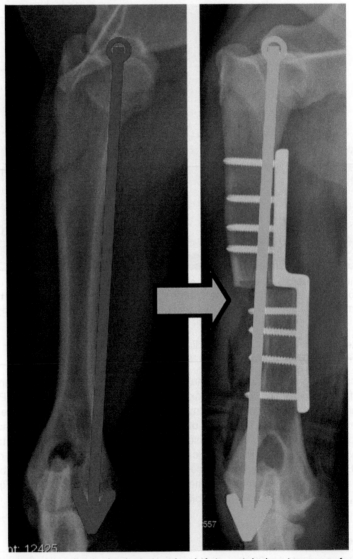

Fig. 3. Craniocaudal radiographs depicting the shift in weight-bearing access from medial (*red arrow* in the left image) to lateral (*green arrow* in the right image) following SHO.

exposure/sclerosis of subchondral bone on both the ulnar and opposing humeral surfaces.

Case Selection

Case selection for this procedure is of utmost importance because the objective of this procedure is to improve the weight-bearing axis of the limb and over time improve the gait of the patient and decrease the secondary effects of MCD. To that goal, patients with advanced degenerative changes are not ideal candidates. Conversely, skeletally immature patients also are not ideal due to open physeal regions that could develop abnormally with the change in force. An ideal candidate is a patient diagnosed arthroscopically with MCD that is skeletally mature (assessed via radiography) and with mild to moderate degenerative changes. A study evaluating dogs with osteochondrosis of the medial humeral condyle that were treated with an SHO procedure showed continued degenerative changes, although this was a small group.[8]

Description of Procedure and Instrumentation

The patient typically is in lateral recumbency, with the affected limb near the table and prepped in a hanging position. A standard medial approach is needed to access the medial aspect of the diaphysis of the humerus. Dissection to the diaphysis of the humerus is important with the distal epicondyle being palpable for a landmark. Retraction of the brachiocephalicus and biceps brachii cranially and the triceps brachii and superficial pectoral muscles caudally using Hohmann retractors is recommended.[9] Care is taken to not disrupt the neurovascular bundle near the distal diaphysis of the humerus. This should be identified and retracted. Once the mid to distal diaphysis is exposed, an appropriate SHO plate is selected. The plate and locking screws are manufactured by New Generation Devices (Glen Rock, New Jersey, USA) as are the drill guides for the locking system.

There are 2 variants of the plates (all same design), 7.5 mm and 10 mm, according to the size of the step desired. Although in general large breed dogs accept the 10-mm plate and medium-sized dogs the 7.5-mm plate, sizing also can be done by planning software, attempting to achieve 50% contact of the cut. A minimum bone overlap of one-third is needed.[9] There is a specific sequence of screw placement (described previously)—in general, the proximal 4 holes use locking screws while cortical screws are initially placed in the center 2 holes of the distal segment of the SHO plate, prior to the mid-diaphyseal transverse bone cut[3] (**Fig. 4**). Once the osteotomy is complete, the 2 cortical screws in the distal fragment are tightened sequentially, drawing the bone to the plate—providing the offset sliding motion of the humerus (**Fig. 5**). The remaining locking screws are placed, and the cortical screws then are converted to locking screws (**Fig. 6**). Closure is performed in normal fashion. Some modifications have been made since this technique first was reported in an attempt to reduce potential short-term complications. In larger dogs, the author (Dr. Benjamino) has added either a cranial or caudal plate and screws (SOP plating system [Orthomed, Huddersfield, West Yorkshire, England]).

Outcome

There have been 2 peer-reviewed articles that have looked at both medium-term and long-term results in dogs that have received an SHO[7,9] (**Fig. 7**). In the study by Wendelburg and Beale[7] (32 cases), 30 dogs exceeded their preoperative ground reactive forces and improvement was noted compared with the contralateral limb. Also, in this study, it was noted that 31 dogs did not have radiographic progression of osteophytosis. These data might be skewed, with a mean follow-up radiographic time of

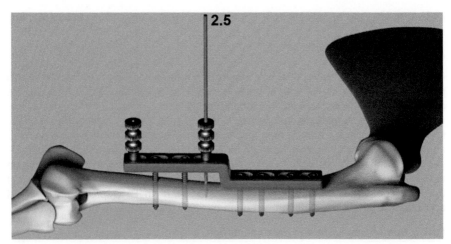

Fig. 4. The proximal portion of the plate is fixed to the humerus with locking screws. Bicortical Cortical screws are placed in holes #6 and #7 before performing the osteotomy.

49 weeks and only 8 dogs having radiographic follow-up greater than 1 year. Most owners (90%) felt there was improvement compared with preoperative lameness. In this case series, there were 10/32 cases with postoperative complications, 6 requiring further surgery.

In the other article, assessing medium-term outcomes (Fitzpatrick and colleagues[9]) (46 dogs/60 elbows), it was reported that lameness improved in all limbs by 12 weeks and resolved in 49 limbs. There were no major complications and 4.17% minor

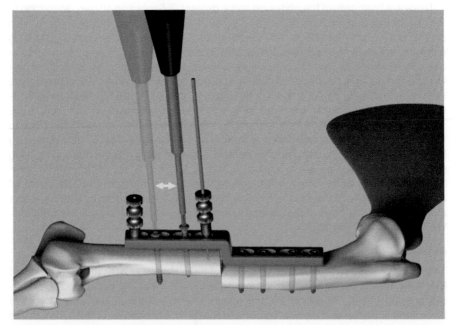

Fig. 5. A transverse osteotomy is made and the cortical screws in the distal segment are sequentially tightened, pulling the distal humerus up to the plate.

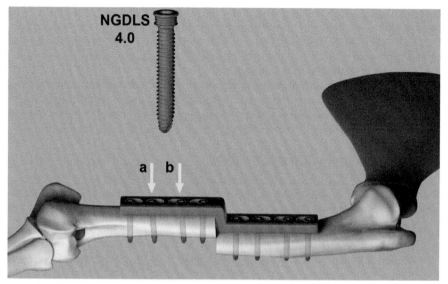

Fig. 6. Locking screws are placed in the remaining holes of the distal segment. The cortical screws (*a,b*) are replaced with locking screws for additional stability. (*Courtesy of* New Generation Devices, Glen Rock, New Jersey, USA).

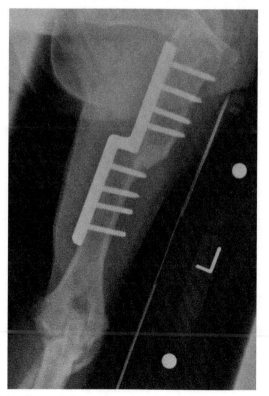

Fig. 7. Craniocaudal radiograph 3 months postoperative SHO showing complete healing.

complications cited.[9] In this article, there had been a change in application of the plate, which contributed to the decreased morbidity, according to the investigators. One potentially unintended secondary outcome associated with the SHO is alteration of limb alignment in the frontal plane of the thoracic limb, as demonstrated in a cadaveric study by Breiteneicher and colleagues.[10]

Overall, the SHO has been shown to be a reasonable option in the patient that has confirmed MCD (based on arthroscopy) (**Fig. 8**). There are some studies that have shown marked improvement in patient lameness, generally occurring after 8 weeks postoperatively. The authors do find this procedure to be useful in the select patient.

PROXIMAL ABDUCTING ULNAR OSTEOTOMY
Rationale

The PAUL technique was developed on the basis of several observations and biomechanical analysis of the canine elbow joint[11]:

- A consequence of MCD, a subset of elbow dysplasia, is medial collapse of the contact mechanics of the elbow joint.
- Medial collapse overloads the medial compartment, exacerbating existing lameness and joint pain.
- A slight abduction, by 4° to 6°, of the ulna results in an unloading of the medial compartment, alleviating pain.

In 2007, Ingo Pfeil and Slobodan Tepic theorized that proximal osteotomy of the ulna fixed by a special plate would shift, abduct, and rotate the ulna, which would lead to lateralization of the paw, thus, unloading of the medial compartment (Pfeil I, personal communication. KYON Symposium, November 12, 2010, Zurich). The proposed biomechanics of PAUL are similar to high tibial osteotomy for treatment of varus deformity of the knee and medial compartment syndrome in humans (**Fig. 9**) as an alternative to unicompartmental knee joint replacement, which may be carried out later on in cases of progressive OA. This procedure in people consists of a medial

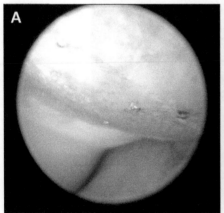 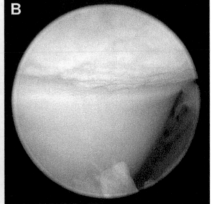

Fig. 8. Arthroscopic images of the medial humeral condyle: (*A*) preoperative and (*B*) 1-year pro-operative SHO depicting cartilage regrowth. (*From* Fitzpatrick N, Yeadon R, Smith T, et al. Techniques of application and initial clinical experience with sliding humeral osteotomy for treatment of medial compartment disease of the canine elbow. Vet Surg. 2009 Feb;38(2):261-78; with permission.)

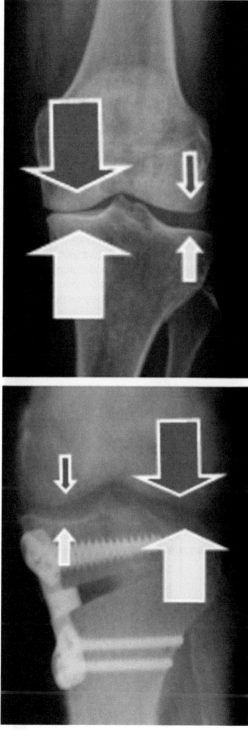

Fig. 9. High tibial osteotomy for treatment of varus deformity of the knee and medial compartment syndrome in humans.

open wedge osteotomy of the tibial plateau and elevation of the tibial plateau medially to allow the distal limb to move laterally. This loads the lateral compartment of the knee and unloads the medial compartment. The PAUL plate produced by KYON is a straight plate with a step of 2 mm to 3 mm and is applied to the lateral surface of the proximal ulna (**Fig. 10**). This is theorized to raise the ulna on the medial humeral condyle and result in a lateral shift of the distal limb, with increased load on the lateral compartment and decreased load on the medial compartment (**Fig. 11**). According to KYON, the amount of achieved abduction is approximately 4° with the 2-mm step plate and 6° with the 3-mm plate, plus 4° to 5° attributable to the natural curvature of the ulna, which is straightened by the plate. The final lateral shift is approximately 8° with the 2-mm step plate and 11° with the 3-mm step plate. In 2019, a new PAUL plate was released by KYON, called PAUL II, which utilizes a different locking screw design.

Case Selection

Dogs at skeletal maturity up to 9 years, not responsive to conservative management and having arthroscopically confirmed MCD (without significant pathology in the lateral compartment), are candidates for PAUL osteotomy. Arthroscopic confirmation is done immediately before PAUL surgery or at a previous operation at the time of conventional joint débridement. PAUL is offered to dog owners as a palliative treatment of

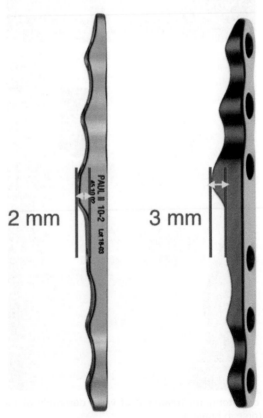

Fig. 10. PAUL II stepped plate available with 2 mm offset (*left*) and 3 mm offset (*right*) and utilizes a conical locking screw design.

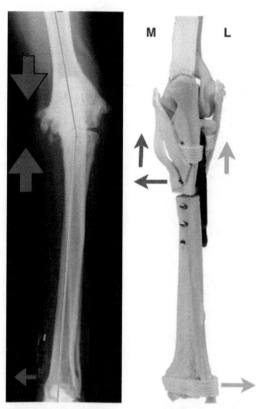

Fig. 11. The stepped plate of PAUL raises the ulna on the medial humeral condyle and results in a lateral shift of the distal limb with increased load on the lateral compartment and decreased load on the medial compartment.

MCD. The authors do not recommend PAUL when arthroscopy shows MCD without significant involvement of the remaining medial compartment. PAUL also is contraindicated when the lateral compartment shows cartilage erosion or in dogs greater than 9 years of age because of irreversible joint changes.

Preoperative Planning

The craniocaudal radiographic view with the olecranon well centered over the humeral condyle is used to evaluate the mechanical medial elbow angle (mMEA). A line from the center of the humeral condyle and the center of the antebrachiocarpal joint is traced and the medial angle between that line and the elbow joint reference line (tangent to the humeral condyles) is measured (**Fig. 12**). The mMEA has a normal range of $81.5° \pm 2.5°$ (Pfeil I, personal communication, KYON Symposium 2010, Zürich, Switzerland). In cases of an mMEA less than or equal to 80°, a 3-mm step PAUL plate is used, and, in cases of an mMEA greater than 80°, a 2-mm step PAUL plate is used. In older dogs with severe OA, a 2-mm step plate could be indicated even with mMEA less than 80° because loss of elasticity of the interosseus ligament may be a limiting factor.

Implant size selection is determined by superimposing a template over the conventional craniocaudal (CrCd) and mediolateral (ML) radiographs or using plug-in software

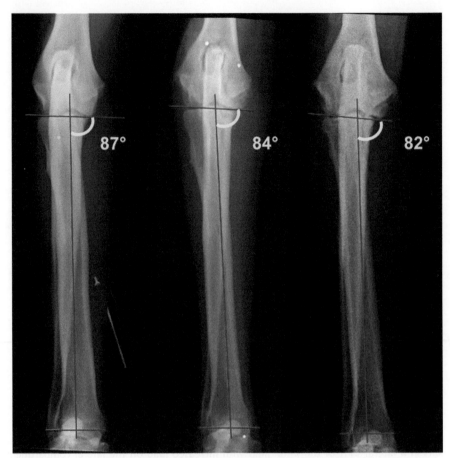

Fig. 12. The craniocaudal radiographic view with the olecranon well centered over the humeral condyle is used to evaluate the mMEA. A line from the center of the humeral condyle and the center of the antebrachiocarpal joint is traced and the medial angle between that line and the elbow joint reference line (tangent to the humeral condyles) is measured.

on digital images. It is recommended to use the largest plate suitable to fit the curvature of the ulna in the ML view, avoidance of the interosseous ligament, and sufficient ulna diameter at the location of the most distal screw. The following are general guidelines for patient weights and implant sizes:

- Dog weight less than 20 kg: PAUL plate size 8
- Dog weight 20 kg–25 kg: PAUL plate size 9
- Dog weight 25 kg–45 kg: PAUL plate size 10
- Dog weight greater than 45 kg: PAUL plate size 11

After the implant size is selected, the osteotomy location can be determined. Two measurements, D1 and D2, are calculated on a calibrated radiograph for reference in surgery. Measurement D1 refers to the distance from the radial head to the preferred osteotomy location, which generally is between 3 cm and 4.5 cm. D2 refers to the distance from the olecranon to the preferred osteotomy location. The proximal tip of the plate should be just below the level of the radial head (**Fig. 13**).

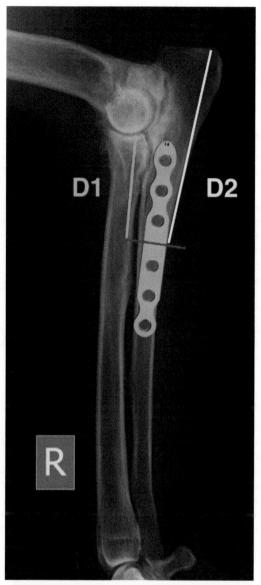

Fig. 13. Implant size selection is determined by superimposing a template over the conventional CrCd and ML radiographs or using plug-in on digital images.

Surgical Technique

Surgical approach
With the patient positioned in dorsal or lateral recumbency, a lateral approach to the proximal ulna is made.

Osteotomy of the ulna
Ulnar osteotomy is carried out perpendicular to the bone with a straight thin and sharp saw blade, from lateral to medial, recognizing that the radius lies adjacent to the ulna.

To reduce the gap at the osteotomy, 5° to 10° of inclination of the osteotomy in the sagittal plane from distal to proximal can be helpful. Excessive inclination of the osteotomy should be avoided; otherwise, the third screw may be too close to the osteotomy.

Plate position/closure

The bone plate is applied such that the top of the plate is at the level of the humeroradial joint. Closure is routine.

Postoperative Radiographs

Position of the osteotomy and implants is confirmed with orthogonal radiographs.

ML and craniocaudal radiographs are taken and the positions of the plate and of the ulna osteotomy are evaluated (**Fig. 14**):

- Plate alignment
- Screw direction, perpendicular to plate and parallel to each other
- Screw #6 screw centered in the distal ulna
- Location of the osteotomy, as planned
- Caudal tilt to the proximal segment
- Step from the proximal to distal segment

Postoperative Care

Soft padded bandage for 2 days to 3 days can be applied to reduce seroma formation.

Follow-up radiographs are obtained every few weeks to months until evidence of osseous union is noted.

Complications

Intraoperative complications

Mainly due to mistakes in the surgical execution
- Plate is not centered distally, which could interfere with the radius during pronation and supination causing pain.
- Plate is not parallel to the distal ulnar segment, which could cause the proximal part of the plate to be too caudal, with less bone purchase, or too cranial, interfering with the radius and possibly causing radial subluxation.
- Osteotomy is not centered in between holes 3 and 4, resulting in excessive correction when the plate is more proximal or less correction when it is more distal (**Fig. 15**).
- Plate is not fixed parallel to the sagittal plane, reducing the efficacy of the procedure.
- Screws are too short, not purchasing enough in the trans cortex, reducing the stability of the fixation.
- There is accidental damage to the radius when the osteotomy of the ulna is performed from caudal to cranial.

Postoperative complications

Among 116 cases with follow-up evaluation of 2 months, the authors observed 5 major complications requiring revision (4%), all requiring plate removal because of loosening, infection, or stress shielding (plates too big in small dogs). In the same group of cases, there were 3 minor complications not requiring surgical revision, 2 partial screw breakages not affecting the osteotomy healing, and 1 asymptomatic stable nonunion.[12]

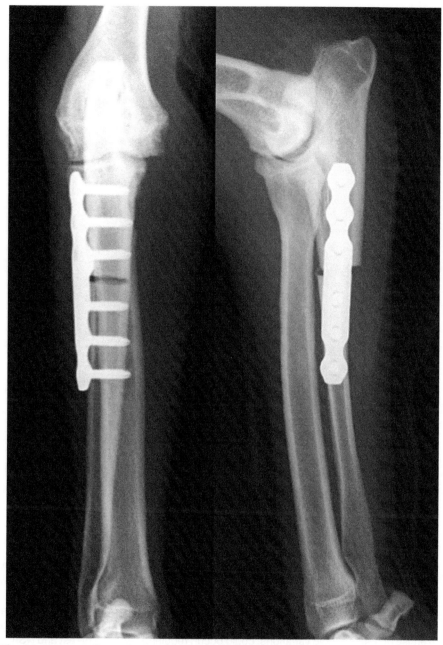

Fig. 14. Postoperative orthogonal radiographs depicting proper osteotomy and implant placement.

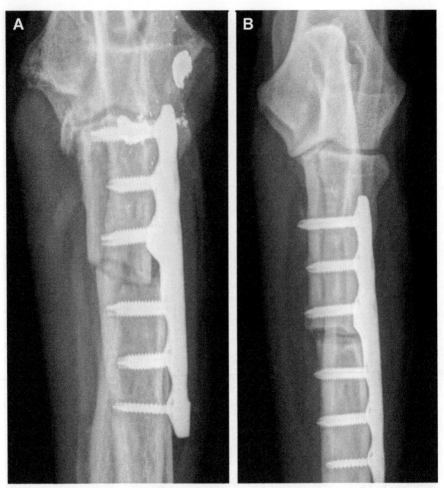

Fig. 15. Craniocaudal radiograph views depicting improper osteotomy and implant position: (*A*) too proximal and (*B*) too distal.

Functional Outcome

The expected functional outcome after PAUL is in relation to the severity of the preoperative severity of OA and the age of the dog. Owners should be aware that elbow OA will not be reversed, but that in most cases it will not progress significantly. A reduction of joint pain is expected due to elimination of the friction in the medial elbow compartment, which provides a reduction in lameness, less need of NSAIDs, and more mobility. Nevertheless, relapses of lameness due to environmental factors, like strong exercise of meteorologic variations, could occur, requiring few days of rest and NSAID therapy.

PAUL-treated elbows were rechecked postoperatively with clinical measures and radiographs (**Fig. 16**). Of the 130 treated elbows, 116 had a recheck between 2 months and 6 months, 49 were rechecked between 6 months and 12 months, and 33 were rechecked 1 to 7 years postoperatively.[12] Lameness was assessed subjectively on a 4-point grading scale: 0—no lameness; 1—mild lameness at walk and trot; 2—moderate lameness; 3—severe lameness; and 4—non–weight-bearing lameness. No

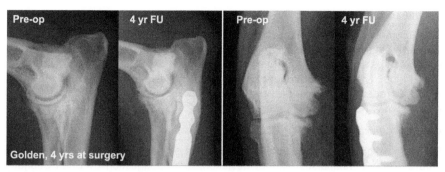

Fig. 16. Minimal progression of radiographic evidence of DJD in this case at 4-year follow-up.

patients were sound (grade 0) and no patients were non–weight bearing (grade 4) preoperatively; 92% had lameness of grade 2 to grade 3 preoperatively. At 6 months postoperative, only 9% were subjectively assessed with grade 2 lameness. There was no grade 3 or grade 4 lameness; 51% were sound and 40% had mild grade 1 lameness. Of the 33 cases followed more than 1 year, 68% were sound (no lameness), 21% had grade 1 lameness, 9% had grade 2 lameness, and 2% had grade 3 lameness.

To get the clients' perspectives, 28 of the dogs also were assessed preoperatively and postoperatively with the Liverpool Osteoarthritis in Dogs client questionnaire. Client impressions paralleled clinician assessment, with improvement in activities of daily living and quality of life 1 or more years after surgery.

A Gait4Dogs pressure-sensitive walkway was used to assess vertical ground reaction forces and contact area of the weight-bearing paw as the patients walked across the mat in 29 dogs preoperatively and beyond 1 year postoperatively. Pressure-sensitive data confirmed the subjective clinician and owner assessments.

Daitan, GSD, M, 4 yrs, before and 1 year after Right PAUL

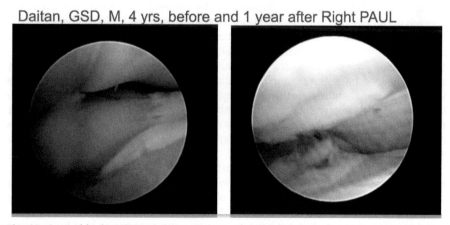

Fig. 17. Second-look arthroscopy in a German shepherd dog at 12 months postoperative. The formation of fibrocartilage in the medial compartment 12 months after PAUL was noted, where erosion (modified Outerbridge score grade 4) was present before surgery.

Second-Look Arthroscopy

Pfeil I (personal communication, Kion Symposium 2010, Zürich, Switzerland), in a second arthroscopy evaluation in a Bernese mountain dog, 7 months after PAUL, observed the formation of fibrocartilage in the medial compartment. Similarly, in second-look arthroscopy in a German shepherd dog, the authors observed the formation of fibrocartilage in the medial compartment 12 months after PAUL, where full erosion was present before surgery (**Fig. 17**).

Ongoing Clinical Studies

Standing weight-bearing radiographs are performed before and after PAUL to measure the elbow mechanical axis of deviation, upon suggestion by Brian Saunders (Texas A&M, College Station, Texas, USA). Preliminary results showed that PAUL reduces elbow mechanical axis of deviation and lateralizes and externally rotates the manus.

SUMMARY

Long-term results indicate that approximately 89% had full restoration of weight bearing or were only occasionally lame. The risk of major complications after PAUL requiring surgical revision was small (4%) and easily resolved, mainly requiring plate removal. Long-term follow-up evaluations up to 9 years have not revealed excessive wear of the lateral compartment due to the intended mechanical axis shift and load redistribution from the medial compartment. The new PAUL plate, with 4.0-mm conical locking screws, showed an overall increased strength to better withstand the strong forces transmitted to the osteotomy by the triceps muscle, promoting quicker bone healing of the ulnar osteotomy.

CANINE UNICOMPARTMENTAL ELBOW ARTHROPLASTY
Rationale

In the late 2000s, the CUE arthroplasty was conceived and developed by James L. Cook, DVM, MS, DACVS, and Kurt Schultz, DVM, MS, DACVS, in association with Arthrex engineer, Josh Karnes.[13] The original concept was to aid in the treatment of clinically symptomatic elbow joint pain and lameness caused by MCD in the canine elbow. MCD is defined as full-thickness articular cartilage loss of the medial humeral condyle and corresponding medial coronoid region of the ulna.[14,15] Subchondral bone devoid of protective articular cartilage allows constant stimulation of subchondral bone nociceptors, leading to debilitating elbow pain. Applying the concept of a unicompartmental rather than a total joint resurfacing procedure more closely maintains physiologic load transmission and distribution throughout the joint, while also preserving anatomic joint stabilizers, thereby mitigating the likelihood of lateral articular cartilage overload, malalignment, instability, and/or luxation. The CUE implant eliminates or limits bone-on-bone disease while maintaining the natural joint stabilizers of the native elbow, thus improving functional weight bearing and elbow joint range of motion and reducing pain and lameness.

The principles behind the development of the CUE implants and procedure included being bone sparing and cementless as well as being a safe procedure with low morbidity. Concerns about limb alignment should not be a significant factor, because the implant has continuous contact throughout gait range of motion. There is diminished stimulation of subchondral bone nociceptors and enhancement of the potential to promote fibrocartilage ingrowth by replacing bone-on-bone contact with implant contact through a functional range of motion of 90° to 150°. The CUE was intended to be a straightforward and repeatable procedure, with simplicity of instrumentation, limited implant inventory needs, and acceptable price point.

Implant Design

The CUE implants consist of both humeral and ulnar components (**Fig. 18**). The humeral component has a curvilinear double-snowman shape composed of a cobalt-chrome alloy surface with high strength and durable wear characteristics. This is mounted to a BioSync-titanium base, which has both high corrosion resistance and outstanding biocompatibility.[16] The implants are available in both medium and large sizes, which cover patient weight ranges from approximately 25 kg to 75 kg. The ulnar component originally was designed as an on-growth ultra high molecular weight polyethylene (UHMWPE) plug, which, due to its small size and point contact, minimizes the chance of secondary polyethylene wear products. A second-generation G2 implant was introduced in 2017, which allowed for the incorporation of a BioSync-titanium ingrowth base attached to an UHMWPE weight-bearing surface.

Instrumentation

The CUE implant system instrumentation is relatively simple in design and concept. The system comprises 2 sizes, medium and large, of both humeral and ulnar Beathe pin guides and reamer guides along with implant impaction instrumentation.

Preoperative Guides for Patient Selection

As with any joint replacement or resurfacing procedure, patient selection is critical to success. The patient should be in relatively good health with minimal comorbidities, illness, or evidence of skin infection. Candidates typically are between 3 years and 10 years of age, in a weight range of between 25 kg to 75 kg, and have elbow arthrosis with corresponding MCD and significant secondary chronic pain and lameness not responsive to medical management (**Fig. 19**). The degree of medial joint collapse and periarticular osteophytosis can range from mild to severe; however, an ideal candidate is in the mild to moderate category with a relatively normal lateral joint compartment (radial head and lateral humeral condyle) usually confirmed arthroscopically. There currently is not an implant templating or sizing guide.

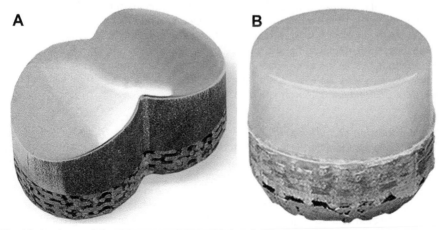

A   **B**

Fig. 18. Implants of the CUE system: (*A*) CUE humeral component and (*B*) CUE ulnar component. (*Courtesy of* Arthrex, Inc., Naples, FL.)

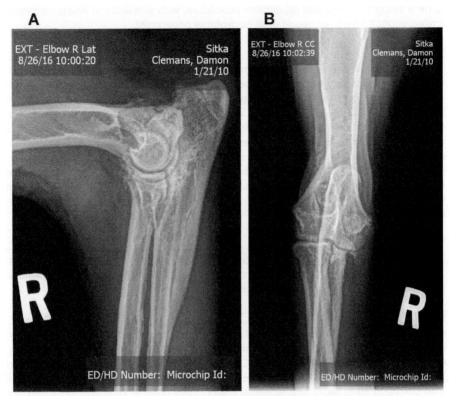

Fig. 19. (*A, B*) Preoperative orthogonal radiographs depicting MCD.

Canine Unicompartmental Elbow Technical Procedure

Approach

Cook and Shultz[18] initially described the approach to the medial elbow as a tenotomy of the medial flexor tendons to allow for adequate exposure of the articulating weight bearing surfaces of the medial humeral condyle and ulna. This quickly evolved to an epicondylar osteotomy with retraction of the flexor tendon origin to gain adequate exposure to the medial humeral condyle and medial coronoid regions. A caudomedial approach (CMA) to the elbow based on a modification of Aman and Wendelberg's[17] initial work toward medial unicompartmental elbow replacement may eliminate the need for epicondylar osteotomy (**Fig. 20**).

Implant location and placement

The ulnar implant location initially is determined after access to the joint through one of the procedures, discussed previously. Depending on the size of the patient and the medial coronoid process, a medium or large ulnar Beathe pin guide is used to place a single pin tangential from the base of the medial coronoid through the caudal spine of the ulna. The elbow joint is reduced while pin tip marks are made in full extension and 135° and 90° of flexion. This ensures proper alignment for humeral implant reaming and ultimate implant orientation and placement. The ulnar socket then is reamed with the appropriate medium or larger reamer.

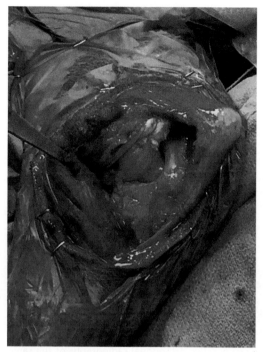

Fig. 20. Modified CMA to the elbow joint.

A humeral guide then is placed along the sagittal line created by the previously made pin marks, described previously. The caudal aspect of the guide should just cover the caudal-most pin mark. Two Beathe pins are placed to allow for proper reamer guide placement and reaming.

After careful cleaning of both the ulnar and humeral bone sockets, implant templating instruments are used to assure proper bone socket depth prior to implantation. Implantation of the ulnar socket is recommended first, followed by placement of the humeral implant. The joint then is reduced and elbow range of motion confirmed.

Closure

If an epicondyle osteotomy was required, reattachment and stabilization using Kirschner wire and single 3.5 mm bone screw is performed. Soft tissue reattachment of the flexor carpi ulnaris muscle origin to the ulna (CMA), followed by routine soft tissue and skin closure.

Radiographs

Orthogonal radiographs are obtained immediately postoperatively and at recheck intervals, as indicated (**Fig. 21**).

Postoperative Management

It is recommended that patients be placed in a soft padded or soft cast bandage for 2 weeks to limit risk of seroma formation. Activity should be limited to (progressive) leash walk activity for 8 weeks to allow for adequate implant bone integration, osteotomy, and soft tissue healing. Gradual increase in leash activity should occur over the

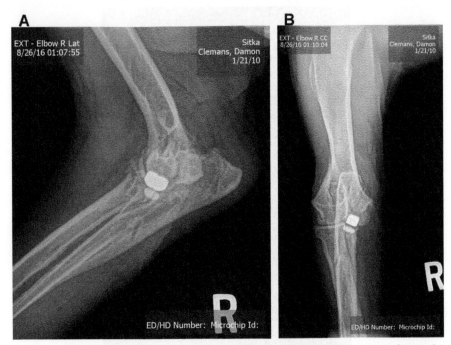

Fig. 21. (*A, B*) CUE postoperative orthogonal radiographs of the same patient depicted in **Fig. 19.**

following 8 weeks to 16 weeks. Patients typically can resume full activity by 12 weeks to 16 weeks postoperatively.

Outcomes

Published outcomes for the CUE arthroplasty currently are limited to the initial article by Cook and colleagues,[18] which described the mid-term to long-term (4-6 months) outcomes with respect to function and complications. This article shows full and acceptable functional outcome of 91% and what is considered an acceptable major/catastrophic complication rate, of 11.7%.

Biomechanically Anatomic, Nonconstrained, and Compartmental Unicompartmental Elbow Replacement

Compartmental joint disease has long been recognized in the human knee joint. The unicompartmental joint replacement for the human knee has been successfully performed since the 1970s. The nonconstrained compartmental prosthetic arthroplasty in the human knee has been reported to have 10 year or greater survivorship rates of more than 96%.[19]

Development of the KYON Biomechanically Anatomic Non-constrained Compartmental partial elbow replacement (BANC PER) began in 2006 with well-defined objectives. The design objectives for the development of the KYON elbow replacement system can be summarized as a BANC arthroplasty. To be biomechanically anatomic, the prosthetic arthroplasty must provide a normal sagittal hinge range of motion arc (SROMA) of the antebrachium about a precisely normal center of rotation, along with allowing for normal protonation and supination throughout the gait (**Fig. 22**).

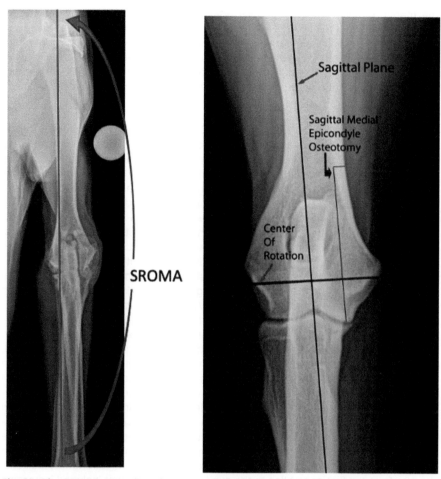

Fig. 22. The SROMA extending through the mechanical axis of the antebrachium

Cadaveric testing continued through 2011, when biomechanical load to failure testing of the first-generation design was compared with paired normal thoracic limbs.[20] Clinical cases of the PER began in 2011.

Design Considerations and Development

Constraint of a prosthetic arthroplasty can be classified as constrained, semiconstrained, or nonconstrained. The elbow joint contains 3 separate articulation compartments, which include the humeroulnar, humeroradial, and radioulnar (RU) articulations with respect to constraint. Constraint is a mechanical link or coupling of the prosthesis between the implanted bones of the joint or between the articulation compartments of the elbow. Constraint causes normal joint movements to transfer significant stresses to the implant-bone interface and has been associated with loosening and metal failure responsible for high failure rates.[21]

The elbow joint also can be described as a 2-compartment joint with respect to the anatomy of the humeral condyles. The lateral capitulum (lateral condyle) articulates with the radial head and the lateral coronoid of the ulna within the lateral compartment.

The medial trochlea (medial condyle) articulates with the ulna within the medial compartment. The KYON BANC PER system is compartmental, allowing it to replace just the affected medial compartment of the elbow, while having no constraint of the radial head as it rotates within the radial notch of the ulna during normal pronation and supination. The original design allows for conversion to a BANC TER if needed, although this may not be required and has not yet been attempted in clinical cases.

Implant Design

Since the first clinical case in 2011, the BANC PER implant has undergone 5 design modifications. The implants consist of a cylindrical medial humeral component with a UHMWPE conical disc press fitted over it and a semicircular medial ulnar component made of titanium, which articulates with the humeral implant. This allows for replacement of the medial condyle of the humerus and the medial coronoid of the ulna as well as the medial aspect of the trochlear notch and anconeal process. The polyethylene ring acts as a meniscus between the metal implants, allowing it to distribute motion and friction between both the circular metal barrel of the humeral implant and the articulation of the metal ulnar component. The humeral implant is held in place with a large diameter transcondylar screw with an internally threaded screw head (**Fig. 23**). The medial epicondyle osteotomy is compressed into the medial ingrowth plate of the humeral component using an epicondylar screw placed through a medial epicondylar advanced locking plate (ALPS) on the medial surface of the humerus. The ulnar implant is compressed into the milled bone bed with radially positioned cortical screws. Stability of the implants is achieved with osseointegration over time. The first-generation device had a ridged titanium bony on-growth surface; however, with the third-generation device, this was substituted for electron beam melting (EBM) of the titanium components. In the third-generation device, the EBM surface was welded onto the existing implant, which maintained stability while encouraging boney ingrowth. To facilitate larger-scale manufacturing, however, this design was altered from a welded EBM bone ingrowth surface to the entire implant, manufactured as a trabecular EBM, weakening the resulting fourth-generation construct. The most recent implant (fifth generation) has remedied this and allowed for improved osseointegration without compromising implant integrity and strength. Additional changes from the first generation to the current model of implant included increasing

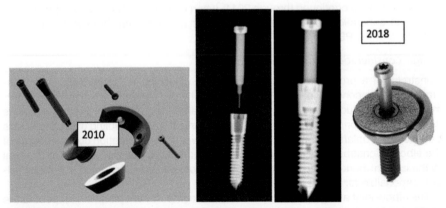

Fig. 23. Implants of the KYON BANC unicompartmental elbow replacement system. (*Courtesy of* KYON Veterinary Surgical Products, Boston, MA.)

the diameter of the transcondylar and epicondylar screws. Following fracture of the screw at the epicondylar-implant interface in the first clinical case using the original implant, the diameter of both components was increased, from 3.8 mm to 7 mm for the transcondylar screw and from 3.0 mm to 4.5 mm for the epicondylar component. This allowed for decreased risk of fatigue fracture and partial pullout or bending of the epicondylar or transcondylar fixation screws.

Indications and Preoperative Planning

Indications for the BANC PER include dogs with severe lameness and OA secondary MCD of the elbow that is refractory to medical or other surgical management. As such, CT scan and elbow arthroscopy are recommended prior to BANC PER to evaluate the status of the lateral compartment. Although patients with intact articular cartilage in the lateral compartment make the most ideal candidates for BANC PEA, anecdotally, even patients with severe wear in the lateral compartment seem to benefit from the replacement of the medial compartment. In addition to advanced imaging, precisely positioned preoperative orthogonal view radiographs are essential for accurate preoperative planning and implant sizing. Medial-lateral views of the elbow are used to template the diameter of the milling reamer and the humeral/ulnar implant using available mylar templates or computer software. Current sizing includes large dog implants (30 mm, 32 mm, and 34 mm) that typically can accommodate an average Labrador retriever to some of the giant breeds. Medium-sized dog implants (24 mm, 26 mm, and 28 mm) currently are being considered for future development.

Surgical Technique

The patient is positioned in oblique dorsal recumbency with a sterile Mayo stand or thin instrument table placed at a right angle to support the forelimb and the BANC SROMA board.[22] Sagittally placed pins are inserted into the proximal humerus and mid-humerus and then are anchored to the SROMA board using posts and clamps. The sagittal distal radius then is inserted just lateral to the extensor carpi radialis groove, and the limb is put through range of motion. SROMA points are marked at full flexion, mid-flexion, and full extension by using posts and clamps at the level of the distal radius pin as it travels through the SROMA. The distal radius is attached to the positioning board with a post and clamp. A connecting bar then is placed between the 2 clamps and serves as the means of achieving appropriate positioning of the guides (**Fig. 24**).

A CMA to the elbow with medial epicondyle ostectomy is performed. The limb then can be mounted to the BANC SROMA board. The use of purpose-specific saw guides and drill guides allows for accurate milling to accept the humeral and ulnar BANC prostheses (**Fig. 25**).

Following insertion of the prosthesis, the media epicondyle ostectomy is reduced and stabilized with ALPS (KYON) plate and screws (**Fig. 26**). The remainder of closure is routine.

Postoperative Evaluation and Management

Patients are hospitalized for 2 days to ensure adequate comfort and mobility. A soft padded bandage is placed postoperatively and maintained for 2 weeks with a bandage change recommended at 1 week. Activity restriction is essential for adequate bony healing and to prevent implant-related complications. Strict activity restriction is recommended for 2 months, allowing for controlled walking only, followed by gradual increased in controlled activity for 1 month (month 3

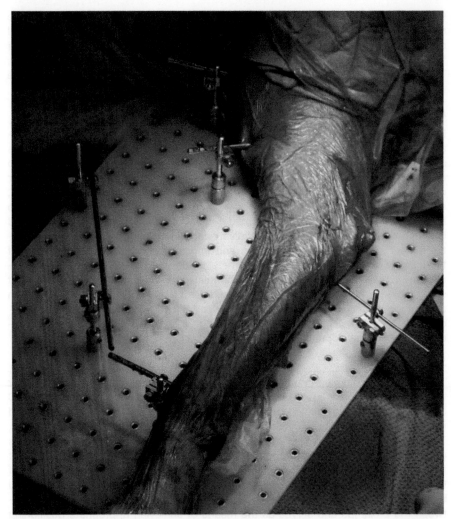

Fig. 24. The humerus and radius are attached to the SROMA board with all post clamps at the level of the SROMA. The connecting rod serves as a sagittal line guide for the paddles of the sagittal saw guide and the transverse drill guide.

postoperatively). This usually involves lengthening the duration of leash walks every 3 days to 5 days for 2 weeks, followed by controlled trotting and jogging for an additional 2 weeks. By 3 months to 4 months they are permitted to have off-leash activity. Immediate postoperative orthogonal radiography is essential to evaluate appropriate implant alignment and positioning as well as reduction and fixation of the epicondylar and ulnar osteotomies (**Fig. 27**). Further radiographic follow-up is recommended at 2 weeks, 1 month, 2 months, 3 months, 4 months, 6 months, and 1 year postoperatively, followed by annual radiographic reassessment. This allows for monitoring of bony ingrowth and signs of implant failure during confinement, rehabilitation, and free activity. Yearly radiographs allow screening for implant associated complications, such as fatigue fracture or aseptic loosening.

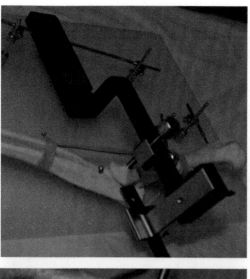

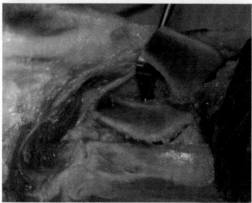

Fig. 25. The sagittal saw guide is used to produce the osteotomy of the medial epicondyle. The medial epicondyle is retracted cranially to the level of the trochlea of the medial humeral condyle.

Clinical Outcome and Complications

Since the first clinical case in 2011, a total of 15 BANC PER procedures have been performed in the United States, with several more performed in Europe. Various modifications were made to address any concerns with implants, instrumentation, and surgical technique. The progressive improvement of older generations of implants, instrumentation, and surgical technique has led to the gradual evolution of the prosthesis to its current version.

Patient outcomes generally have shown a significant improvement in gait and elbow pain. Most patients throughout the history of the KYON partial joint replacement returned to normal athletic activity, free of lameness or pain (base on owner evaluation and follow-up examinations), and have discontinued the use of NSAIDs following the procedure. There was a short period during evolution of the implant, which resulted in 4 cracked or broken implants observed from 1 month to 12 months postoperatively. This occurred after converting the titanium of the ulnar and humeral component to

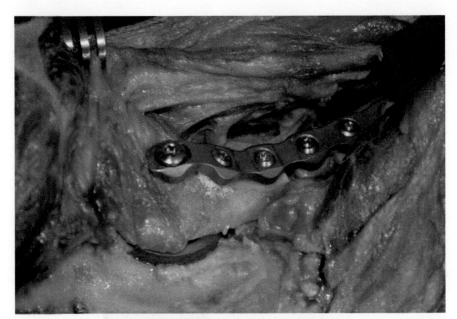

Fig. 26. The epicondyle screw is compressed into the transcondylar screw head and the medial epicondyle osteotomy stabilized with ALPS plate and screws.

an EBM manufacturing process in order to configure a trabecular mesh with the objective of improved osseointegration. These dogs accounted for all of the major complications in the 9-year series of cases in the United States. Although 2 dogs with cracked implants never showed clinical signs of lameness or pain secondary to the cracked metal, 1 dog required a successful revision to replace the implants and return to normal function, whereas another case (in a 73 kg rottweiler) resulted in a failed revision of the crushed implants. The implant manufacturing process converted back to solid titanium with a thin layer of hydroxyapatite (HA) or EBM mesh to promote bony ingrowth. Long-term data beyond 4 years postoperatively currently are unavailable because earlier patients have died for reasons unrelated to the elbow replacement. Objective force plate data are lacking and need to be collected. The clinical evaluation of short-term and long-term outcomes of the BANC PER, however, is ongoing (Follette and Wendelburg, unpublished, 2021).

Limitations

Limitations of the BANC partial elbow arthroplasty system are inherent to any elbow replacement system in that few acceptable options for revision are available. Although implant revision can be performed successfully, severe cases of failure or infection likely result in arthrodesis or possibly amputation. For this reason, owner education on alternative therapies and risks as well as full disclosure of the limited long-term data on this procedure is essential.

TATE TOTAL ELBOW REPLACEMENT IN DOGS
Rationale

During the past 30 years, functional limitations of conservative management and non-replacement surgeries for the treatment of end-stage canine elbow OA have fueled

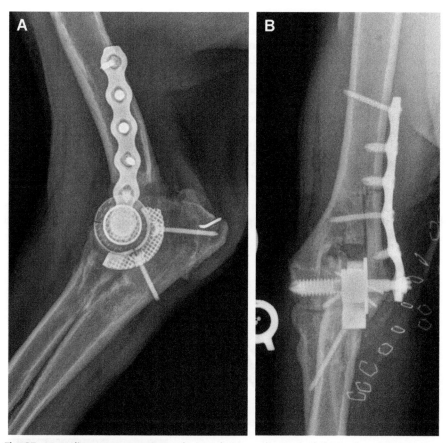

Fig. 27. Immediate postoperative orthogonal view radiographs [A] ML view; [B] CrCd view of patient with BANC PER. (*Courtesy of* KYON Veterinary Surgical Products, Boston, MA.)

growing interest in TER and PER. Clinical use of a TER first was reported by Whittick and colleagues,[23] who in 1964, used a custom-made spherical hinged prosthesis to treat a gunshot-induced comminuted elbow fracture in a cat. To the authors' knowledge, the first clinical canine TER was implanted in 1989 by Chancrin, who used a prototype cemented hinged prosthesis to treat a Labrador retriever affected with end-stage OA (Chancrin J, personal communication, 2008). Subsequently in 1996, Lewis[24] reported on the first clinical results of a hinged TER implanted in 10 dogs. In these first-generation systems, Chancrin and Lewis used cemented, fully constrained hinged designs (linked systems). Because of the rigid mechanical link between the humeral and RU components, most of the forces across the joint were transmitted through the implant to the cement and its interfaces.[25] The high complication rates encountered with these initial designs quickly led to a paradigm shift to unlinked TER designs. Vasseur (Sidebotham CG, personal communication, 2008), Lewis (second and third generations),[24] Cook,[26] and Conzemius[27,28] developed the first unlinked designs in the late 1990s. All encountered unacceptable postoperative morbidity that led either to termination or further refinement of the respective designs. Following iterations of his earlier designs, Conzemius and colleagues[29,30] reported encouraging results after TER in 6 normal dogs, then 2 years later, in 20 dogs afflicted with naturally occurring OA. Minor modifications, including the addition of porous coated surfaces to the lateral and medial aspects of the humeral component as well as curvilinear humeral articular profile, led to Conzemius' fifth TER generation, which became commercially available in 2005 (Iowa State system, BioMedtrix, Whippany, New Jersey).

More recently, a radically novel TER system (TATE Elbow system, BioMedtrix) was developed by Acker and Van Der Meulen[31,32] (**Fig. 28**). Similar to Iowa State System prosthesis, the TATE uses an unlinked, semiconstrained design. Several fundamental differences exist, however, between these 2 systems. Unlike previous conventional stemmed and cemented systems, the cementless TATE implant was designed to use a novel resurfacing concept as well as less invasive surgical approaches. In 2008, Acker and Van Der Meulen[33] reported satisfactory results 6 months after implantation of this resurfacing system in 6 dogs affected with end-stage OA.

In 2003, a UK company (OsteoGen, Bath, United Kingdom) began developing the Sirius, a TER design that is based in part on resurfacing technology for both humeral

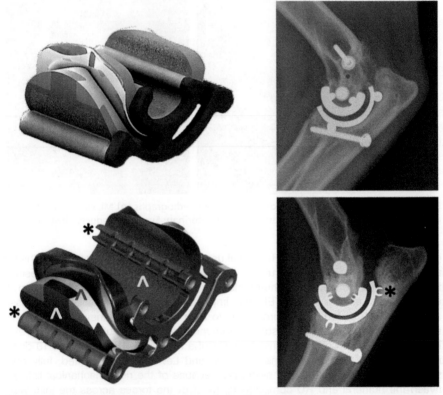

Fig. 28. Computer-generated rendering of the first-generation (*top row*) and second-generation (*bottom row*) TATE prostheses and corresponding postoperative 24 weeks' radiographs. To optimize osteointegration potential, the following iterations were implemented in the second-generation design: (1) hollow primary fixation posts to the surface area of the implant/bone interface (*asterisk*), (2) HA-coated prosthetic surfaces (*yellow ^*), and (3) flattening of the RU UHMWE lining ridge (*red ^*). The latter was intended to reduce prosthetic congruity in order to reduce implant/bone interface shear stresses. The 24 weeks postoperative radiographs show robust osteointegration of the humeral and RU components. (*Courtesy of* BioMedtrix, Whippany, NJ.)

and RU components. Similar to the Iowa State system, and unlike the TATE, however, the humeral component featured a cemented stem. Yet another crucial difference between the TATE and the Sirius prostheses is that the latter relies on RU cortical screws to achieve primary fixation of the RU component. Over the ensuing 15 years, Osteo-Gen continued to develop this novel design in collaboration with Innes and Pettitt, then at the University of Liverpool.[34] Mixed clinical results have led to several iterations of the original designs.

Design Rationale

The TATE Elbow system uses an unlinked semiconstrained 2-component design. In the absence of a rigid mechanical link between the humeral and RU components, the stability of unlinked prostheses is provided by the matching geometry of the prosthetic articulating surfaces and the surrounding soft tissue envelope.[25] Specifically, some of the transarticular forces (eg, the forces in varus-valgus) almost exclusively are counteracted by passive soft tissue constraints (ie, collateral ligaments), whereas other forces (eg, internal/external rotation and ML translation) also are controlled by the geometry of the prosthetic articular surfaces. Although contributing to joint stability, prosthetic constraint has been shown to influence stresses at the bone-implant interface. Interfacial stress distribution is further complicated by the fact that the TATE system features a single RU component that eliminates motion between the radius and the ulna.

Although the ideal prosthesis should allow near-normal joint kinematics of humeroantebrachial and RU joints, such a design would require more complex 3-component systems featuring separate components to replace the radial head and the ulnar notch. Nonetheless, 3-component prostheses have been used in the past (Vasseur, 1993 [Sidebotham CG, personal communication, 2008]; and Lewis, 1996)[24] and subsequently were abandoned due to poor clinical results. Thanks to recent technological advancement in design (resurfacing rather than stemmed or screwed components), materials (titanium rather than cobalt-chrome alloys), and interface surface texture (EBM rather than bead sintering), there is a renewed interest in developing 3-component prostheses. The current TATE design likely was chosen as a compromise between optimal joint kinematics and decreased prosthetic complexity and related risk of implant failure.

Although physiologic RU motion is limited in arthritic elbows, residual motion could be detrimental to the osteointegration of the RU component and thus its long-term stability. To reduce the risk of interfacial failure at the level of the RU component, the surgical procedure includes an RU synostosis.

The original TATE Elbow system uses a cementless resurfacing design consisting of a cobalt-chrome humeral component and a 175° arc UHMWPE RU component featuring a cobalt-chrome metal backing. Both humeral component and RU metal backing feature 2 ML posts for primary fixation and a porous surface for long-term stability via bone ingrowth. The TATE Elbow system was designed to use a relatively less-invasive approach than previous systems, via osteotomy of the medial humeral epicondyle. During implantation, both components are linked by a set plate and are inserted simultaneously as a cartridge implant.

In an effort to optimize bone ingrowth a second-generation TATE Elbow system was released early 2010. This refined design has been progressively replacing the first TATE generation. Design modifications included hollow primary fixation posts and HA coating. In addition, reduced prosthetic constraint in rotation and ML translation was achieved through modification of the RU articular profile.[35,36] Although no cases of implant loosening had been documented with the first-generation TATE when the second-generation design iterations were implemented, the rationale for changes was to promote implant osteointegration. Further modifications were introduced in 2016 and included (1) titanium 3-dimensional (3-D) humeral component and RU metal back, (2) titanium nitride coating of the articular surface of the humeral component, and (3) HA coating of the metal/bone interfaces of both humeral and RU components.

Indications–Contraindications

The primary indication for TER is severe, intractable DJD that is not responsive or poorly responsive to medical management. Although elbow OA is associated most commonly with elbow dysplasia, it also can result from articular fracture, elbow luxation, or angular limb deformities with subsequent elbow incongruity. Because of the limited long-term follow-up available for the currently available systems, it has been recommended that TER be restricted to older dogs with a clearly decreased quality of life on a day-to-day basis, which cannot be managed satisfactorily with medical treatment. Based on their favorable experience with the TATE prosthesis, however, the authors have extended their recommendation for TER to include younger dogs afflicted with intractable end-stage OA. Similarly, due to the risk of potentially severe complications, with limited revision strategies, early TERs were preferentially, yet not exclusively, performed in dogs with unilateral elbow OA. As with the initial age restriction, encouraging results with the TATE prosthesis have led the authors to recommend TER in dogs with severe bilateral elbow OA. As for any total joint replacement, systemic or local infections (eg, local pyoderma, bacterial cystitis, otitis externa, and periodontal disease) increase the risk of postoperative infection and should be identified and addressed before surgery. Chronic elbow luxation is a relative contraindication to TER. The compromised periarticular soft tissue envelope may increase the risk of postoperative luxation with the currently available, unlinked, systems. Finally, severe malunion may preclude the use of the resurfacing TATE Elbow system. Neurologic dysfunction and skeletally immature dogs represent other potential contraindications.

Preoperative Evaluation

Comprehensive physical, orthopedic (including goniometry), and neurologic examinations are mandatory to fully assess functional alterations in the affected elbow joint, to rule out other potential causes of thoracic limb lameness, and to document concurrent abnormalities.

Radiography then is used to confirm the diagnosis and assess the severity of the periarticular osteophytosis. Standard, accurate craniocaudal and ML views with concomitant use of a magnification phantom are mandatory, because these films are used with acetate or digital templates to select an appropriately sized prosthesis. When extensive periarticular osteophytosis is present, a computed tomography (CT) scan with 3-D reconstruction of the elbow is useful for surgical planning. Poor identification of anatomic landmarks during the implantation surgery can result in an improperly aligned implant and can have disastrous effects on the outcome.

Surgical Technique

The elbow joint is approached through a medial epicondyle osteotomy. The elbow axis of rotation (AOR) is identified with the use of dedicated instruments. A datum pin, inserted along the AOR, serves as a reference throughout the procedure. The elbow is flexed at approximately 90° and then is locked in place using an alignment plate screwed into the humerus, radius, and ulna. Next, a drilling guide is loaded onto the AOR pin and is used to drill 4 transverse holes (2 in the humerus, 1 in the radius, and 2 in the ulna) that accommodates the ML posts in the matching prosthetic components. Using a custom end mill, the proximal (humeral) and distal (RU) articular surfaces are removed simultaneously along a 200° arc concentric to the AOR. A cartridge implant then is press-fitted into the open joint space. A set plate used to link the components during impaction is removed, and the elbow range of motion is assessed. If cranial or caudal impingements are present, osteophytes are débrided with the use of rongeurs or a high-speed burr. The medial epicondyle is reduced and fixed with transcondylar and epicondylar lag screws or a bone plate. Routine closure in layers concludes the procedure.

Postoperative Evaluation and Management

ML and craniocaudal elbow radiographic views are obtained to assess proper implant alignment and positioning as well as osteotomy reduction and fixation. Subsequent radiographic evaluations are recommended at 6 weeks, 12 weeks, 24 weeks, and 52 weeks, then yearly thereafter, to assess bone ingrowth as well as implant stability and/or failure (eg, aseptic loosening). Postoperative radiographs are shown in **Fig. 29**. A soft padded bandage is applied for a few days after surgery. Professional physical rehabilitation, after an initial 6-week period of restricted activity, is strongly encouraged.

Clinical Outcome–Complications

To date, although clinical and experimental studies are ongoing, no objective data are available on the TATE Elbow system. This dearth of information may be explained by the relatively recent release of this prosthesis and by the limited number of cases performed by any given surgical group. The only report currently available required the compilation of 32 clinical cases (33 elbows) by 7 surgeons from a mix of 5 academic institutions and specialized private practices.[37] In that retrospective study, the long-term clinical outcomes after TATE Elbow replacement was evaluated subjectively by means of radiographs as well as via surgeon and owner questionnaires; objective evaluation, such as force plate analysis or kinematic gait assessment, was not performed. Although surgeons reported 76% of full (24%) or acceptable (52%) function, 24% of the cases had unacceptable clinical outcomes. This evaluation was corroborated somewhat by the 19 owners (67%) who provided feedback. Of these, 12 (63%) were very satisfied with the procedure, 5 (26%) were somewhat disappointed, and 2 (11%) had no opinion.

Despite a surprisingly high rate of major (15 cases [45%]) or catastrophic (5 cases [15%]) complications, this report concluded that the TATE procedure provided a significant reduction in pain severity in most cases, although mobility scores were unchanged over time. Infections occurred in 10 cases (30%) up to 12 months postoperatively. Finally, the investigators reported suboptimal implant positioning in 97% of the cases, while acknowledging that this finding had no impact on clinical outcome. Nonetheless, such high complication rates are unusual in orthopedic surgery. Although the nature of these complications (infection and implant malposition) suggests surgical and/or technical errors, it may highlight the difficult learning curve associated with this procedure, despite the availability of a precise, dedicated instrumentation designed to normalize surgical steps. Considering that most cases[16] were performed by a single surgeon (Burton N, personal communication, VOS meeting 2016.) it might be assumed that the remaining investigators may have contributed a substantially lower number of cases and, therefore, may have been in the early phase of the learning curve. As suggested previously, the limited number of cases performed by any given surgical group and the lack of objective outcome measures may contribute to the dearth of peer-reviewed publications. Conversely, the question is,

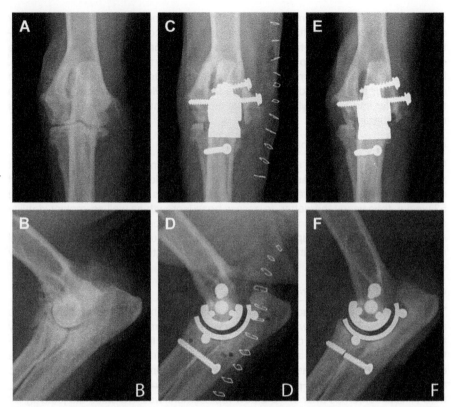

Fig. 29. Preoperative (*A, B*) and postoperative (*C, D*) radiographs showing proper positioning of a TATE prosthesis as well as the bone implant interface 21 months later (*E, F*). The proximal screws are used to stabilize the medial epicondyle. Lagged between the radius and the ulna, the distal screw is used to maintain stability during healing of a surgical RU synostosis. Note the fractured RU screw and the mild local bone resorption around the ulnar post. (*Courtesy of* L. Déjardin, DVM, East Lansing, MI. and BioMedtrix, Whippany, NJ.)

how might the compilation of a few cases from numerous sources affect the interpretation of the findings of the clinical reports?.

What follows is a synthesis of subjective data provided by fellow surgeons who have performed at least 5 procedures. The authors strongly emphasize that this information is anecdotal in nature and, therefore, should be assessed cautiously.

It is estimated that the TATE prosthesis has been implanted in approximately 250 cases worldwide since July 2007. In 2009[38] and then 2010,[39] the authors reported subjective data compiled through feedback from the 6 centers, where more than 5 cases had been performed (total of 73 elbows at the time). Three severe complications, consisting of 2 humeral fractures and 1 implant loosening, were recorded, all within 5 weeks postoperatively (rate of 4%). Of these, 2 cases were associated with secondary infection and 1 case with secondary ulnar fracture. Two cases were euthanized by the referring veterinarian without reevaluation by the primary surgeon, and 1 was amputated because of concomitant deep infection (**Fig. 30**).

Although recent biomechanical studies have demonstrated that implant intrinsic stability is lower in both TATE Elbow generations than in the Iowa State system (first commercially available TER system), luxations have not been reported in any TATE cases. This finding suggests that weakening of the joint's passive constraints, as a result of lateral collateral ligament desmotomy during implantation of the Iowa State system, offsets the potential benefit (stability) of more congruent designs. Similarly, primary ulnar fractures, another complication seen with the Iowa State system,[30,40,41] have not been observed with either TATE Elbow generations.

A variety of minor complications, including pin migration, screw loosening, fracture and/or clinically inconsequential delayed union of the medial epicondylar fragment, skin dehiscence, and neuropraxia were seen in approximately 8% of the cases. Successful revisions consisted of pin removal, screw retightening, primary repair, and local wound care. Iatrogenic intraoperative complications due to surgical error (transection of the ulnar nerve and trochlear fracture) were described by Acker in 1 dog, which remains ambulatory nearly 3 years postoperatively.

The authors have limited knowledge of 20 additional cases treated elsewhere with the assistance of a trained surgeon. In that subgroup, the authors are aware of 4 severe complications (20%). Humeral fractures were reported in 2 cases, 1 of which was successfully repaired, whereas the other resulted in an amputation because of associated methicillin-resistant *Staphylococcus aureus* infection. The remaining 2 cases developed infection; 1 patient underwent successful arthrodesis and the other was lost to follow-up.

Since their 2010 report, to the authors' knowledge, approximately 45 and 10 additional cases have been treated with a TATE by the Acker (65 cases) and Michigan State University (20 cases) groups, respectively. Although no further postoperative major complications have been reported by Acker, clinical outcome on these cases is lacking. In 1 of the 10 additional cases operated by the authors' team, milling difficulties during surgery led to the presence a greater than 1-mm gap along the ulnar

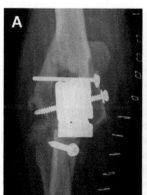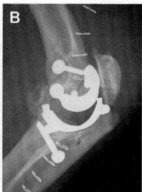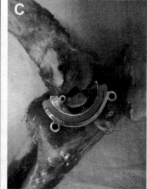

Fig. 30. Radiographs (*A, B*) and photograph (*C*) of a gross specimen 2 weeks after implantation of a TATE Elbow system. Failure occurred 7 days postoperatively and was attributed to an intraoperative technical error that resulted in iatrogenic widening of the axis of rotation drill hole at the center of the trochlea. Based on owner testimony, the authors believe that this led to an initial condylar fracture between the 2 humeral component posts, followed by an olecranon fracture during a sudden subsequent fall. Although osteosynthesis might have been attempted immediately after the fracture occurred, deep infection was present by the time we became aware of the incident. Because elbow arthritis was unilateral in this dog, amputation rather than arthrodesis was elected. (*Courtesy of* L. Déjardin, DVM, East Lansing, MI. and BioMedtrix, Whippany, NJ.)

bone interface of a first-generation TATE prosthesis. Limited osteointegration of the RU component was observed at 6 months and was followed by premature loosening, with debonding of the sintered beads along the RU/bone interface, 36 weeks postoperatively. Amputation eventually was performed 2 years postoperatively due to the lack of clinical improvement.

Objective data regarding functional outcome following TATE implantation still are lacking at this point in time. Subjective clinical evaluation from the authors' group (unpublished data on 21 elbows in 20 cases) suggest that limb function improves over time after an initial aggravation at 6 weeks to 12 weeks. Although dogs appear pain-free and show improved range of motion, mainly in extension, subtle to mild lameness may persist. These findings agree with those reported by De Sousa and colleagues.[37] As part of an ongoing prospective clinical study led by Michigan State University, objective force plate analysis is being conducted on 14 of these 20 dogs up to 6 years following implantation of a TATE Elbow system. In all cases, the peak vertical force of the affected front limb was significantly lower than the normal reported range of 105% to 125% of body weight at the trot.[42] By 6 months to 12 months following surgery, the peak vertical ground reaction force (PVGRF) of the operated limb was greater than that of the contralateral side. Continued improvement was seen at 2 years, as the peak vertical force of the operated limbs had returned to a normal reported value of approximately 115% of body weight. Although these data highlight the slow functional recovery following TATE Elbow replacement, it is worth noting that mean PVGRF of the operated side became significantly greater than that of the affected side approximately 1 year after surgery (unpublished, ongoing data collection).

Prospective experimental and clinical evaluations of the TATE Elbow system are ongoing and may provide some needed objective data in the near future. The objectives of this research program are to characterize functional outcomes and expectations further, to identify potential pitfalls, and, if deemed necessary, to refine the implant design and/or surgical technique.

Ongoing Design Evolution

Starting in 2019, BioMedtrix initiated the development of a third-generation TATE prosthesis along with a simplification of both instrumentation and surgical technique. Although this new design is fundamentally similar to that of the second generation, components modifications were introduced to improve immediate and long-term stability. These include (1) deformable fixation posts that can be expanded to enhance primary fixation and (2) EBM surface treatment of the titanium humeral and RU components intended to promote bone ingrowth (**Fig. 31**). Identification of the AOR as well as determination of the milling depth and amplitude originally were achieved using a condylar clamp and a caliper while the elbow was secured to the surgical table via an articulated positioning arm. Although effective, this instrumentation was relatively complex. The new, simplified instrumentation relies on CT based, 3-D printed, patient-specific instrumentation (PSI) to accurately identify the AOR and position the elbow joint (**Fig. 32**). Subsequently, the joint is locked in place using a modified alignment plate prior to milling at a depth predetermined from CT data. Finally, capitalizing on the total ankle replacement experience, the milling technique also has been refined. First, milling is conducted in 2 increments, starting with a narrower milling bit followed by a final size bit. The purpose of this stepwise approach is to enhance milling accuracy while reducing the risk of thermal damage to the bone and therefore promote osteointegration of the prosthesis. Second, the milling arm and alignment plate feature high-power magnets that provide a tight linkage between these instruments during

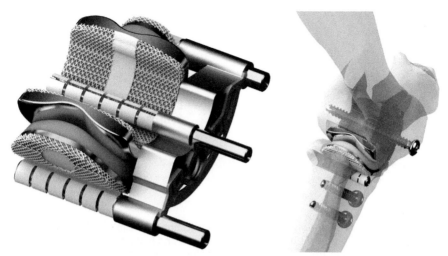

Fig. 31. Computer-generated image of the third-generation TATE prosthesis (*left*) and 3-D rendering of the prosthesis in situ. Although most design changes of the second generation were maintained, additional iterations were made to simplify the surgical technique while further improving primary and secondary fixation. The humeral component features a single-fixation post rather than 2 as in the second-generation TATE. To improve immediate stability, a cam system allowing expansion of the posts has been added. To promote bone ingrowth and, therefore, the long-term stability of the prosthesis, EBM now is used as a surface treatment of the titanium humeral and RU components. In addition, deleterious shear stresses at the RU bone/implant interface are reduced by eliminating prosupination using 2 RU lag screws to create a synostosis. (*Courtesy of* BioMedtrix, Whippany, NJ.)

milling (Sidebotham CG, personal communication, 2008). By virtually eliminating vibrations, precisely milled walls can be obtained reliably, which further improves the potential for rapid and successful osteointegration of the prosthesis. At this time, the third-generation TATE has been tested successfully in bone models and ex vivo specimens, and a limited clinical trial is ongoing at Michigan State University.

Limitations of Total Elbow Replacement

A major limitation of TER is the absence of effective revision options in cases of failure. Unfortunately, because end-stage elbow OA often is a bilateral condition, amputation is not a valid option in most cases, and arthrodesis remains the main alternative. Although some fractures or luxations may be repaired successfully, others may require explantation and arthrodesis because of the limited bone stock available for implant fixation or continuous joint instability. Infection is and likely will continue to be the most challenging complication because antibiotic therapy alone unlikely is effective as long as the prosthesis is implanted. As with intractable fractures and luxations, cases of infection might be treated by explantation and arthrodesis. Alternatively, in cases of unilateral end-stage OA, amputation may represent a safer alternative to arthrodesis. Although the purpose of arthrodesis is to eliminate pain, variable alterations in limb function, or even quality of life, should be considered carefully if painful contralateral ankylosis is present or in cases that may require bilateral elbow arthrodesis. With unilateral arthrodesis, however, limb function has been described as acceptable in most cases, despite continuous limb circumduction. Because of these limitations, owner education is critical and must be thorough and

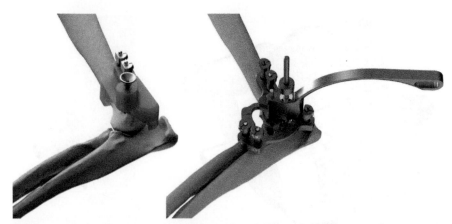

Fig. 32. A CT-based PSI is printed to improve identification of the joint axis of rotation. The PSI block (*left*) locks on the distal aspect of the humerus and features a guide hole accurately aligned with the axis of rotation. Milling accuracy has been enhanced by using high power magnets imbedded in the milling arm and alignment plate (*right*). The tight linkage between these instruments virtually eliminates vibrations during milling. As a result, precisely milled walls can be reliably obtained, which further improves the potential for rapid and successful osteointegration of the prosthesis.

objective. Fair disclosure of alternative treatments and realistic expectations, particularly with regard to complications and revisions, should be presented to anyone contemplating TER.

Despite an enormous amount of work from forward-thinking surgeons, such as Whittick, Chancrin, Lewis, Vasseur, Conzemius, Acker, and others, as well as engineers, the ideal prosthetic design remains elusive. Based on early experiences and failures, however, substantial improvements in both design and surgical procedures have been made in recent years. Nonetheless, questions regarding optimal articular surface constraint and long-term periprosthetic osteolysis or osteointegration remain unanswered. Similarly, long-term objective clinical trials and retrieval analyses are desperately needed. Furthermore, limited revision options will continue to constitute one of the most serious hurdles to be overcome in the foreseeable future. Although further advancements are required before TER gains widespread acceptance as a reliable treatment option for end-stage elbow OA in dogs, novel ideas and promising, although imperfect, clinical results likely will continue to generate interest and much needed research in this open and challenging field.

SUMMARY

The elbow joint is a complex joint. Erosion of the articular cartilage of the medial compartment, resulting in DJD and OA secondary to incongruity associated with elbow dysplasia or trauma, is the most common cause of lameness of the forelimb of mature dogs in the authors' orthopedic practices.

In cases of early detection and mild cartilage loss (modified Outerbridge scores of I–II), PAUL and SHO have shown to decrease or even reverse arthroscopic evidence of cartilage loss. In more advanced, severe irreversible cartilage loss and DJD (modified Outerbridge scores of III–IV), resurfacing with CUE, partial elbow joint replacement (eg, BANC), or total joint replacement (eg, TATE) may be a more appropriate consideration.

External beam radiation has had some positive effect in palliating signs of elbow OA/DJD in the short term.[43] Recently, conversion electron therapy that targets macrophages and synoviocytes delivered by intra-articular injection (Synovetin OA) has been approved for use in dogs with elbow OA with a proposed benefit of up to 1 year.[44] Although these treatment modalities may benefit patients that are not considered good surgical candidates, long-term results are not published for either.

CLINIC CARE POINTS

- Erosion of the articular cartilage of the medial compartment of the elbow secondary to incongruity associated with elbow dysplasia or traumatic injury has been termed, *MCD* or *medial compartment syndrome.*

- Mild to moderate cartilage loss may be managed successfully with PAUL or SHO by shifting the weight-bearing axis more laterally.

- In severe cases of cartilage loss of the medial compartment, management with resurfacing by CUE or PER with the unicompartmental BANC prosthesis is more appropriate.

- TER may be warranted in cases of severe and end-stage OA or global cartilage loss.

- External beam radiation and intra-articular conversion electron therapy may be short-term options for improving comfort in patients not deemed suitable for surgical management.

DISCLOSURE

K.L. Wendelburg holds a US patent for the Unicompartmental Partial Elbow Replacement System and Surgical Technique as well as honoraria from KYON for teaching the surgical technique.

REFERENCES

1. Schulz KS. Diagnostic assessment of the elbow (when in doubt, scope the elbow). Proc 14th Annual American College of Veterinary Surgeons Symposium, Denver, CO, October 2004.
2. Slattery C, Kweon CY. Classifications in brief. Clin Orthop Relat Res 2018; 476(10):2101–4.
3. Fitzpatrick N, Yeadon R, Smith T, et al. Techniques of application and initial clinical experience with sliding humeral osteotomy for treatment of medial compartment disease of the canine elbow. Vet Surg 2009;38(2):261–78.
4. Fitzpatrick N, Yeadon R. Working algorithm for treatment decision making for developmental disease of the medial compartment of the elbow in dogs. Vet Surg 2009;38(2):285–300.
5. Fujita Y, Schulz KS, Mason DR, et al. Effect of humeral osteotomy on joint surface contact in canine elbow joints. Am J Vet Res 2003;64(4):506–11.
6. Mason DR, Schulz KS, Fujita Y, et al. Measurement of humeroradial and humeroulnar transarticular joint forces in the canine elbow joint after humeral wedge and humeral slide osteotomies. Vet Surg 2008;37(1):63–70.
7. Wendelburg KM, Beale BS. Medium and long term evaluation of sliding humeral osteotomy in dogs. Vet Surg 2014;43(7):804–13.

8. Quinn R, Preston C. Arthroscopic assessment of osteochondrosis of the medial humeral condyle treated with debridement and sliding humeral osteotomy. Vet Surg 2014;43(7):814–8.

9. Fitzpatrick N, Bertran J, Solano MA. Sliding humeral osteotomy: medium-term objective outcome measures and reduction of complications with a modified technique. Vet Surg 2015;44(2):137–49.

10. Breiteneicher AH, Norby B, Schulz KS, et al. The effect of sliding humeral osteotomy (SHO) on frontal plane thoracic limb alignment: an ex vivo canine cadaveric study. Vet Surg 2016;45(8):1095–107.

11. Wind AP. Elbow incongruity and developmental elbow diseases in the dog. J Am Anim Hosp Assoc 1986;22:712–30.

12. Vezzoni A. Elbow Techniques Update: PAUL. Proceedings of the 27th Annual Scientific Meeting of the European College of Veterinary Surgeons. 2018.

13. Franklin S, Schulz KS, Karnes J, et al. Theory and development of a unicompartmental resurfacing system for treatment of medial compartment disease of the canine elbow. Vet Surg 2014;43(7):765–73.

14. Schulz K, Krotschek U. Canine elbow dysplasia. In: Slatter D, editor. Textbook of small animal surgery. 3rd edition. Philadelphia: Saunders; 2003. p. 19–1954.

15. Vermote KA, Bergenhuyzen AL, Gielen I, et al. Elbow lameness in dogs of six years and older: arthroscopic and imaging findings of medial coronoid disease in 51 dogs. Vet Comp Orthop Traumatol 2010;23(1):43–50.

16. Cook J, Kuroki K, Bozynski CC, et al. Evaluation of Synthetic osteochondral implants. J Knee Surg 2014;27(4):295–302.

17. Aman AM, Wendelberg, KL. Poster session, ACVS symposium. A Novel Approach to the Medial Aspect of the Canine Elbow via Parasagittal osteotomy of the Medial Ridge of the Olecranon.

18. Cook J, Schulz KS, Karnes GJ, et al. Clinical outcomes associated with the initial use of the Canine Unicompartmental Elbow (CUE) Arthroplasty System. Can Vet J 2015;56(9):971–7.

19. Pandit H, Jenkins C, Gill HS, et al. Minimally invasive Oxford phase 3 unicompartmental knee replacement: results of 1000 cases. J Bone Joint Surg Br 2011;93(2):198–204.

20. Smith ZF, Wendelburg KL, Wendelburg KL, et al. In vitro biomechanical comparison of load to failure testing of a canine unconstrained medial compartment elbow arthroplasty system and normal canine thoracic limbs. Vet Comp Orthop Traumatol 2013;26(5):356–65.

21. Morgan H, Battista V, Leopold SS. Constraint in primary total knee arthroplasty. J Am Acad Orthop Surg 2005;13(8):515–24.

22. Wendelburg K Medial compartment elbow replacement surgical guide. Elbow surgical technique, Ver. 181114.

23. Whittick WG, Bonar CJ, Reeve-Newson JA. Prosthesis for elbow fracture. Can Vet J 1964;5:56.

24. Lewis RH: Development of elbow arthroplasty (canine) clinical trials, ACVS symposium 1996,110.

25. Armstrong AD, King GJW, Yamaguchi K. Total elbow arthroplasty design. In: Williams GR Jr, Yamaguchi K, Ramsey ML, et al, editors. Shoulder and elbow arthroplasty. Philadelphia: Lippincott Williams & Willkins; 2005.

26. Cook JL, Lower J: Elbow athroplasty system, Patent US007419507B2. USA, 2008.

27. Conzemius MG, Aper RL. Development and evaluation of semiconstrained arthroplasty for the treatment of elbow osteoarthritis in the dog. Vet Comp Orthop Traumatol 1998;11:A54.
28. Conzemius MG. Total elbow replacement in the dog: development and evaluation. Thesis. Ames (IA): Iowa State University; 2000.
29. Conzemius MG, Aper RL, Hill CM. Evaluation of a canine total-elbow arthroplasty system: a preliminary study in normal dogs. Vet Surg 2001;30(1):11.
30. Conzemius MG, Aper RL, Corti LB. Short-term outcome after total elbow arthroplasty in dogs with severe, naturally occurring osteoarthritis. Vet Surg 2003; 32(6):545.
31. Acker RL, Van Der Meulen GT: Joint prosthesis, Patent US20080154384A1, USA, 2008.
32. Acker RL, Van Der Meulen GT: Joint prosthesis and method of implanting same, Patent US20070073408A1, USA, 2007.
33. Acker R, Van Der Meulen GT: Tate elbow preliminary trials. Presented at: 35th Veterinary Orthopedic Society (VOS) Annual Conference, March 8-15, 2008, Big Sky, MT.
34. Lorenz ND, Channon S, Pettitt R, et al. Ex vivo kinematic studies of a canine unlinked semi-constrained hybrid total elbow arthroplasty system. Vet Comp Orthop Traumatol 2015;28(1):39–47.
35. Déjardin LM, Guillou RP, Sawyer MJ, et al: Effect of articular design on rotational constraint of two unlinked canine total elbow prostheses. Presented at: 3rd World Veterinary Orthopedic Congress (WVOC), September 15–18, 2010, Bologna, Italy. CD-ROM.
36. Guillou RP, Demianiuk R, Déjardin LM, et al: Effect of articular design on mediolateral constraint and stability of two unlinked canine total elbow prostheses. Presented at: 38th Annual Meeting of the Veterinary Orthopedic Society (VOS). 2011.
37. De Sousa RJ, Parsons KJ, Owen MR, et al. Radiographic, Surgeon and Owner Assessment of the BioMedtrix TATE Elbow Arthroplasty. Vet Surg 2016;45(6): 726–35.
38. Déjardin LM, Guillou RP: Total elbow replacement in dogs: recent design evolution and early results with the TATE system. Presented at: 18th Annual Scientific Meeting, European College of Veterinary Surgeons, July 2009, Nantes, France.
39. Déjardin LM, Guillou RP: TATE total elbow replacement: results and complications. Presented at: 3rd World Veterinary Orthopedic Congress (WVOC). September 2010, Bologna, Italy.
40. Conzemius MG. Nonconstrained elbow replacement in dogs. Vet Surg 2009; 38(2):279.
41. Conzemius MG: Total elbow replacement: facts, fiction and opinions. Presented at: ACVS Veterinary Symposium, October 2007, Chicago, IL.
42. Lascelles BD, Roe SC, Smith E, et al. Evaluation of a pressure walkway system for measurement of vertical limb forces in clinically normal dogs. Am J Vet Res 2006; 67(2):277.
43. Kapatkin AS, Nordquist B, Garcia TC, et al. Effect of single dose radiation therapy on weight-bearing lameness in dogs with elbow osteoarthritis. Vet Comp Orthop Traumatol 2016;29(4):338–43.
44. Donecker JM, Stevenson NR. Radiosynoviorthesis: A new therapeutic and diagnostic tool for canine joint inflammation. Technical Bulletin. Exubrion Therapeutics, July 2019.

Printed and bound by CPI Group (UK) Ltd, Croydon, CR0 4YY

14/10/2024

01773715-0002